GENERAL DISCLAIMER
The contents of this book are intended to provide useful information
to the general public. All materials, including text and images,
are for informational purposes only and are not a substitute
for medical diagnosis, advice, or treatment for specific medical
conditions. All readers should seek expert medical care and consult
their own physicians before commencing any regimen for any
general or specific health issues. The author and publishers do not
recommend or endorse specific treatments, procedures, advice,
or other information found in this book and specifically disclaim
all responsibility for any and all liability, loss, or risk, personal or
otherwise, which is incurred as a consequence, directly or indirectly,
of the use or application of any of the material in this publication.

Thunder Bay Press
An imprint of Printers Row Publishing Group
10350 Barnes Canyon Road, Suite 100, San Diego, CA 92121
www.thunderbaybooks.com • mail@thunderbaybooks.com

Thunder Bay Press
Publisher: Peter Norton
Associate Publisher: Ana Parker
Senior Developmental Editor: April Graham Farr
Editor: Kelly Larsen
Senior Product Manager: Kathryn C. Dalby
Production Team: Jonathan Lopes, Rusty von Dyl

Produced by Moseley Road Inc., www.moseleyroad.com
President: Sean Moore
Art and Editorial Director: Lisa Purcell
Production Director: Adam Moore
Editor: Audra Avizienis
Designer: Philippa Baile, oiloften.co.uk
Photography: Naila Ruechel, www.nailaruechel.com

Library of Congress Cataloging-in-Publication data available on request.

ISBN: 978-1-64517-045-7

Printed in China

23 22 21 20 19   1 2 3 4 5

ULTIMATE GUIDE TO
YOGA

WITH DETAILED INSTRUCTIONS AND ANATOMICAL ILLUSTRATIONS FOR 161 YOGA POSES

Nancy J. Hajeski

THUNDER BAY
P·R·E·S·S

San Diego, California

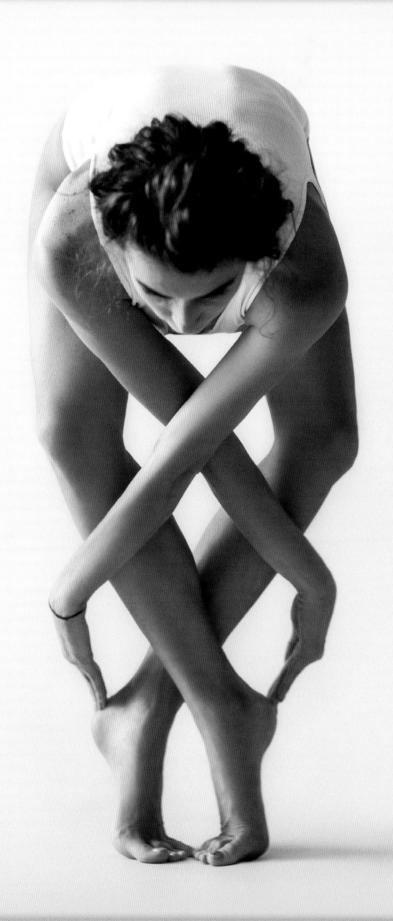

CONTENTS

Nourishing Body, Mind, and Spirit

Yoga can truly claim to offer something positive to students of almost any age—from rambunctious children to stressed or sedentary adults . . . even to seniors with joint issues or mobility problems.

No other low-impact discipline is as good for stretching and strengthening your muscles, tendons, and ligaments, while offering beneficial effects for your brain, heart, lungs, digestive tract, and other organs. It's also healthy for your psyche. Yoga poses, or postures, are typically achieved through a powerful triumvirate of breath control, meditative concentration, and studied movements. Limbs are never jerked or thrust into place, heads never loll, torsos are never wrenched—although they can be effectively twisted. Poses are held in stillness for a prescribed amount of breaths, aided by heightened balance skills and by activating muscles through torsion or flexion.

Ideally, one yoga posture should flow effortlessly into the next: standing poses hinging into forward bends, reclining poses arching up into backbends, arm supports extending into shoulderstands or headstands. A series of yoga poses should almost appear to be a dance—one performed with graceful, collected holds and supple transitions.

It is no surprise that during the "age of fitness" in the latter part of the twentieth century, yoga was one of the many exercise modalities that grew in popularity. But while other novelty workout disciplines lost their luster, yoga has only strengthened its position as one of the most versatile and beneficial disciplines for increasing fitness and stamina, improving balance, toning the body, and relieving tension, anxiety, stress, and a variety of physical conditions. And because yoga is so diverse and opens itself to so many interpretations, it allows students to progress at their own individual pace, from one week to the next, or even during the same class—all within their own comfort zones.

Yoga's advocates, including many hard-core trainers, know it can easily be integrated into any type of exercise regimen, perhaps alternating with high-intensity or cardio workout days, or be used on its own to create an encompassing sense of well-being and an aura of glowing health.

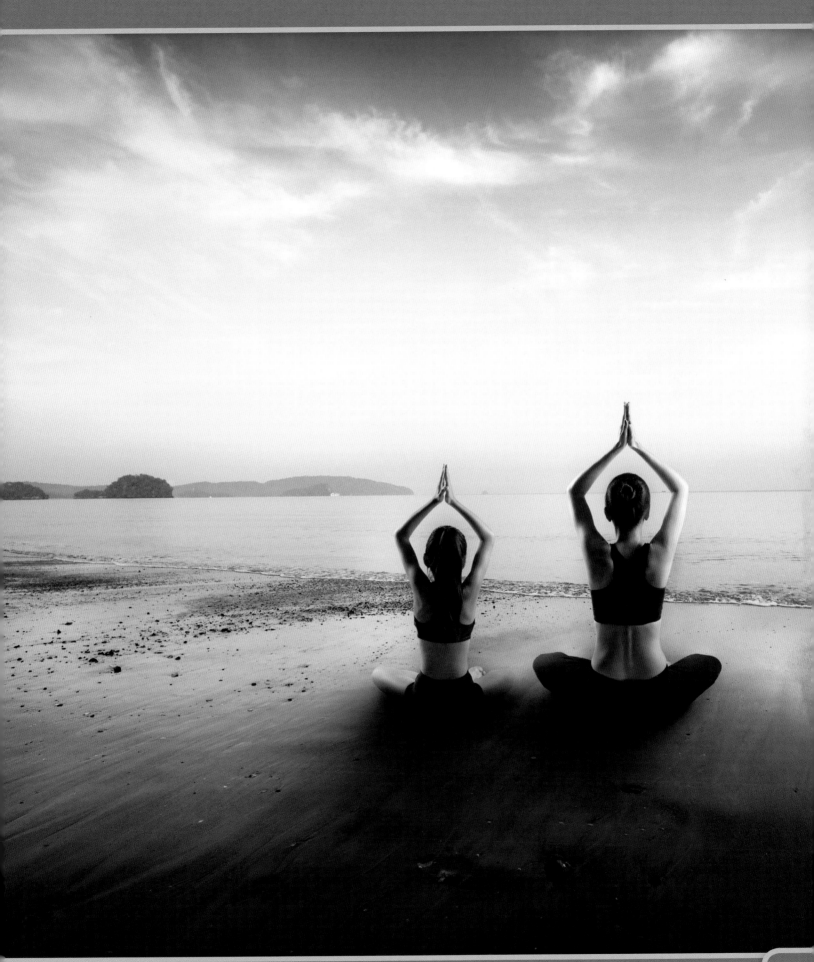

History of Yoga

The word yoga comes from the Sanskrit word *yug*, meaning to "unite" or "yoke." Its essential purpose is the unification of body, mind, and spirit into a harmonious whole. This is accomplished through a three-tiered approach: physical postures, or asanas; breath control methods, or pranayamas; and concentration on spiritual mindfulness, or enlightenment, known as meditation.

The early practice of yoga, known as preclassical yoga, began more than 5,000 years ago in the Indus Valley in northern India. The Indus-Sarasvati civilization developed yoga as a system of physical exercises as well as a path toward spiritual growth. It was refined by the Brahmans, priests who studied the holy Vedas, and by mystic seers called *rishis*. Their refinements were documented in the Upanishads, a massive work containing more than 200 scriptures. The most notable of these yogic scriptures is the *Bhagavad Gita*, written around 500 BC. The Upanishads also reworked the concept of ritual sacrifice found in the Vedas, focusing instead on the sacrifice of the ego along three pathways: knowledge, action, and wisdom.

Classical yoga took the somewhat confusing or contradictory ideas, beliefs, and techniques of the earlier era and coalesced them into one doctrine. This was primarily the work of the sage Patanjali, whose *Yoga-sutras* from the second century became the first systematic presentation of yoga. He organized yoga into an "eight-limbed path" that provided the stages needed to achieve *samadhi*, or enlightenment. Patanjali is often called the father of yoga, and his sutras continue to influence modern yoga practices.

Several centuries after Patanjali's sutras, in the postclassical period, a group of yoga masters posited that the physical body was the key to enlightenment and prolonged life. As a result, they developed tantric yoga; its focus on mind-body connections led to the creation of the popular variation called hatha yoga.

In the modern era, around the turn of the twentieth century, several yoga masters traveled beyond India to spread their teachings. Swami Vivekananda's appearance at the 1893 World's Parliament of Religions in Chicago gained him a great deal of followers. What is recognized as yoga today, with its many asanas, developed in India during the Modern Yoga Renaissance, quite probably as a result of blending Western-style gymnastics with traditional hatha yoga postures. Fostered by gurus such as Yogendra, Kuvalayananda, Seetharaman Sundaram, and Krishnamacharya, modern yoga first appeared in the 1920s. Yet it was not until 1947, when Indra Devi opened her highly successful "yoga studio to the stars" in Hollywood, that yoga truly entered the mainstream in the West.

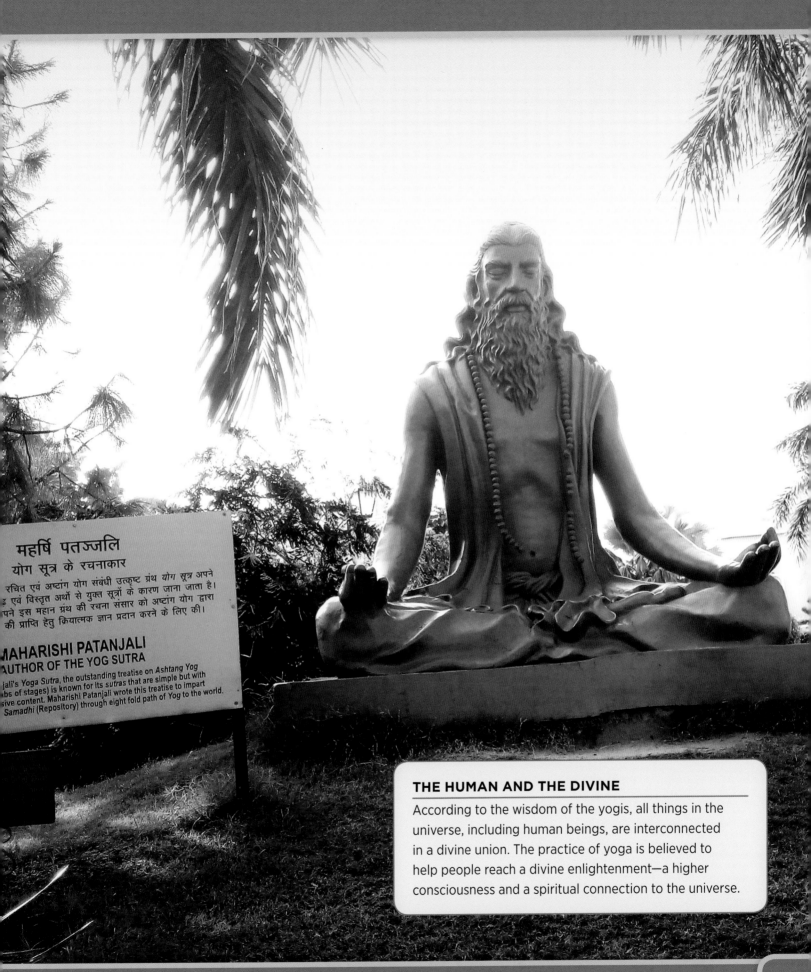

महर्षि पतज्ज्लि
योग सूत्र के रचनाकार

रचित एवं अष्टांग योग संबंधी उत्कृष्ट ग्रंथ योग सूत्र अपने
एवं विस्तृत अर्थों से युक्त सूत्रों के कारण जाना जाता है।
पने इस महान ग्रंथ की रचना संसार को अष्टांग योग द्वारा
की प्राप्ति हेतु कियात्मक ज्ञान प्रदान करने के लिए की।

MAHARISHI PATANJALI
AUTHOR OF THE YOG SUTRA

jali's Yoga Sutra, the outstanding treatise on Ashtang Yog
bs of stages) is known for its sutras that are simple but with
sive content. Maharishi Patanjali wrote this treatise to impart
Samadhi (Repository) through eight fold path of Yog to the world.

THE HUMAN AND THE DIVINE

According to the wisdom of the yogis, all things in the universe, including human beings, are interconnected in a divine union. The practice of yoga is believed to help people reach a divine enlightenment—a higher consciousness and a spiritual connection to the universe.

Variants

Over time, many types of yoga evolved that focused on different aspects of the yoga experience—breathing, muscle control, stamina, stretching, spiritual renewal, and cleansing. Today, most of these variations are available at gyms or yoga studios. Although these modalities tend to incorporate the same basic poses, each variation might place a different emphasis on each posture.

Hatha is the general term for a slow-paced, gentle form of yoga that makes for an excellent introduction to the discipline.

Vinyasa, which refers to breath-synchronized movement, is a more demanding form of yoga. It is based on a series of poses called Sun Salutations, during which movements are matched to your breaths.

Ashtanga, which means "eight limbs" in Sanskrit, is more physically demanding. In this intense, fast-paced discipline, a set of poses is performed in the same order, requiring constant movement from one pose to the next. Ashtanga is the inspiration behind classes called Power Yoga.

Iyengar yoga focuses on how the body should be precisely positioned to gain the most from each pose while avoiding injury. It utilizes props such as bands, blankets, and blocks and involves holding one pose for a longer period rather than moving quickly into the next pose.

Kundalini yoga utilizes breathing and physical movement to free the energy in the lower body and allow it to move upward. It employs rapid, repetitive movement that might be accompanied by call-and-response chants from the teacher.

Bikram yoga, which is based on the teachings of Bikram Choudhury, takes place in a room heated to 95–100°F (35–38°C). This allows a loosening of tight muscles and the cleansing effect of sweating. Not surprisingly, *Bikram* is often advertised in gyms as hot yoga.

Yin yoga is a slow, studied variation that incorporates minutes-long holds that target fascia, or connective tissue. Yin yoga provides elasticity and length to limbs and restorative meditative qualities.

Restorative yoga is a slow-moving discipline with longer holds that are meant to tap into the parasympathetic nervous system, fostering deep relaxation. It is used to ease insomnia and anxiety. Athletes may perform restorative yoga postures on recovery days. Props can include bolsters, blankets, and blocks.

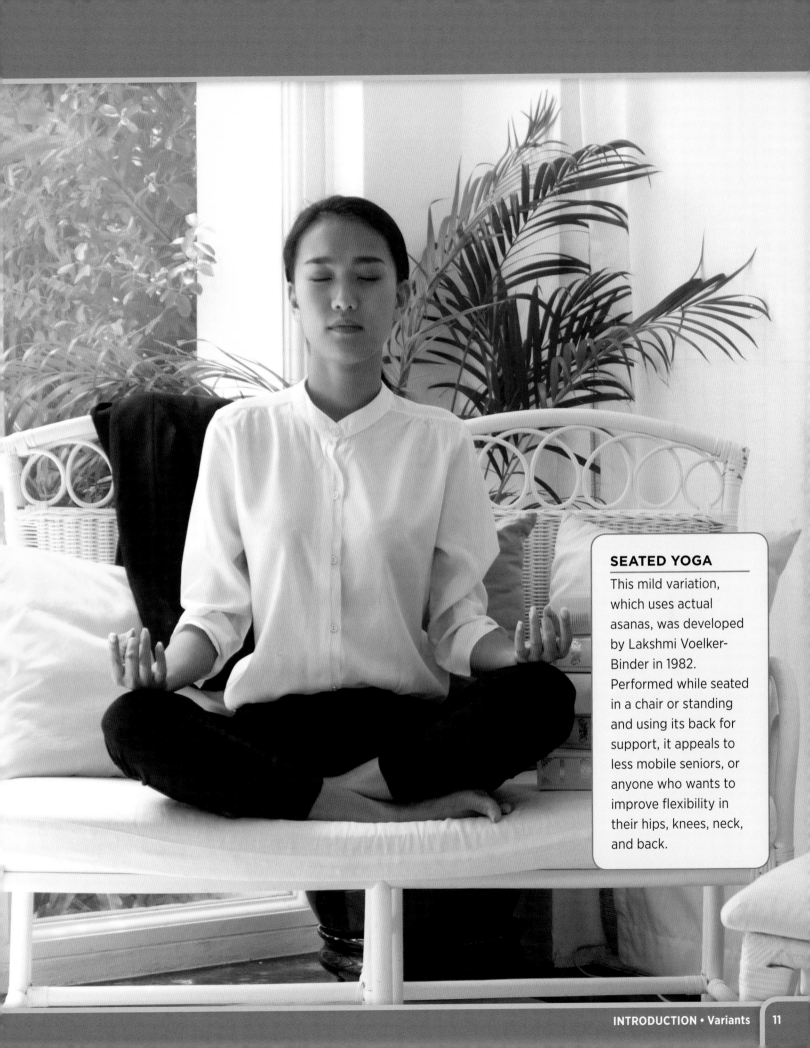

SEATED YOGA

This mild variation, which uses actual asanas, was developed by Lakshmi Voelker-Binder in 1982. Performed while seated in a chair or standing and using its back for support, it appeals to less mobile seniors, or anyone who wants to improve flexibility in their hips, knees, neck, and back.

The Yoga Class

Even for those who spend hours a week at the gym, a yoga class may seem like foreign territory at first. Below are some of the things the uninitiated can expect. And always remember that in yoga, it is the student who determines the extent of any pose, not the teacher.

In a typical yoga class, the students will be spread out in organized rows and positioned at least arm's-length apart. You will start by unrolling your mat so that the edges curl down toward the floor, and removing your shoes and socks—yoga is traditionally performed barefoot, in order to engage your toes, heels, and muscles of your feet.

If your class is in a gym or health club, your instructor will likely focus primarily on the physical aspects of yoga. If you are in a dedicated yoga studio, there will probably me more emphasis on all three aspects of yoga: body, mind, and spirit. Your teacher might go over breathing methods, the pranayamas; lead a call-and-response chanting session; introduce you to the basics of meditation; or read a passage from an inspiring text. How much of this supplementation occurs will be based on which yoga discipline your teacher practices. It is up to you to determine whether you want a class that is strictly physical or one that incorporates a more spiritual approach.

If this is your first class, introduce yourself and inform the teacher if you have any problems or if you are pregnant or recovering from an injury or surgery, for instance. Assuming you have enrolled in a beginner-intermediate class—there is no point to "cutting in line" in yoga—you will start with some warm-up poses and move on to more taxing positions. At any point, you can modify the pose to your own comfort level or ask the teacher for a less difficult variation. If you need to rest, you can assume Child's Pose: knees bent, torso folded down, your chin on the floor, and your arms relaxed out in front of you or along your sides.

At the end of your session, you will rest in Corpse Pose for several minutes, lying flat on your back, with your arms and legs slightly outspread. At this point, you will likely experience a heightened awareness of your body as the outer world recedes. Do not rise too quickly from Corpse Pose—the change can be jarring. Once you are upright again, thank your instructor, and gather up your supplies.

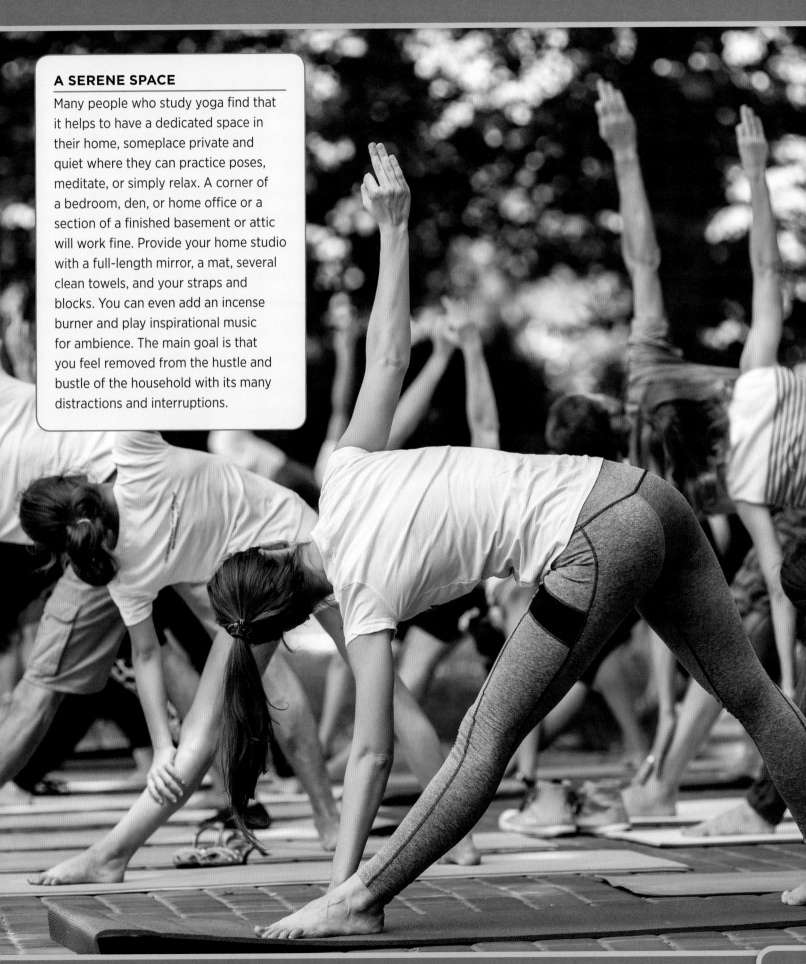

A SERENE SPACE

Many people who study yoga find that it helps to have a dedicated space in their home, someplace private and quiet where they can practice poses, meditate, or simply relax. A corner of a bedroom, den, or home office or a section of a finished basement or attic will work fine. Provide your home studio with a full-length mirror, a mat, several clean towels, and your straps and blocks. You can even add an incense burner and play inspirational music for ambience. The main goal is that you feel removed from the hustle and bustle of the household with its many distractions and interruptions.

Tools

As with any sports or exercise program, yoga requires some basic equipment—the proper clothing, a mat, and a few props or aids. The good news is, with the exception of the mat, the other things you require can probably be sourced at home.

CLOTHING

The basic requirement for yoga clothing is simply that it should feel comfortable. It need not be anything fancy from the sporting goods store, just something relatively stretchy that is not confining. A comfy T-shirt and running pants are fine, as are a tank top and gym shorts. Jeans or cords are generally too stiff to accommodate the bending and twisting movements. You don't need to worry about special footgear—yoga is traditionally performed barefoot.

MAT

You can buy inexpensive yoga mats for less than $20, but it might be worthwhile to invest a bit more than that. A good mat can make a difference in how you assume and hold poses: your mat should be sturdy and slightly tacky to the touch. While it is true that you may be able to use a studio mat free of charge or for a small fee, you will probably want your own for sanitary reasons—some people sweat a lot during yoga sessions. Plus, mats are quite light and easy to carry to and from class.

PROPS

If a yoga pose is too difficult to complete, or if you find a position too painful to maintain, there are a number of props or aids that can be employed to ease you into a pose. Some of these props are also used in restorative yoga to remove stress from your body.

- Blocks can help achieve poses, deepen your stretches, and ensure correct alignment while holding a pose. In a pinch, a thick book can be substituted for a block.
- Folded blankets can be elevate your buttocks in poses where your hips and thighs are opened.
- Webbing straps can help you reach down to your feet or raise your legs as well as allow holds behind your back if you are knotted up or recovering from an injury. They also align your posture and help maintain the structure of a pose. A long towel can be used in place of a strap.
- Bolsters are like firm body pillows; they are often used in restorative yoga to foster relaxation, soften posture, and open your body.

Other useful props to consider include a meditation pillow, a yoga wedge, a neck pillow, yoga knee pads, a Swiss ball, toe spreaders, and yoga gloves.

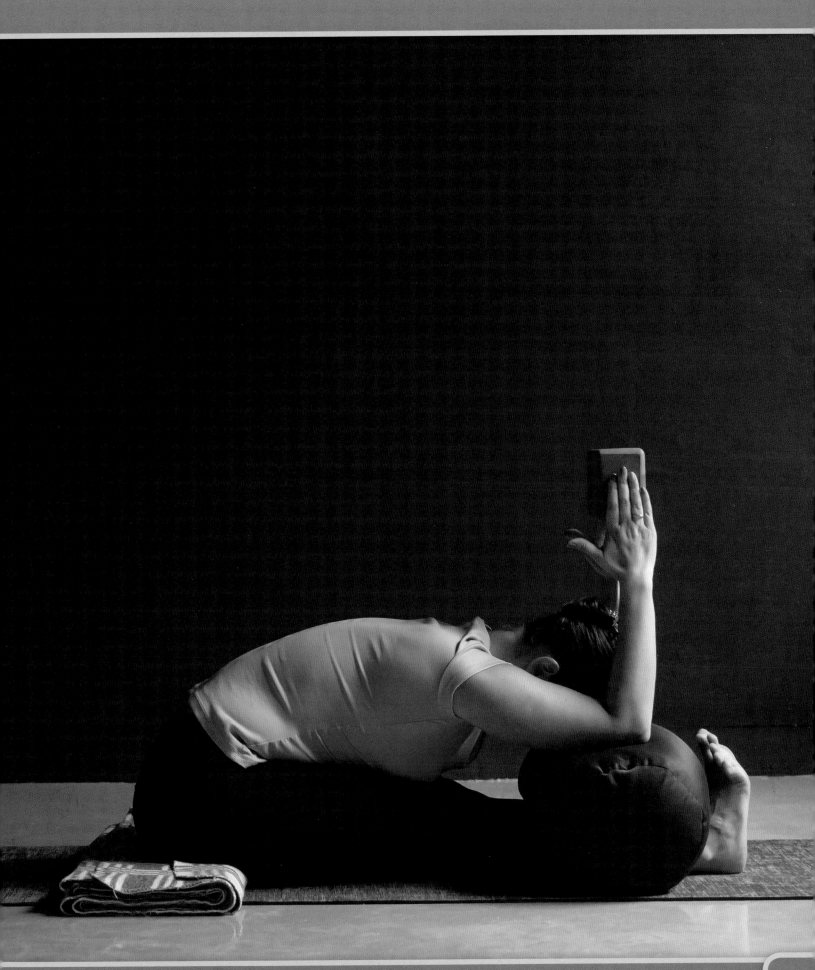

Yoga Lingo

Yoga has its roots in the centuries-old Indian Vedas, and many of the words describing the poses and body positioning are in Sanskrit, the language of ancient India. Yoga students quickly become familiar with words such as asana, pranayama, and mudra. When pronounced correctly, these words create distinct inhalations and exhalations that are similar to those employed in meditative mantras.

ASANA: a "seat," or a physical posture of yoga.

ASHRAM: a hermitage; a monastic community or a religious retreat, especially in India and Southeast Asia.

ASHTANGA: the eight-limbed yogic path.

AYURVEDA: the ancient Indian science of health.

BAKTI: devotion, as in Bakti yoga.

BANDHA: internal muscular "locks" that, when engaged, support the toning and lifting of strategic areas of the body. The three major bandhas of Hatha yoga are:

- Mula Bandha: the pelvic floor muscles
- Uddiyana Bandha: the abdominals up to the diaphragm
- Jalandhara Bandha: the throat

CHAKRA: meaning a "wheel"; one of seven energy centers in your body located between the base of your spine and the top of your head.

- Root chakra (Muladhara): the base of your spine
- Sacral chakra (Svadhisthana): the lower abdomen
- Solar plexus chakra (Manipura): the upper abdomen
- Heart chakra (Anahata): the center of your chest
- Throat chakra (Vishuddha): the throat area
- Third eye chakra (Ajna): the forehead, between your eyebrows
- Crown chakra (Sahasrara): the very top of your head

CORE: the core is often thought of as the abdominal muscles, but it's more accurate to think of it as an apple core, running from the top of your head to the inner arches of your feet.

DOSHA: a physical body type; in Ayurvedic medicine there are three doshas: pitta ("fire"), vata ("wind"), and kapha ("earth").

DRISHTI: focal point of gazing during meditation or yoga practice—and quite useful during balancing poses.

GURU: teacher or master; one who illumines the darkness.

HATHA YOGA: from ha ("sun") and tha ("moon"), hatha yoga seeks to unify opposites—body and mind —and describes any of the physical practices of yoga.

KIRTAN: a community gathering that includes chanting, music, and meditation.

MANTRA: "a tool or instrument of thought"; sounds, syllables, words, or groups of words that are repeated with the goal of creating a positive transformation; a sacred thought or a prayer.

MEDITATION: the focusing and calming of the mind, often through breath work, to reach a deeper level of consciousness.

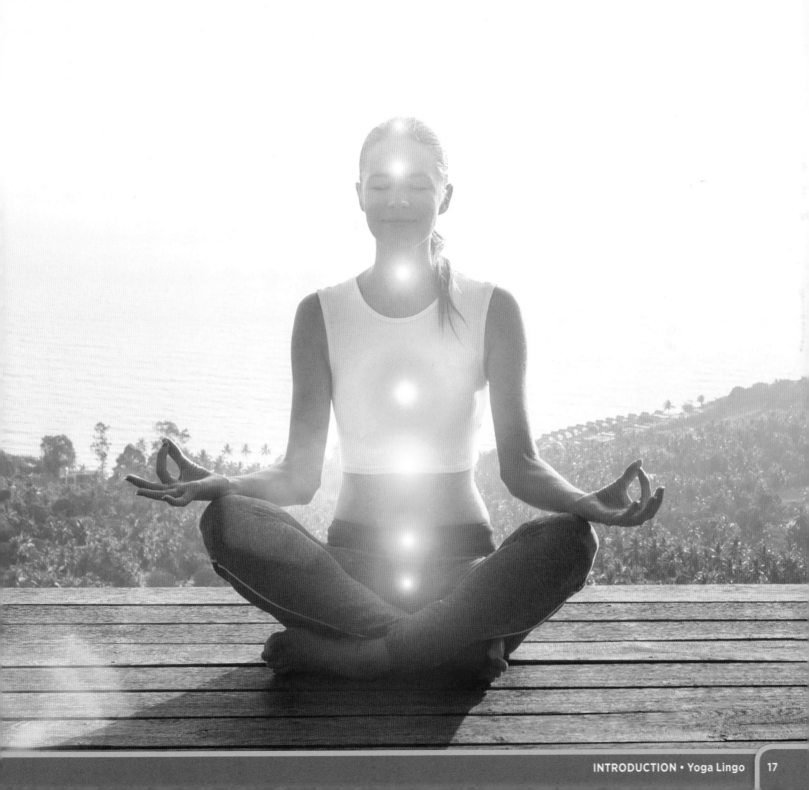

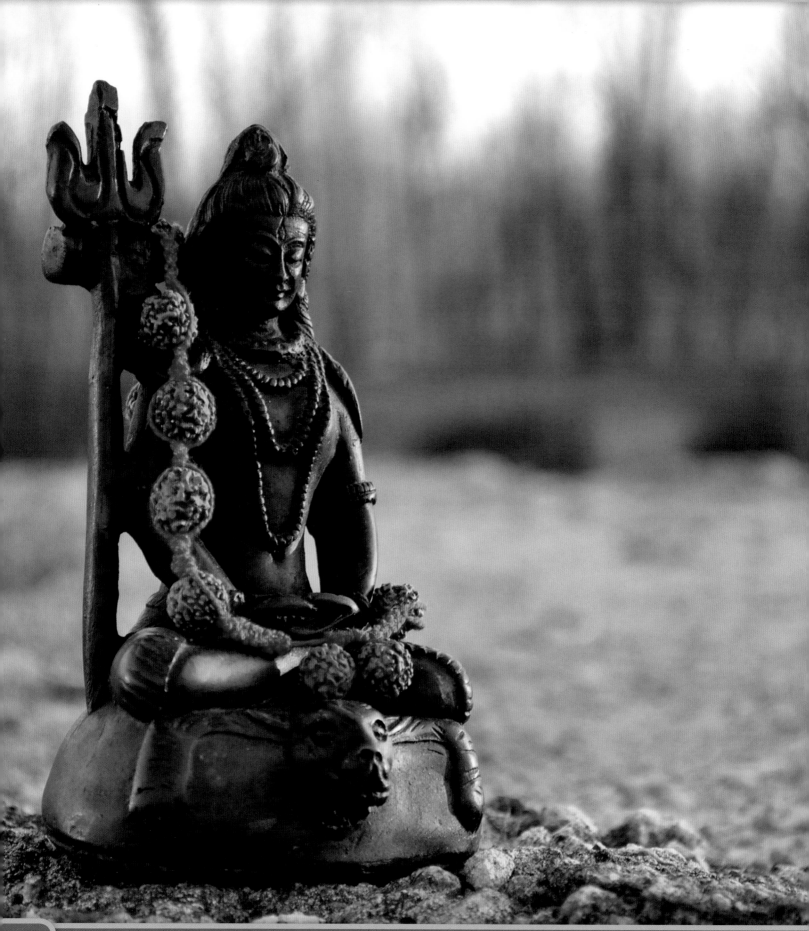

MUDRA: a "seal," or hand gesture, that influences the energies of the body or mood. Most often the hands and fingers are held in a mudra to aid concentration, focus, and connection to yourself. The most common mudras are Anjali (palms pressed together at the heart) and Gyan (forefinger and thumb forming a circle, the other three fingers stretching away).

NADI: the energy channels through which *prana*, or life force, flows. Pranayama uses the breath to direct and expand the flow of prana in the nadis.

NAMASTE: Sanskrit word commonly spoken at the end of a yoga class. One thoughtful interpretation: I honor that place in you where the whole universe resides; and when I am in that place in me and you are in that place in you, there is only one of us.

OM: a mantra usually chanted at the beginning and end of a yoga class. It is said to be the origin of all sounds and the seed of creation and is often referred to as the "universal sound of consciousness."

PATANJALI: an ancient sage who is said to have compiled the *Yoga-sutras*, a guide on how to live in order to advance along a spiritual path toward enlightenment.

PRANA: life energy, or life force.

PRANAYAMA: breath awareness used to facilitate inner stillness and awareness.

PROPS: tools such as mats, blocks, blankets, and straps used to extend your range of motion or facilitate achieving a pose.

SAMADHI: a state of complete enlightenment.

SAVASANA, OR CORPSE POSE: the ultimate relaxation pose, typically at the end of yoga class.

SHAKTI: female energy.

SHANTI: a word meaning "peace" that is often chanted three times in class.

SHIVA: a Hindu deity; male energy.

SURYA NAMASKAR, OR SUN SALUTATIONS: a sequence of dynamic asanas often used to warm up the body at the beginning of a yoga class.

SWAMI: a "master," or Hindu ascetic or religious leader, especially a senior member of a religious order.

TANTRA: the yoga of union between mind and body.

UJJAYI, HISSING BREATH, OR VICTORIOUS BREATH: a type of pranayama in which the lungs are fully expanded and the chest is puffed out; especially associated with the vinyasa style.

UPANISHADS: texts of a religious and philosophical nature, written in India between 800 BC and 500 BC.

VINYASA: movement linked with breath; postures are strung together to create a short flow or a long flow.

YANG YOGA: a style of yoga that is rhythmic, repetitive, and energetic and is great for building strength and fitness.

YIN YOGA: a series of long-held, passive floor poses that target the fascia, or connective tissue, in the body. A combination of yin and yang keeps students balanced and healthy.

YOGA: from the Sanskrit *yug*, meaning "yoke" or "union"; yoga is an ancient discipline in which physical postures, breath practice, meditation, and philosophical study are used as tools for achieving liberation.

YOGI/YOGINI: a male/female practitioner of yoga.

Hand Gestures

In the practice of meditative yoga, it is believed that each part of the hand has a reflex reaction in a specific region of the brain. Therefore, the mudras, or hand gestures, used in some yoga poses can actually help guide energy flow and channel it to the brain. To this end, there are more than 100 known mudras, which have developed over time. In many seated yoga poses, the hands are relaxed, resting palms faceup on the thighs, in what is called Hands in Lap. But if the pose calls for a mudra, do try to include it.

The following are some of the most widely used mudras.

GYAN, OR CHIN, MUDRA: This is one of the most common mudras. Place the tips of your index finger and thumb together, while your other three fingers stretch away, relaxed. Your index finger stands for the planet Jupiter, which represents knowledge and expansion. This is an especially beneficial mudra to employ when seeking understanding or insight.

ANJALI, OR PRAYER, MUDRA: This gestures involves pressing your palms together, typically at your heart or behind your back. It is used to neutralize the positive (male) and the negative (female) sides of the body. It is often performed before a yoga class and again at the end. Pressing your palms together helps connect and balance the two hemispheres of your brain.

SURYA RAVI MUDRA: form a circle with your ring finger and thumb—or bend your ring finger down to the base of your thumb—keeping the other fingers straight. This pose represents courage and responsibility and is believed to improve digestion and increase metabolism.

SHUNI, OR SHOONYA, MUDRA: for this gesture, place the tips of your middle finger and thumb together, keeping the other fingers straight. This joining represents patience and discernment and is used to improve intuition, awareness, and sensory powers as well as purify emotions.

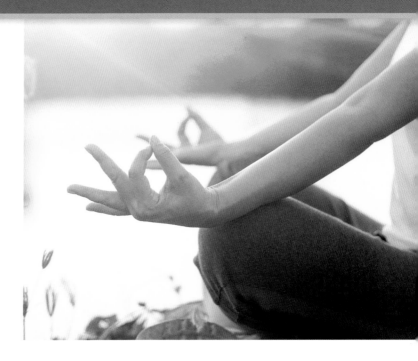

VISHNU MUDRA: curl your index finger and middle finger down toward your palm, while keeping your ring finger and pinkie close together and upright. This mudra is used while practicing the breathing technique known as anuloma viloma.

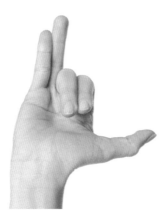

VENUS LOCK: interlace the fingers of both hands, with the right pinkie down for women and the left pinkie down for men. This pose represents both sexuality and sensuality.

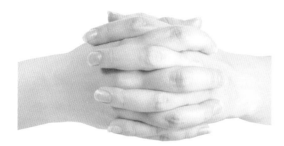

Other common variations include Buddhi Mudra, with your pinkie and thumb forming a circle. The pinkie stands for the planet Mercury, which represents quickness and the power of communication. Prana Mudra, which activates the dormant energy inside you, involves touching your ring finger and pinkie to the tip of your thumb. In Dhyana Mudra, your hands lie quietly, with your right hand resting in your left palm, thumbs touching. This pose deepens concentration. In Apana Mudra, your index and middle fingers touch the thumb, while your outer fingers fan out to the sides. It is used to aid both mental and physical digestion. In Ganesha, or Bear Grip, Mudra, face your right palm toward your heart and your left palm outward, then curl your fingers, grip them together, and pull your arms out to your sides. This mudra stimulates your heart and intensifies concentration.

The Breath of Life

In yogic culture, the practice of controlled breathing is known as pranayama. *Prana* refers to breath's internal energy, or life force; *ayama* refers to extension and control. In addition to drawing in the breath of life, it is also important to eliminate the toxins within the respiratory system. Breath control can restore health and mental clarity, improve physical control, relieve stress, and increase awareness of the body's natural rhythms.

During pranayama, inhalation, or *puraka*, stimulates your respiratory system. Retention, or *kumbhaka*, raises your internal temperature and increases the absorption of oxygen. And exhalation, or *rechak*, contracts your intercostal muscles to eject air full of toxins and impurities. These actions massage your abdominal muscles and tone various organs of your body, facilitating the flow of energy. The effectiveness of pranayama depends on maintaining the proper ratios between inhalation, retention, and exhalation.

Yoga students of all levels can learn how to alter the movement of prana. You can start breath control by familiarizing yourself with, and practicing, the exercises below. They will enable you to draw oxygen deep into your lungs, encourage a connection between your body and mind, and leave you feeling rejuvenated and refreshed.

BEGINNING YOUR PRACTICE

Although it is normal to perform pranayama in a seated position, at this point you should start in Corpse Pose (pages 308–09), lying on your back and focusing only on your breathing. Many people breathe by filling only the top portion of their lungs. Pranayama teaches you how to fill your lungs from bottom to top, using both diaphragmatic and thoracic breathing, in order to nourish them completely.

Draw in even breaths as you concentrate on filling every portion of your lungs with oxygen. Begin at the bottom, expanding your diaphragm to inflate your abdomen; then raise your rib cage as oxygen floods the middle of your lungs. Finally, allow the top of your lungs to fill as your chest expands. Make sure both sides of your chest rise simultaneously.

Now you should be ready to practice pranayama in an upright, seated position. Once you are comfortable— perhaps with your legs folded, and shins crossed—place one hand flat on your chest and the other on your abdominal muscles. This will help you monitor your breath as it enters your body. Close your eyes, lift up from your spine, draw your chin in slightly toward your chest, and listen to your breath as your stomach and rib cage expand and contract. Concentrate on the pathways the oxygen travels, the rhythm of your breathing, and the texture of the sound.

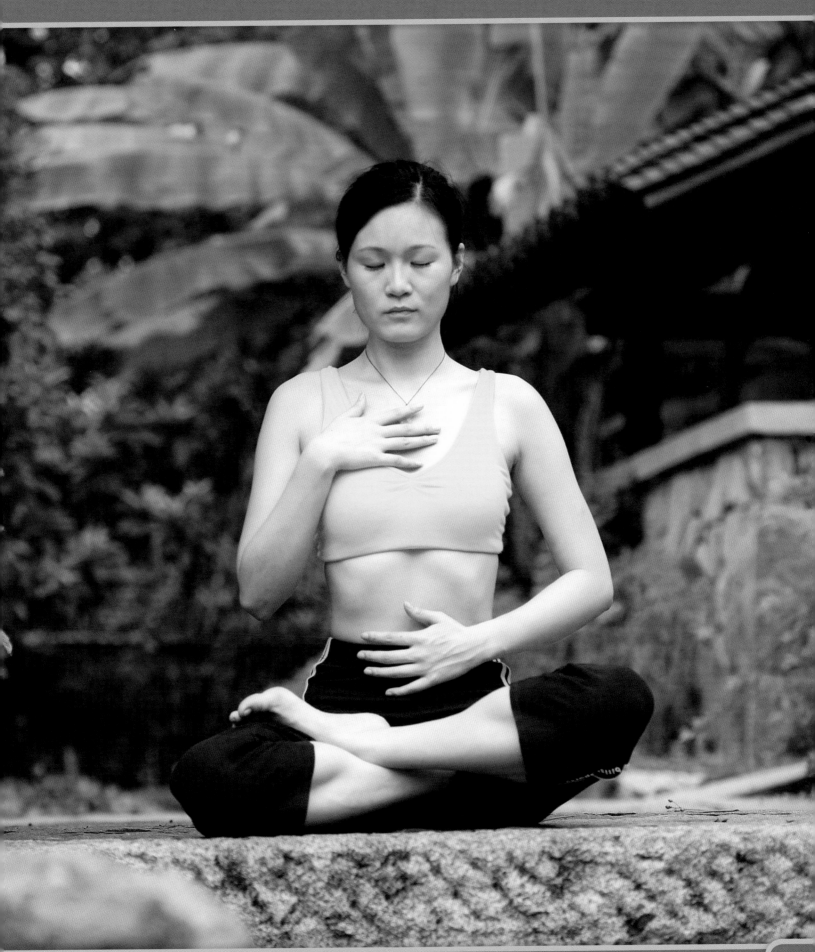

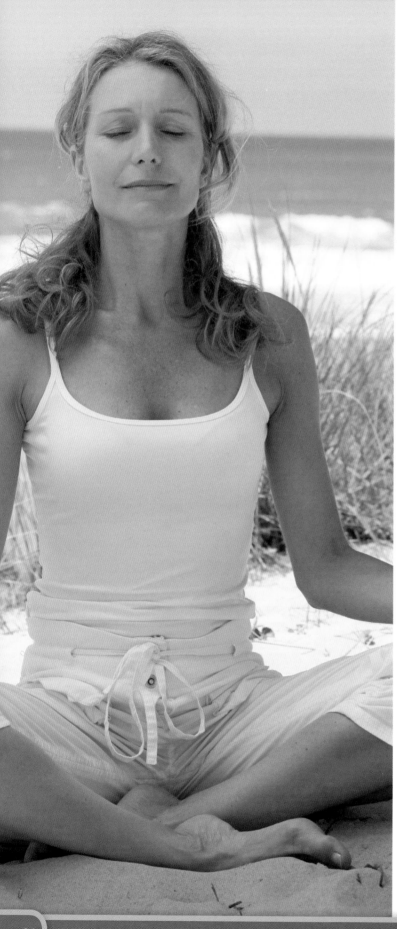

BREATHING EXERCISES

- **SAMAVRITTI, OR THE SAME BREATH**: If there are irregularities to your breathing, focus on taking slower, more even breaths. To achieve samavritti, meaning "the same action," inhale for four counts, then exhale for four. Repeat until you are doing it almost instinctively without the counting. This breathing method can calm the mind and establish a sense of balance and stability.

- **UJJAYI, OR THE VICTORIOUS BREATH:** This is sometimes referred to as the "ocean breath" because of the surflike sound that air makes as it passes through the narrow epiglottal passage in your throat. Maintaining an even rhythm, constrict the epiglottis, and keep your mouth closed as you listen for the hiss at the back of your throat. Ujjayi tones your internal organs, raises your internal temperature, aids in concentration, and calms your mind.

- **KUMBHAKA, OR THE RETAINED BREATH:** This may simply mean the practice of holding your breath, but it is key to pranayama. Begin with ujjayi or samavritti breathing, and after four breaths, hold your breath for four to eight counts. Exhale, allowing your exhalation to last longer than your inhalation. Initially, your retention, or kumbhaka, will be shorter than your other breaths. Eventually, reduce the number of normal breaths in between kumbhaka breaths and increase the number of counts in your inhale, exhale, and kumbhaka retention. Build up to an exhalation that is twice as long as your inhalation, and a kumbhaka breath three times as long. This breathing method strengthens the diaphragm, restores vitality, and purifies the respiratory system. Studies indicate it may even improve cerebral circulation.

• ANULOMA VILOMA, OR ALTERNATE NOSTRIL BREATHING: This breathing method purifies the energy channels through the right and left nostrils, thus stimulating the movement of prana. Position your hands in Vishnu Mudra, with the index and middle fingers curled down. Place your right thumb against the outside of your right nostril, and with your mouth closed inhale through the left nostril. Close the left nostril with your ring finger and hold for a moment. Then raise your thumb, and exhale from the right nostril. Switch hands and repeat on the opposite side. Begin with five cycles, and gradually increase the number. This method lowers your heart rate and reduces stress.

• KAPALABHATI, OR THE SHINING SKULL: This exercise utilizes a rhythmic pumping action in the abdomen to exhale. Loosen your abdominals and fill your diaphragm with air. Then force the air out of your lungs with a quick, explosive exhale. Inhale automatically. Start with two rounds of 10 cycles and work up to four rounds of 20 cycles. This method strengthens the diaphragm, revives energy, and purifies the respiratory system.

• SITHALI, OR THE COILING BREATH: In this method, inhalation occurs through the mouth. To begin, curl the edges of your tongue into a tube, and stick it out slightly. Inhale through the center of your tongue tube. Retain that breath, close your mouth, and exhale through your nose. Continue for five or 10 cycles. Sithali helps to cool and comfort your body.

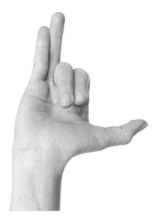

1. Place your fingers in the Vishnu Mudra with your index and middle fingers curled down, keeping your ring finger and pinkie together and pointed up.

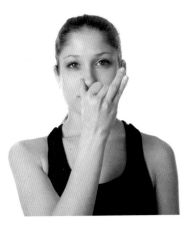

2. Close your right nostril with your right thumb, and inhale through your left nostril.

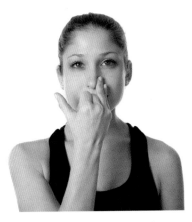

3. Retain your breath, squeezing the left nostril with your ring finger, and then release your thumb as you exhale through your right nostril.

How to Use This Book

Ultimate Guide to Yoga features step-by-step instructions for 161 poses specially selected to fit into an effective and beneficial yoga regimen.

For each pose, you'll find a short overview of the position, photos with step-by-step instructions, tips on proper form, and anatomical illustrations that highlight the targeted muscles. A quick-read panel features key points. There may be pose variations shown in a modification box.

CHAPTER BREAKDOWNS

Chapter One: Standing Poses Build strength and give yourself a secure foundation for safe yoga practice.

Chapter Two: Standing Forward and Side Bends Strengthen your legs, stretch your hamstrings, and stabilize your hips with these weight-bearing poses.

Chapter Three: Seated Forward Bends Experience a healthy stretch along the back of your body, from your neck to your heels, with an emphasis on your hamstrings.

Chapter Four: Backbends Gain tremendous physical and psychological benefits as you invigorate and strengthen your leg, arm, and back muscles.

Chapter Five: Seated Poses and Twists Use these poses to practice breathing exercises or to meditate; they also help prepare you for more complex poses.

Chapter Six: Arm Supports and Inversions Develop strength in your arms, wrists, hands, core, shoulders, and back as you engage your abdominals to stabilize your body.

Chapter Seven: Reclining and Restorative Poses Relax and replenish your body as you cool down at the end of your yoga session.

Chapter Eight: Yoga Sequences Once you've familiarized yourself with the featured poses, turn to this chapter to learn how to flow them together into extended yoga sequences.

KEY

KEY POSE SPREADS

❶ Category
Indicates the difficulty of the pose.

❷ Exercise Info
Provides the name of the pose and some key details that you need to know about the pose.

❸ How to Do It
Offers step-by-step instructions that specify how to achieve the pose.

❹ Step-by-Step Photos
Shows images of the key steps required to complete the pose.

❺ Do It Right
Provides tips to help you perfect your form.

❻ Close-Up
Highlights an important element of the pose.

❼ Fact File
Lists key facts: the Sanskrit name of the pose, the targeted muscles, the benefits, and any cautions that may apply.

❽ Anatomical Illustration
Indicates the key working muscles. May also include an inset showing muscles not illustrated in the main image.

❾ Modification
Shows you modifications of the pose that may be easier or harder, or variations of similar difficulty.

WORKOUT SPREADS

❶ Sequence info
Gives the name of the sequence and some essential details you need to know about it.

❷ Pose Info
Shows the name of the pose, the pages where you can find it, and how many breaths to hold the pose.

❸ Photo Icon
Offers a quick view of the pose.

❹ Fact File
Lists key facts about the sequence: the level of difficulty, the objective, the work-rest ratio, and an estimate of how long it takes to perform.

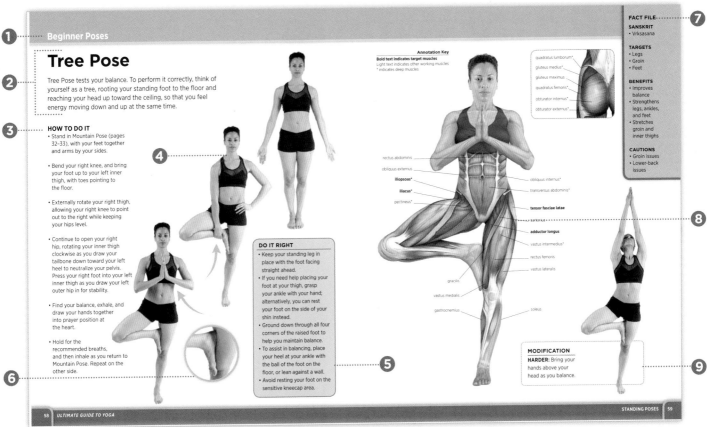

① Beginner Poses

Tree Pose ②

Tree Pose tests your balance. To perform it correctly, think of yourself as a tree, rooting your standing foot to the floor and reaching your head up toward the ceiling, so that you feel energy moving down and up at the same time.

③ HOW TO DO IT
- Stand in Mountain Pose (pages 32–33), with your feet together and arms by your sides.
- Bend your right knee, and bring your foot up to your left inner thigh, with toes pointing to the floor.
- Externally rotate your right thigh, allowing your right knee to point out to the right while keeping your hips level.
- Continue to open your right hip, rotating your inner thigh clockwise as you draw your tailbone down toward your left heel to neutralize your pelvis. Press your right foot into your left inner thigh as you draw your left outer hip in for stability.
- Find your balance, exhale, and draw your hands together into prayer position at the heart.
- Hold for the recommended breaths, and then inhale as you return to Mountain Pose. Repeat on the other side. **⑥**

④

DO IT RIGHT ⑤
- Keep your standing leg in place with the foot facing straight ahead.
- If you need help placing your foot at your thigh, grasp your ankle with your hand; alternatively, you can rest your foot on the side of your shin instead.
- Ground down through all four corners of the raised foot to help you maintain balance.
- To assist in balancing, place your heel at your ankle with the ball of the foot on the floor, or lean against a wall.
- Avoid resting your foot on the sensitive kneecap area.

Annotation Key
Bold text indicates target muscles
Light text indicates other working muscles
* indicates deep muscles

quadratus lumborum*
gluteus medius*
gluteus maximus
quadratus femoris*
obturator internus*
obturator externus*

rectus abdominis
obliquus externus
iliopsoas*
iliacus*
pectineus*
obliquus internus*
transversus abdominis*
tensor fasciae latae
sartorius
adductor longus
vastus intermedius*
rectus femoris
vastus lateralis
gracilis
vastus medialis
gastrocnemius
soleus

⑧

MODIFICATION
HARDER: Bring your hands above your head as you balance. **⑨**

FACT FILE ⑦
SANSKRIT
- Vrksasana

TARGETS
- Legs
- Groin
- Feet

BENEFITS
- Improves balance
- Strengthens legs, ankles, and feet
- Stretches groin and inner thighs

CAUTIONS
- Groin issues
- Lower-back issues

58 *ULTIMATE GUIDE TO YOGA*   STANDING POSES 59

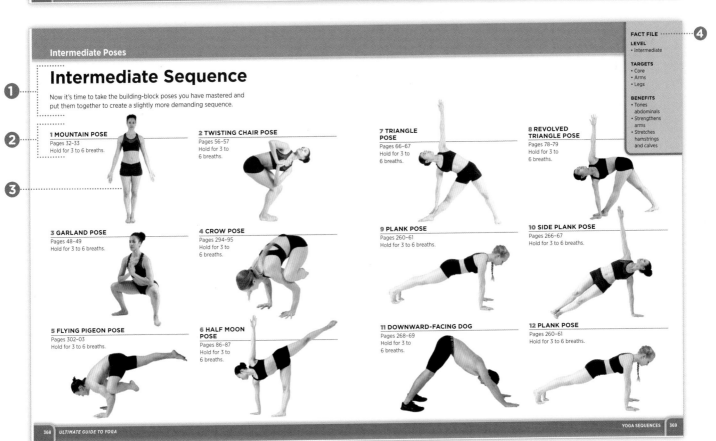

Intermediate Poses

Intermediate Sequence ①

Now it's time to take the building-block poses you have mastered and put them together to create a slightly more demanding sequence.

② ③

1 MOUNTAIN POSE
Pages 32–33
Hold for 3 to 6 breaths.

2 TWISTING CHAIR POSE
Pages 56–57
Hold for 3 to 6 breaths.

3 GARLAND POSE
Pages 48–49
Hold for 3 to 6 breaths.

4 CROW POSE
Pages 294–95
Hold for 3 to 6 breaths.

5 FLYING PIGEON POSE
Pages 302–03
Hold for 3 to 6 breaths.

6 HALF MOON POSE
Pages 86–87
Hold for 3 to 6 breaths.

7 TRIANGLE POSE
Pages 66–67
Hold for 3 to 6 breaths.

8 REVOLVED TRIANGLE POSE
Pages 78–79
Hold for 3 to 6 breaths.

9 PLANK POSE
Pages 260–61
Hold for 3 to 6 breaths.

10 SIDE PLANK POSE
Pages 266–67
Hold for 3 to 6 breaths.

11 DOWNWARD-FACING DOG
Pages 268–69
Hold for 3 to 6 breaths.

12 PLANK POSE
Pages 260–61
Hold for 3 to 6 breaths.

FACT FILE ④
LEVEL
- Intermediate

TARGETS
- Core
- Arms
- Legs

BENEFITS
- Tones abdominals
- Strengthens arms
- Stretches hamstrings and calves

368 *ULTIMATE GUIDE TO YOGA*   YOGA SEQUENCES 369

Full-Body Anatomy

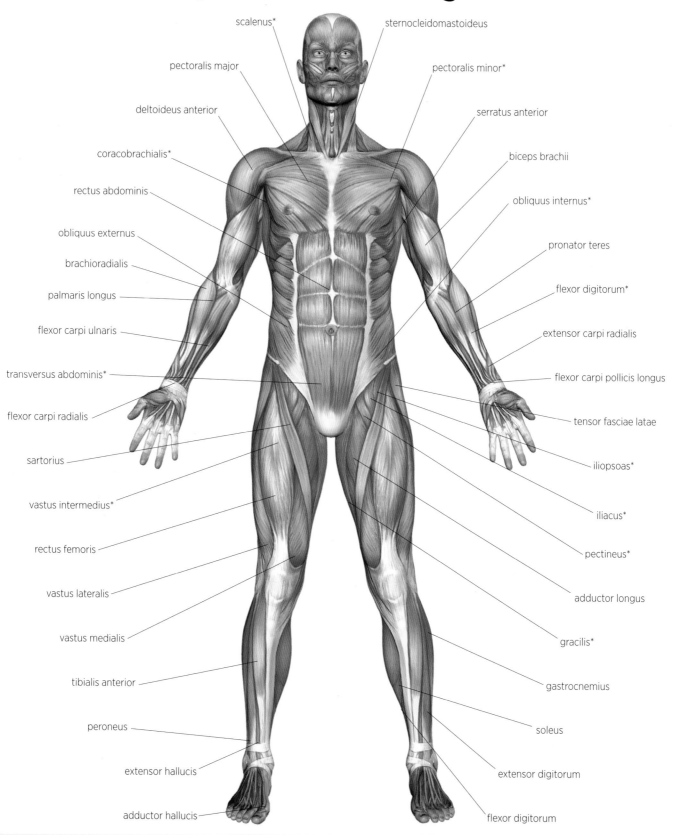

scalenus*
sternocleidomastoideus
pectoralis major
pectoralis minor*
deltoideus anterior
serratus anterior
coracobrachialis*
biceps brachii
rectus abdominis
obliquus internus*
obliquus externus
pronator teres
brachioradialis
flexor digitorum*
palmaris longus
extensor carpi radialis
flexor carpi ulnaris
flexor carpi pollicis longus
transversus abdominis*
tensor fasciae latae
flexor carpi radialis
sartorius
iliopsoas*
vastus intermedius*
iliacus*
rectus femoris
pectineus*
vastus lateralis
adductor longus
vastus medialis
gracilis*
tibialis anterior
gastrocnemius
peroneus
soleus
extensor hallucis
extensor digitorum
adductor hallucis
flexor digitorum

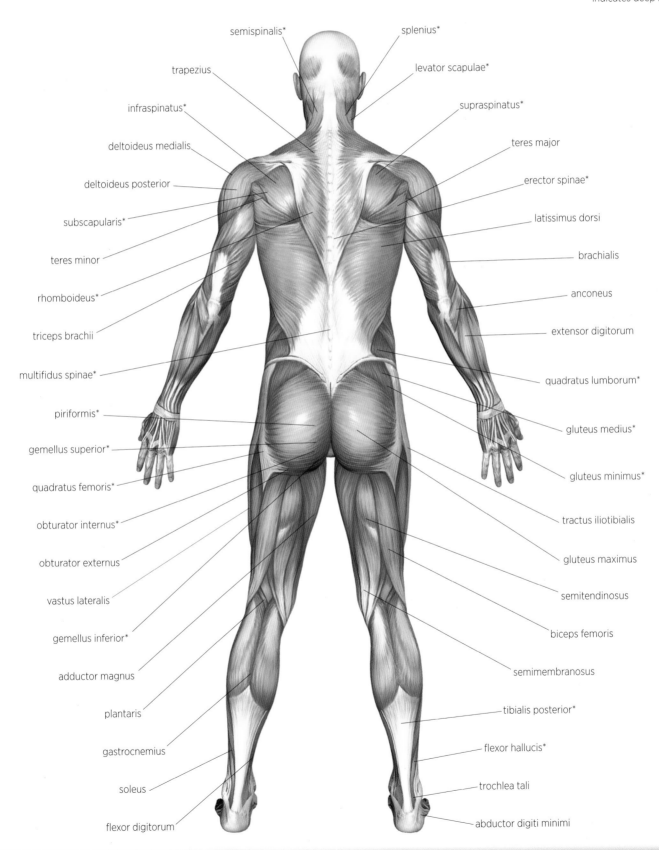

semispinalis*

splenius*

trapezius

levator scapulae*

infraspinatus*

supraspinatus*

deltoideus medialis

teres major

deltoideus posterior

erector spinae*

subscapularis*

latissimus dorsi

teres minor

brachialis

rhomboideus*

anconeus

triceps brachii

extensor digitorum

multifidus spinae*

quadratus lumborum*

piriformis*

gluteus medius*

gemellus superior*

quadratus femoris*

gluteus minimus*

obturator internus*

tractus iliotibialis

obturator externus

gluteus maximus

vastus lateralis

semitendinosus

gemellus inferior*

biceps femoris

adductor magnus

semimembranosus

plantaris

tibialis posterior*

gastrocnemius

flexor hallucis*

soleus

trochlea tali

flexor digitorum

abductor digiti minimi

CHAPTER ONE

STANDING POSES

The classic standing poses are the foundation of your practice, building your awareness of the fundamental movements of yoga. You will typically begin your yoga workout by moving through a series of these poses that energize your body, develop stamina, and revitalize your legs. Standing poses require strength, flexibility, and balance, and they can tell you which areas of your body are weak or unstable. When practicing these poses, key into your body's alignment and strive to find a graceful balance.

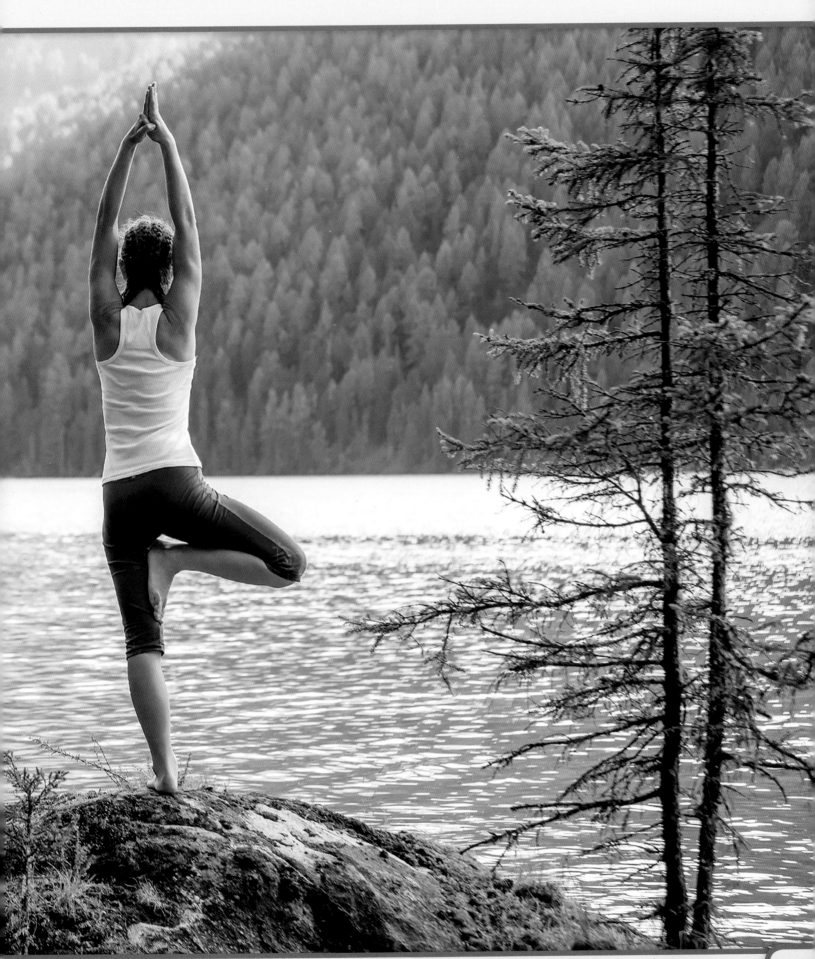

Mountain Pose

Mountain Pose forms the base for all standing poses. This posture may seem simple, but it can actually be quite challenging to achieve the correct alignment. Once you have mastered your form, you will be ready to experiment with more complicated standing poses.

HOW TO DO IT

- Stand with your feet together, with both heels and toes touching.

- Keeping your back straight and both arms pressed slightly against your sides, face your palms outward.

- Lift all your toes and let them fan out, and then gently drop them down to create a wide, solid base.

- Rock from side to side until you gradually bring your weight evenly onto all four corners of both feet.

- While balancing your weight evenly on both feet, slightly contract the muscles in your knees and thighs, rotating both thighs inward to create a widening of the sit bones.

- Tighten your abdominals, drawing them in slightly, maintaining a firm posture.

- Widen your collarbones, making sure your shoulders are parallel to your pelvis.

- Lengthen your neck, so that the crown of your head rises toward the ceiling, and your shoulder blades slide down your back.

- Hold for the recommended breaths.

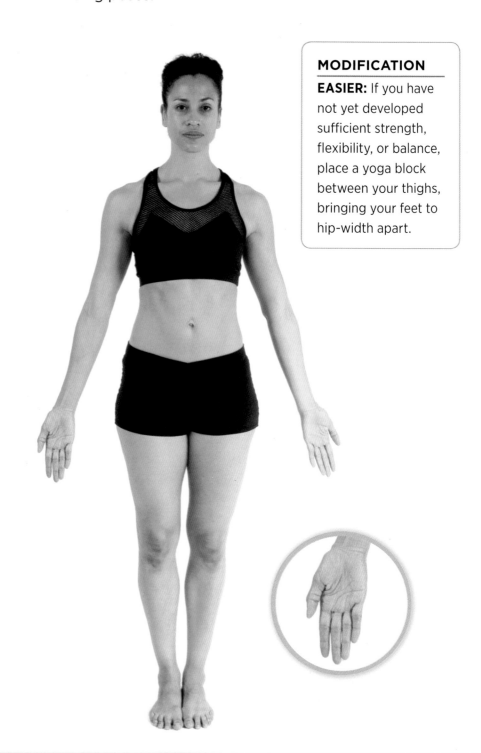

MODIFICATION

EASIER: If you have not yet developed sufficient strength, flexibility, or balance, place a yoga block between your thighs, bringing your feet to hip-width apart.

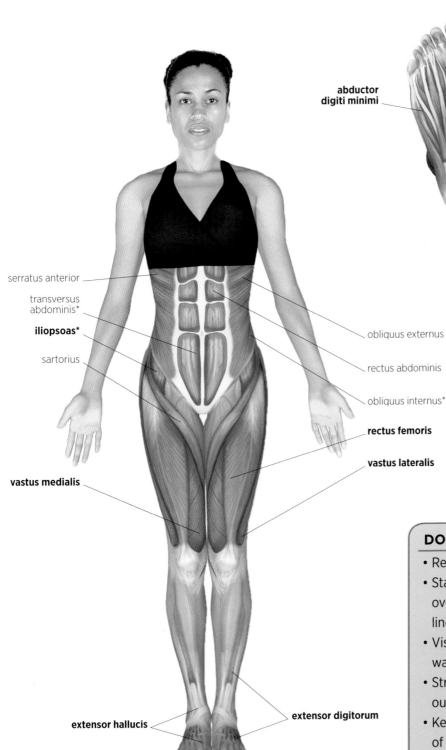

SANSKRIT
• Tadasana

TARGET
• Entire body

BENEFITS
• Improves posture
• Strengthens thighs, knees, and ankles
• Tones abdomen and buttocks
• Relieves sciatica
• Helps to treat flat feet

CAUTIONS
• Headache
• Insomnia
• Low blood pressure

flexor hallucis*

adductor hallucis

flexor digitorum*

abductor digiti minimi

plantar aponeurosis

serratus anterior

transversus abdominis*

iliopsoas*

sartorius

obliquus externus

rectus abdominis

obliquus internus*

rectus femoris

vastus lateralis

vastus medialis

extensor hallucis

extensor digitorum

Annotation Key
Bold text indicates target muscles
Light text indicates other working muscles
* indicates deep muscles

DO IT RIGHT
• Release any tension in your facial area.
• Stand completely straight with shoulders stacked over hips, hips stacked over knees, and knees in line with feet.
• Visualize your pelvis as a bowl of soup—you don't want to spill it forward or backward.
• Stretch your arms straight, with energy reaching out of your fingertips.
• Keep your chin parallel to the floor and the crown of your head pressing upward.
• Avoid arching your lower back.
• Avoid pushing your ribs forward.
• Avoid overtucking your pelvis.
• Avoid holding your breath.

Prayer Pose

Prayer Pose, like Mountain Pose, is a base position for many standing poses, and you will often assume it at the beginning and end of your yoga practice. Move into this centering posture as part of the Sun Salutation series or assume it as a transitional move in other flows. You can also sit or squat when practicing Prayer Pose.

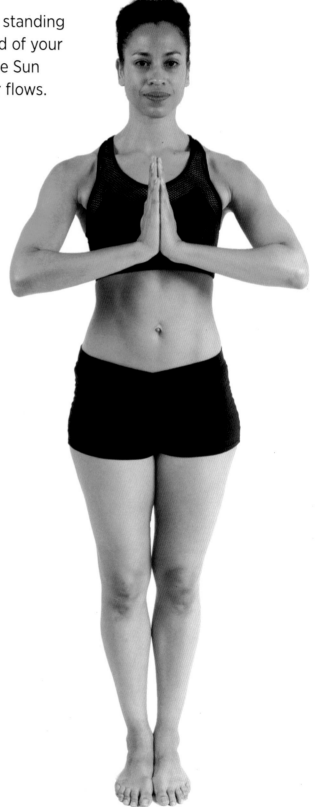

HOW TO DO IT

• Begin in Mountain Pose (pages 32–33), with your arms at your sides.

• Exhale and draw your hands together and down into prayer position at the heart.

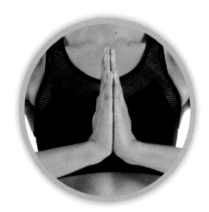

• Release any tension from your neck and shoulders, and then gently close your eyes. Hold for the recommended breaths.

DO IT RIGHT

• Release any tension in your facial area.
• Stand completely straight with shoulders stacked over hips, hips stacked over knees, and knees in line with feet.
• Visualize your pelvis as a bowl of soup—you don't want to spill it forward or backward.
• Stretch your arms straight, with energy reaching out of your fingertips.
• Keep your chin parallel to the floor and the crown of your head pressing upward.
• Avoid arching your lower back.
• Avoid pushing your ribs forward.
• Avoid overtucking your pelvis.
• Avoid holding your breath.

SANSKRIT
• Pranamasana

TARGET
• Entire body

BENEFITS
• Improves
  posture
• Strengthens
  thighs, knees,
  and ankles
• Tones abdomen
  and buttocks
• Relieves sciatica
• Helps to treat
  flat feet

CAUTIONS
• Headache
• Insomnia
• Low blood
  pressure

Annotation Key

Bold text indicates target muscles
Light text indicates other working muscles
* indicates deep muscles

abductor
digiti minimi

flexor hallucis*

adductor
hallucis

flexor
digitorum*

plantar aponeurosis

serratus anterior

transversus
abdominis*

iliopsoas*

sartorius

obliquus externus

rectus abdominis

obliquus internus*

rectus femoris

vastus lateralis

vastus medialis

extensor hallucis

extensor digitorum

MODIFICATION

HARDER: To
assume Reverse
Prayer, bring your
arms behind you,
with your fingers
pointing downward
and your palms
together. Rotate
your arms so that
your fingers point
up to the sky.

Upward Salute

Upward Salute is a joyous pose, worthy of its place as the second pose in Sun Salutation A (page 39). Performed correctly, it stretches your entire body.

HOW TO DO IT

• Begin in Mountain Pose (pages 32–33), with your arms at your sides.

• Inhale as you reach your arms out to your sides, and continue lifting until you are standing with your arms above your head. Your hands should be shoulder-width apart.

• Straighten your arms, and rotate your shoulders open externally so that the palms of your hands face each other, spreading up through your fingertips.

• Gaze forward. Hold for the recommended breaths.

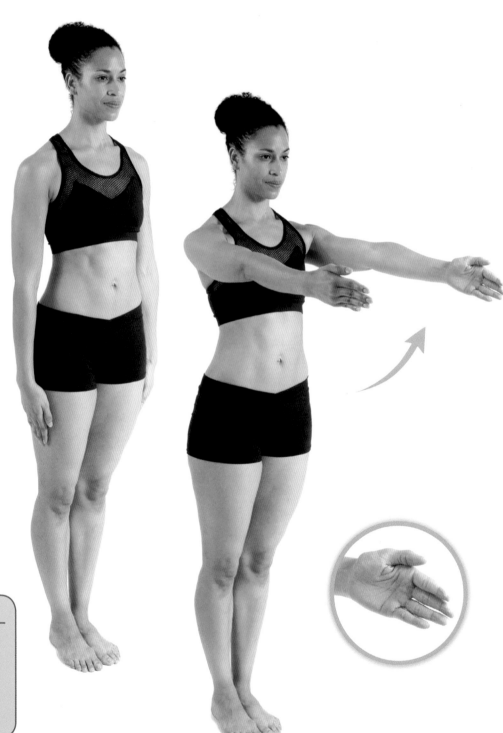

DO IT RIGHT

• Stretch your arms completely straight from your elbows.
• Soften any tension in your shoulders.
• Avoid tensing your shoulders up toward your ears.

SANSKRIT
- Urdhva Hastasana

TARGETS
- Entire body

BENEFITS
- Offers a full-body stretch, especially the arms, shoulders, and abdomen

CAUTIONS
- Neck issues
- Shoulder issues

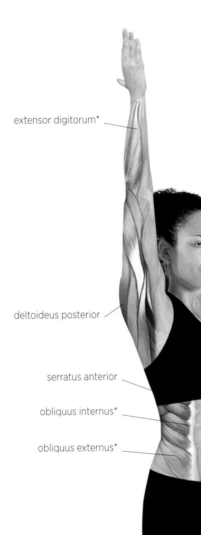

extensor digitorum*

biceps brachii

deltoideus posterior

deltoideus anterior

serratus anterior

obliquus internus*

obliquus externus*

Annotation Key

Bold text indicates target muscles
Light text indicates other working muscles
* indicates deep muscles

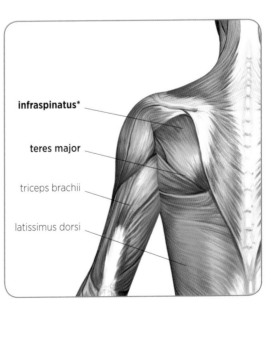

infraspinatus*

teres major

triceps brachii

latissimus dorsi

Volcano Pose

A variation of Upward Salute, Volcano Pose is also known as Upward Hand Pose. It is a base pose that helps boost energy, making it a great pose to include in yoga sequences.

HOW TO DO IT

- Begin in Mountain Pose (pages 32–33), with your arms at your sides.

- Gently raise your arms to the ceiling.

- Tilt your head back to bring your gaze up to your thumbs. Hold for the recommended breaths.

DO IT RIGHT

- Stretch your arms completely straight from your elbows.
- Soften any tension in your shoulders.
- Avoid tensing your shoulders up toward your ears.

FACT FILE

SANSKRIT
- Urdhva Hastasana

TARGETS
- Entire body

BENEFITS
- Offers a full-body stretch, especially the arms, shoulders, and abdomen

CAUTION
- Neck issues
- Shoulder issues

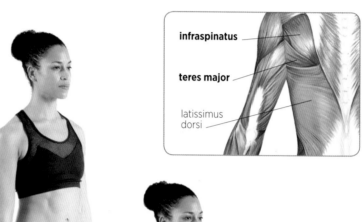

infraspinatus

teres major

latissimus dorsi

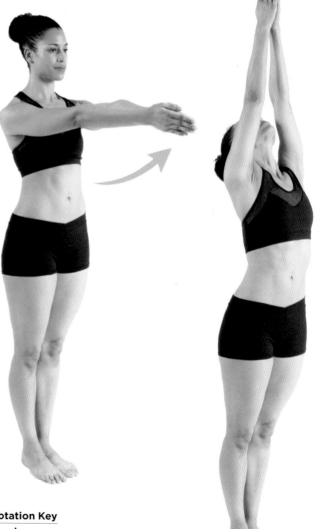

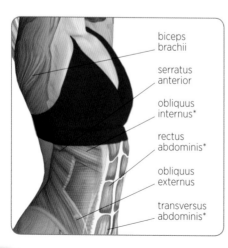

biceps brachii

serratus anterior

obliquus internus*

rectus abdominis*

obliquus externus

transversus abdominis*

Annotation Key

Bold text indicates target muscles
Light text indicates other working muscles
* indicates deep muscles

Sun Salutation A

As its name suggests, this graceful standing bend is often part of a Sun Salutation variation, following Upward Salute or Volcano Pose. It creates space in the lower back and hip flexors, preparing you to move into a forward bend.

HOW TO DO IT

- Begin in Mountain Pose (pages 32–33), with your arms at your sides.

- Move into Upward Salute (pages 36–37).

- Keeping your arms extended, drop your shoulders back in as deep a backbend as you can comfortably assume. Hold for the recommended breaths.

DO IT RIGHT

- Perform it on a deep exhalation.
- Begin with small moves, tilting backward only as far as you can go while maintaining your balance.
- Stretch your arms completely straight from your elbows.
- Soften any tension in your shoulders.
- Avoid tensing your shoulders up toward your ears.

FACT FILE

SANSKRIT
- Surya Namaskarasana

TARGETS
- Entire body

BENEFITS
- Offers a full-body stretch, especially the arms, shoulders, and abdomen

CAUTIONS
- Neck issues
- Shoulder issues
- Lower-back issues

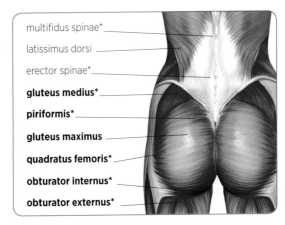

multifidus spinae*
latissimus dorsi
erector spinae*
gluteus medius*
piriformis*
gluteus maximus
quadratus femoris*
obturator internus*
obturator externus*

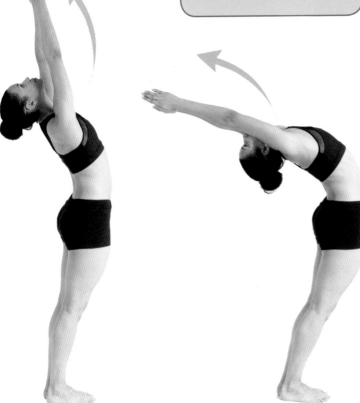

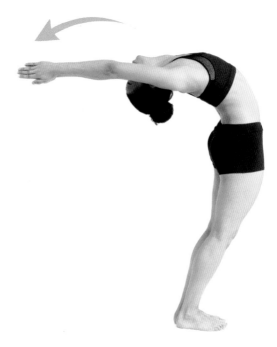

Wide-Stance Upward Salute

This version of Upward Salute will help you hone your balance, calling for you to take a wider stance, which is a more stable foot position than those with feet together. Wide-Stance Upward Salute is particularly suitable for yoga newbies, elders who may be prone to falls, or for women in later stages of pregnancy.

HOW TO DO IT

- Stand with your legs and feet parallel and shoulder-width apart. Bend your knees very slightly.

- Tighten and lift the muscles above your kneecaps, and tuck in your tailbone.

- Inhale deeply and reach your arms up toward the ceiling, keeping them long and in parallel with your body. Focus your energy on the middle of your palms, which should be facing inward. Turn your gaze upward as you stretch.

- Hold for the recommended breaths.

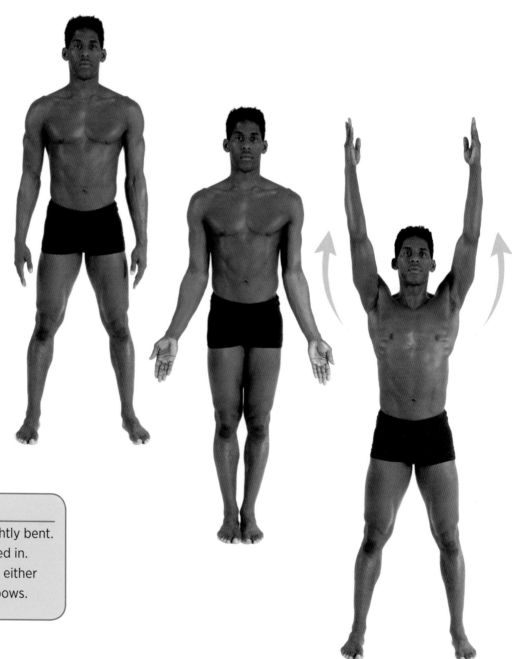

DO IT RIGHT
- Keep your elbows slightly bent.
- Keep your pelvis tucked in.
- Avoid hyperextending either your lower back or elbows.

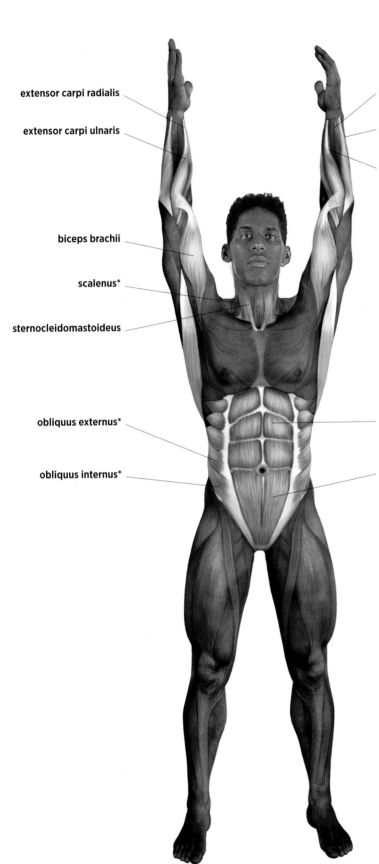

extensor carpi radialis

extensor carpi ulnaris

biceps brachii

scalenus*

sternocleidomastoideus

flexor carpi radialis

flexor carpi ulnaris

palmaris longus

obliquus externus*

obliquus internus*

rectus abdominis

transversus abdominis*

FACT FILE

SANSKRIT
• Urdhva Hastasana

TARGETS
• Entire body

BENEFITS
• Offers a full-body stretch, especially the arms, shoulders, and abdomen
• Aligns the spine and corrects posture problems
• Restores balance to the body and the mind

CAUTIONS
• Neck issues
• Shoulder issues

Annotation Key
Bold text indicates target muscles
Light text indicates other working muscles
* indicates deep muscles

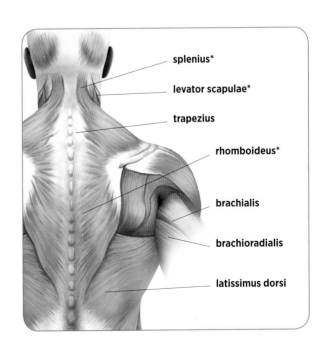

splenius*

levator scapulae*

trapezius

rhomboideus*

brachialis

brachioradialis

latissimus dorsi

Palm Tree Pose

Taking its name from the shape your body resembles while in the pose, Palm Tree Pose is another variation of Upward Salute. It is an excellent transitional posture in yoga flows. It allows you to move easily into a bend in any direction.

HOW TO DO IT

• Begin in Mountain Pose (pages 32–33), with your arms at your sides.

• Inhale as you reach your arms out to your sides, and then raise them above your head to clasp your hands together, palms facing upward. Keep your elbows bent so that your arms form gentle curves.

• Hold for the recommended breaths.

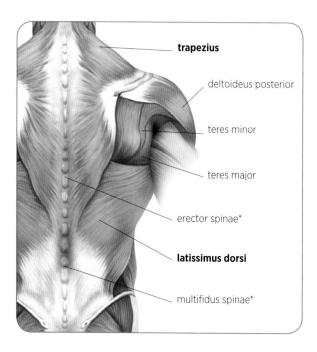

trapezius

deltoideus posterior

teres minor

teres major

erector spinae*

latissimus dorsi

multifidus spinae*

Annotation Key

Bold text indicates target muscles
Light text indicates other working muscles
* indicates deep muscles

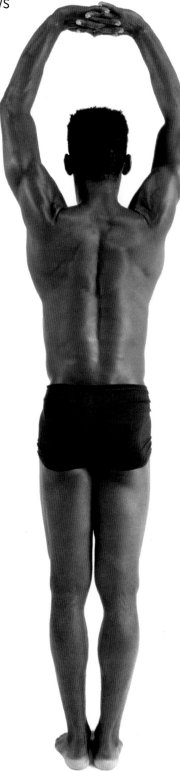

FACT FILE

SANSKRIT
• Urdhva Hastasana

TARGETS
• Entire body

BENEFITS
• Offers a full-body stretch, especially the arms, shoulders, and abdomen

CAUTION
• Neck issues
• Shoulder issues

DO IT RIGHT

• Elongate your arms and shoulders as much as possible.
• Soften any tension in your shoulders.
• Avoid tensing your shoulders up toward your ears.

Palm Tree Side Bend

A stand-alone pose by itself, Palm Tree Side Bend Pose is also a great warm-up move that prepares the body for more intense yoga poses.

HOW TO DO IT

- Begin in Palm Tree Pose (opposite page).

- Leaning from the hips, slowly drop your torso to the right.

- Keeping a smooth flow, lean your torso to the left.

- Continue alternating sides for the recommended repetitions or breaths.

FACT FILE

SANSKRIT
- Urdhva Hastasana

TARGETS
- Entire body

BENEFITS
- Offers a full-body stretch, especially the arms, shoulders, and abdomen
- Stretches the abdominals and obliques

CAUTIONS
- Neck issues
- Shoulder issues
- Lower-back issues

Annotation Key

Bold text indicates target muscles
Light text indicates other working muscles
* indicates deep muscles

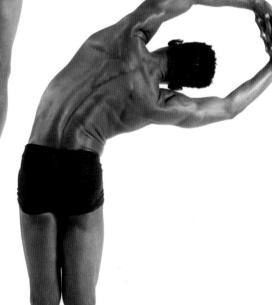

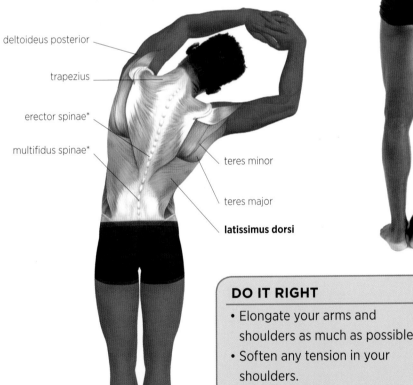

deltoideus posterior

trapezius

erector spinae*

multifidus spinae*

teres minor

teres major

latissimus dorsi

DO IT RIGHT

- Elongate your arms and shoulders as much as possible.
- Soften any tension in your shoulders.
- Avoid tensing your shoulders up toward your ears.
- Avoid bending forward or backward at the torso.

Standing Side Bend

A useful warm-up move, Standing Side Bend offers an energizing upper-body stretch. When performing this pose, concentrate on the lengthening of your sides. Focus on keeping your feet planted and your lower body strongly rooted and stable, like a tree with branches leaning over in the wind.

HOW TO DO IT

- Begin in Mountain Pose (pages 32–33), with your arms at your sides. Turn your palms inward to rest against your thighs.

- Inhale and reach your left arm out to the side, and then raise it above your head, keeping your arm straight as you lean to the right.

- Exhale and return to Mountain Pose, and then repeat with your right arm raised.

- Continue alternating sides for the recommended repetitions or breaths.

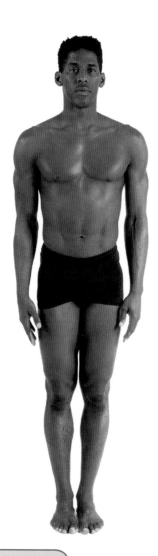
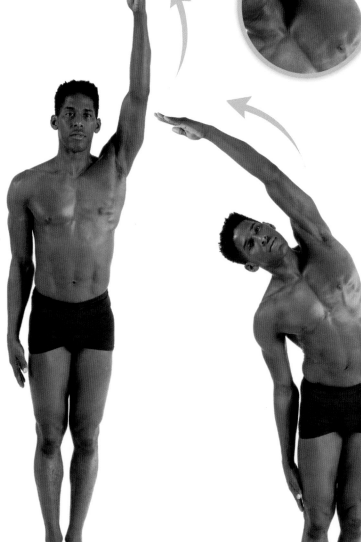

DO IT RIGHT

- Elongate your arms and shoulders as much as possible.
- Soften any tension in your shoulders.
- Avoid tensing your shoulders up toward your ears.
- Avoid bending forward or backward at the torso.

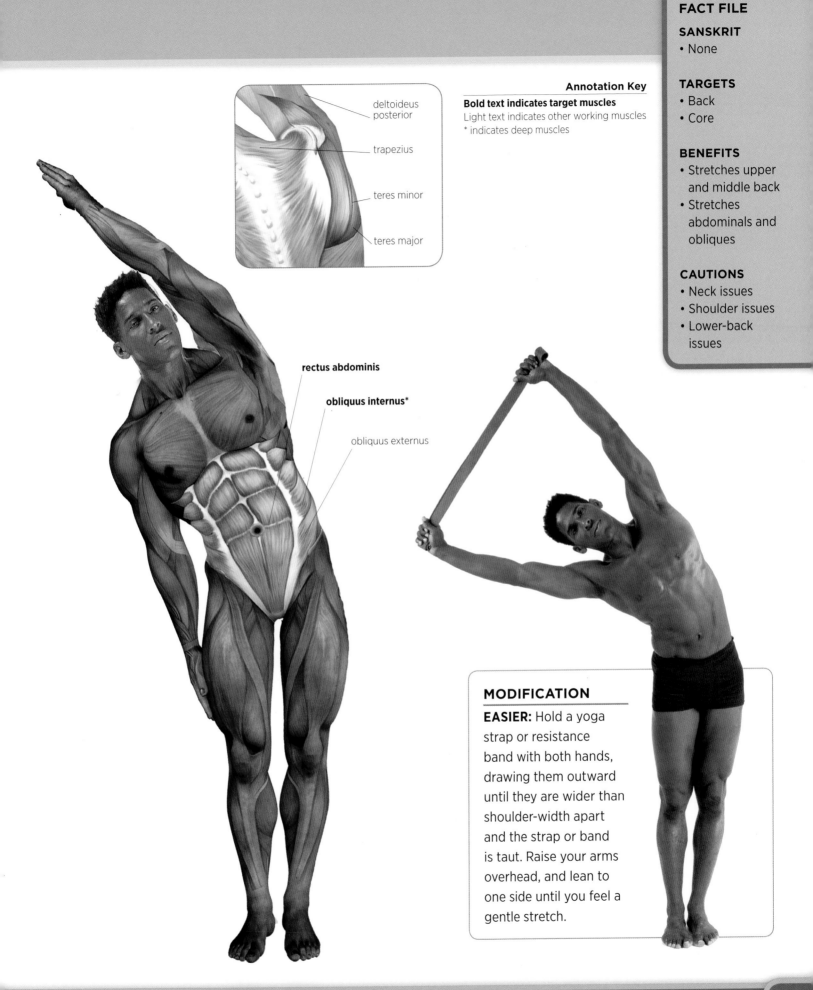

FACT FILE

SANSKRIT
• None

TARGETS
• Back
• Core

BENEFITS
• Stretches upper and middle back
• Stretches abdominals and obliques

CAUTIONS
• Neck issues
• Shoulder issues
• Lower-back issues

deltoideus posterior

trapezius

teres minor

teres major

Annotation Key
Bold text indicates target muscles
Light text indicates other working muscles
* indicates deep muscles

rectus abdominis

obliquus internus*

obliquus externus

MODIFICATION

EASIER: Hold a yoga strap or resistance band with both hands, drawing them outward until they are wider than shoulder-width apart and the strap or band is taut. Raise your arms overhead, and lean to one side until you feel a gentle stretch.

Gate Pose

Gate Pose offers a stretch similar to that of Standing Side Bend (pages 44–45), but you begin by kneeling rather than standing.

HOW TO DO IT

• Kneel on the floor. Stretch your left leg out to the left, and press your foot into the floor. Keeping your right knee directly below your right hip, align your left heel with your right knee. Turn your pelvis slightly to the right as you turn your upper torso back to the left. Point your kneecap toward the ceiling, turning your left leg out.

• Inhale and bring your arms out to the side, parallel to the floor, palms down. Bend to the left, and place your left hand on your shin. Contract the left side of your torso and stretch to the left.

• Slide your hand from your outer right hip to your lower right ribs, inhale, and then sweep your right arm upward over the back of your right ear.

• Hold for the recommended breaths, and then release the stretch. Bring your left knee back beside the right, and repeat on the other side.

DO IT RIGHT
• Avoid dropping your torso toward the floor.

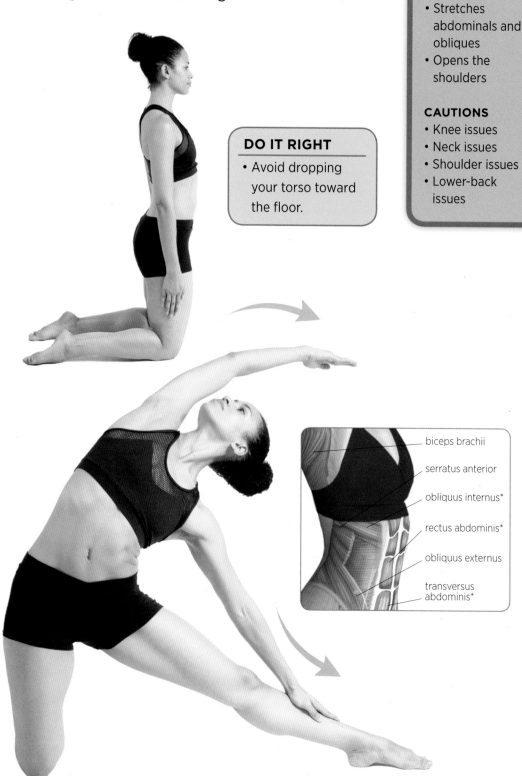

biceps brachii

serratus anterior

obliquus internus*

rectus abdominis*

obliquus externus

transversus abdominis*

Annotation Key

Bold text indicates target muscles
Light text indicates other working muscles
* indicates deep muscles

FACT FILE
SANSKRIT
• Parighasana

TARGETS
• Back
• Core

BENEFITS
• Stretches spine
• Stretches abdominals and obliques
• Opens the shoulders

CAUTIONS
• Knee issues
• Neck issues
• Shoulder issues
• Lower-back issues

Lord Shiva Cycle of Life Dance Pose

A graceful, dramatic pose, Lord Shiva Cycle of Life Dance Pose offers more than a side stretch. Coming into this pose is a fantastic way to work on stability and balance.

HOW TO DO IT

- Begin in Palm Tree Pose (page 42), stretching your arms upward while extending your shoulders, chest, and lower back.

- Cross your left leg behind your right, keeping both feet flat on the floor.

- Lean your torso back and to the right, so that you are now facing the ceiling.

- Hold for the recommended breaths, release the stretch, and repeat on the other side.

FACT FILE

SANSKRIT
- Tandavasana

TARGETS
- Entire body

BENEFITS
- Offers a full-body stretch, especially the arms, shoulders, and belly
- Stretches the abdominals and obliques

CAUTIONS
- Neck issues
- Shoulder issues
- Lower-back issues
- Knee issues

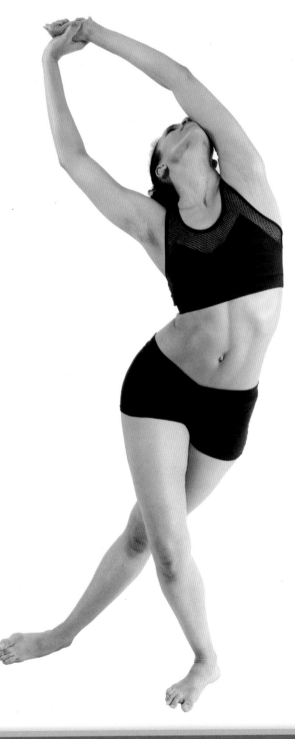

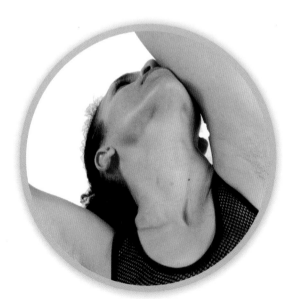

Garland Pose

An efficient hip and thigh opener for everyone, Garland Pose is especially beneficial for pregnant women. You can practice this posture throughout your entire pregnancy.

HOW TO DO IT

- Stand in Mountain Pose (pages 32–33), facing the front short edge of your mat. Separate your feet wider than hip-width apart.

- Bend your knees as deeply as you can, letting your feet turn out, squatting down until your hips are lower than your knees.

- Join your hands in a prayer position in front of your heart. Hold for the recommended breaths.

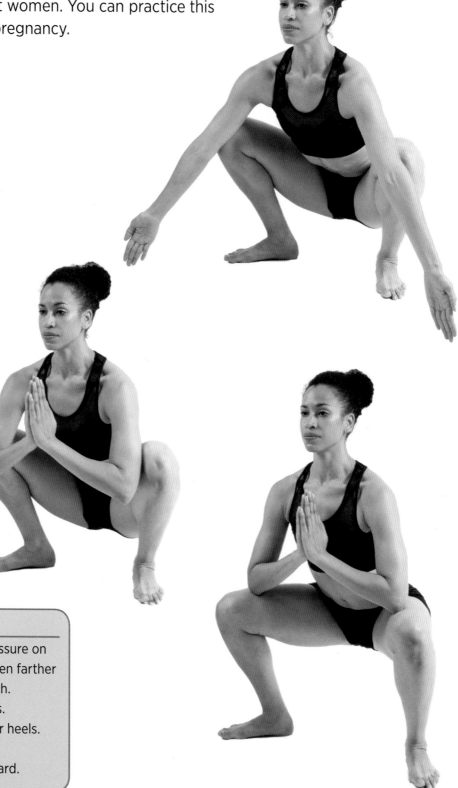
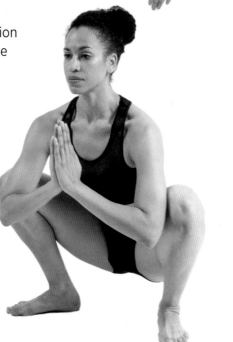

DO IT RIGHT

- Use your elbows to apply gentle pressure on your knees, encouraging them to open farther and deepening the inner thigh stretch.
- Push your knees toward your elbows.
- If desired, place a blanket under your heels.
- Broaden across your collarbones.
- Avoid rounding your shoulders forward.

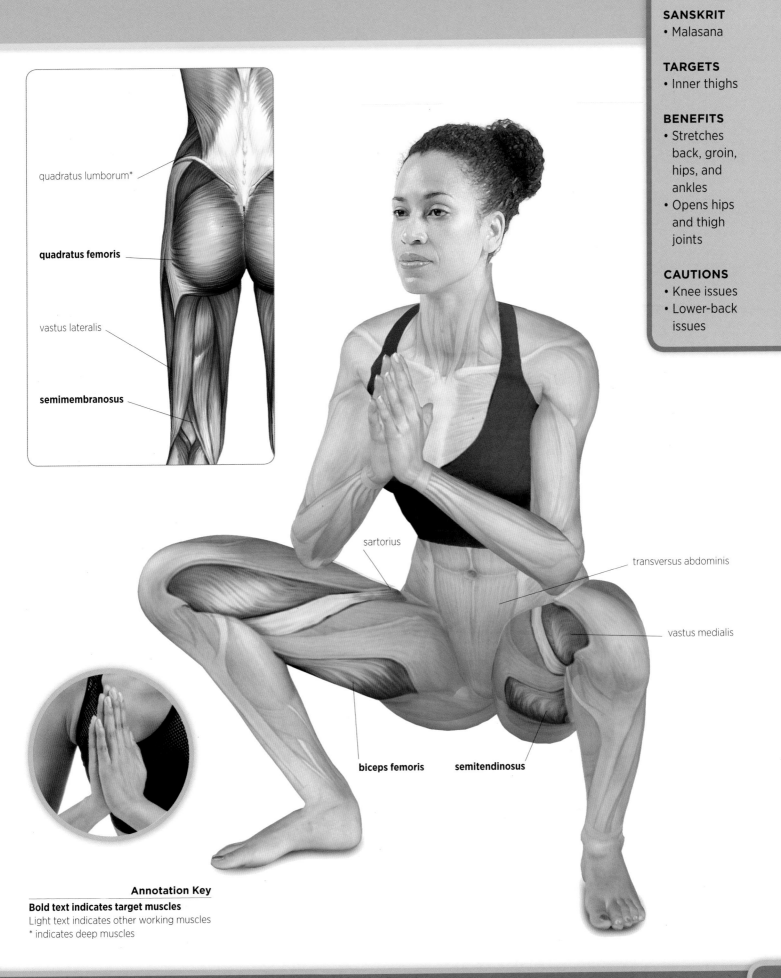

SANSKRIT
• Malasana

TARGETS
• Inner thighs

BENEFITS
• Stretches back, groin, hips, and ankles
• Opens hips and thigh joints

CAUTIONS
• Knee issues
• Lower-back issues

quadratus lumborum*

quadratus femoris

vastus lateralis

semimembranosus

sartorius

transversus abdominis

vastus medialis

biceps femoris

semitendinosus

Annotation Key
Bold text indicates target muscles
Light text indicates other working muscles
* indicates deep muscles

Horse Pose

Also known as Sumo Squat or Plié Squat, Horse Pose is an energy-boosting posture that builds lower-body strength and flexibility.

HOW TO DO IT

- Stand in Mountain Pose (pages 32–33), with your feet together and arms by your sides. Step your feet out about one-leg's-width apart. Turn your heels in, pointing your toes slightly outward.

- Inhale and reach your arms overhead to bring your palms together.

- Exhale and bend your knees so that your thighs are as close to perpendicular with the floor as possible, while pulling your hands to your chest into prayer position, sliding your shoulder blades downward. Hold for the recommended breaths.

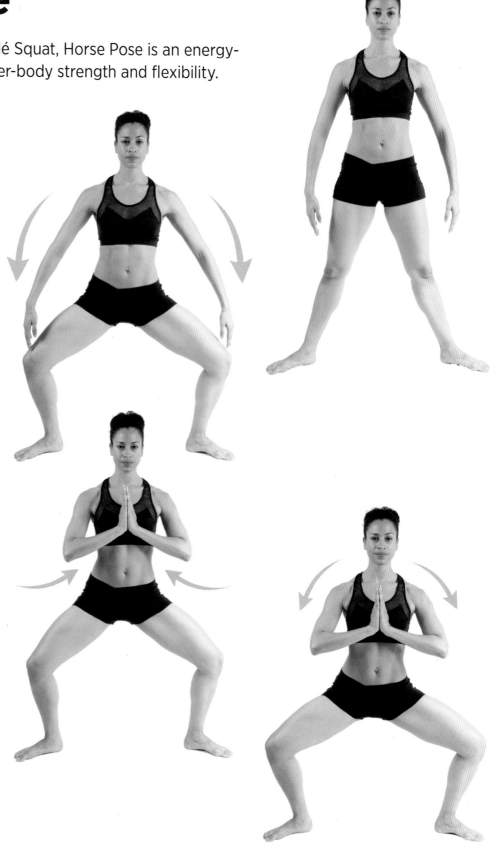

DO IT RIGHT

- Keep your abdominals pulled in.
- Keep your knees soft.
- Move gracefully and with control.
- Avoid turning your toes out to the point where it is uncomfortable.
- Avoid twisting to either side.
- Avoid arching your back or hunching forward.

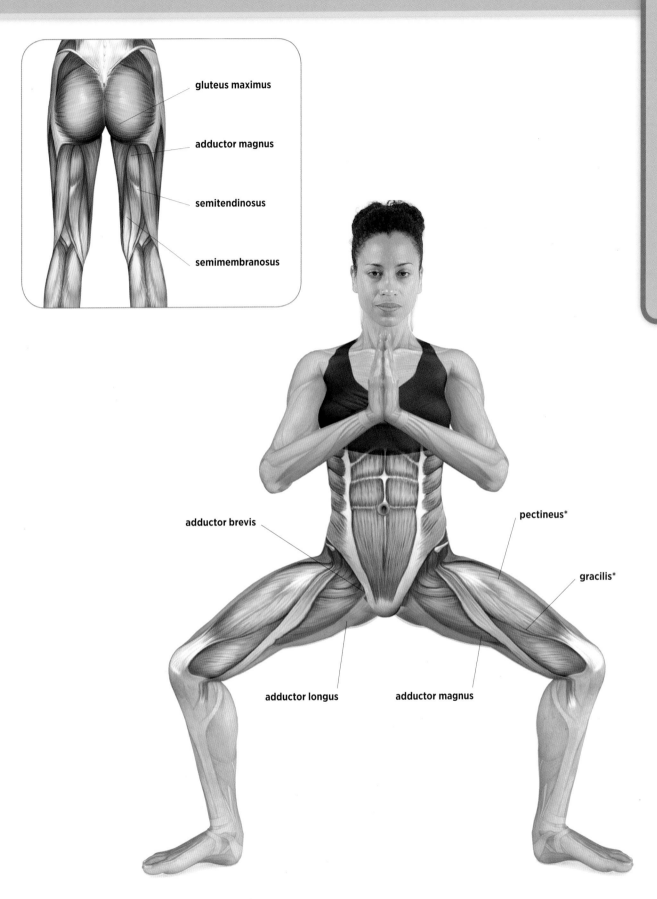

gluteus maximus

adductor magnus

semitendinosus

semimembranosus

FACT FILE

SANSKRIT
• Vatayanasana

TARGETS
• Hamstrings
• Hips
• Knees
• Quadriceps

BENEFITS
• Tones hip
  adductors
• Improves
  lateral
  movement

CAUTIONS
• Hip issues
• Knee issues

adductor brevis

pectineus*

gracilis*

adductor longus

adductor magnus

Horse Pose with Palms Up

This version of Horse Pose also boosts energy and builds lower-body strength and flexibility. The arm position adds a further challenge to your shoulders while helping you hone your sense of balance.

HOW TO DO IT

• Stand in Mountain Pose (pages 32–33), with your feet together and arms by your sides. Step your feet out about one-leg's-width apart. Turn your heels in, pointing your toes slightly outward.

• Inhale and reach your arms out to the sides.

• Exhale and bend your knees so that your thighs are as close to perpendicular with the floor as possible, turning your palms upward and sliding your shoulder blades downward. Hold for the recommended breaths.

DO IT RIGHT

• Keep your abdominals pulled in.
• Keep your knees soft.
• Move gracefully and with control.
• Avoid turning your toes out to the point where it is uncomfortable.
• Avoid twisting to either side.
• Avoid arching your back or hunching forward.

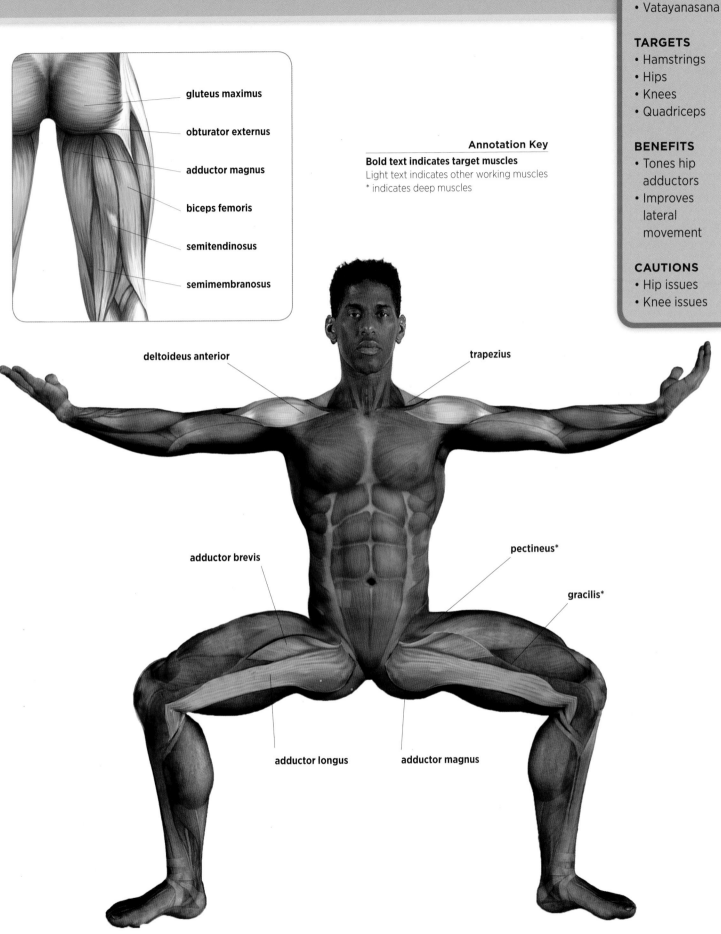

SANSKRIT
• Vatayanasana

TARGETS
• Hamstrings
• Hips
• Knees
• Quadriceps

BENEFITS
• Tones hip adductors
• Improves lateral movement

CAUTIONS
• Hip issues
• Knee issues

gluteus maximus

obturator externus

adductor magnus

biceps femoris

semitendinosus

semimembranosus

Annotation Key
Bold text indicates target muscles
Light text indicates other working muscles
* indicates deep muscles

deltoideus anterior

trapezius

adductor brevis

pectineus*

gracilis*

adductor longus

adductor magnus

Chair Pose

Also known as Awkward Pose, Chair Pose is an element of many yoga flows. It takes quite a bit of strength, but you can easily control its intensity, bending your knees just a few inches or all the way down so that your hips are in line with your knees.

HOW TO DO IT

• Stand in Mountain Pose (pages 32–33), with your feet together and arms by your sides.

• Inhale as you bring your arms into Upward Salute (pages 36–37), reaching above your head so that your arms are parallel to each other. Rotate your outer upper arms inward and reach up through your fingertips.

• Exhale and bend your knees. Both ankles, inner thighs, and knees should be touching. Bring your weight onto your heels, shift your hips back, and draw your knees right above your ankles. Hold for the recommended breaths.

DO IT RIGHT
• Find a neutral position by drawing your tailbone down as you roll your inner thighs toward the floor.
• Keep your feet together.
• Keep your heels on the floor.
• Avoid overtucking your pelvis.
• Avoid overarching your lower back.
• Avoid knocking your knees inward.

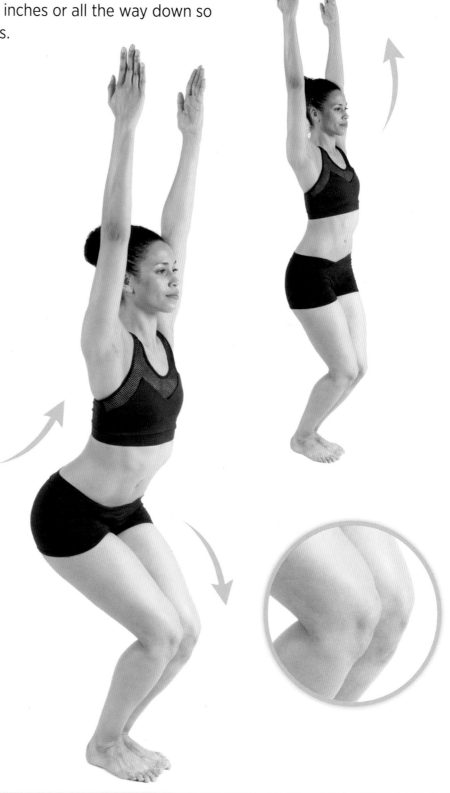

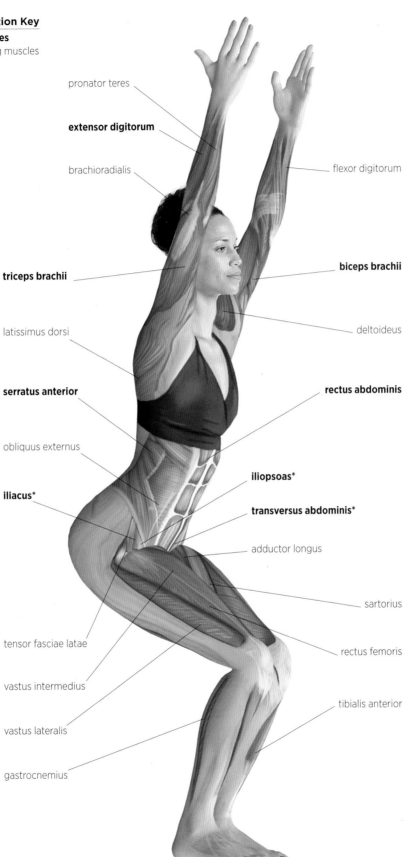

Annotation Key

Bold text indicates target muscles
Light text indicates other working muscles
* indicates deep muscles

pronator teres

extensor digitorum

brachioradialis

flexor digitorum

triceps brachii

biceps brachii

latissimus dorsi

deltoideus

serratus anterior

rectus abdominis

obliquus externus

iliopsoas*

iliacus*

transversus abdominis*

adductor longus

tensor fasciae latae

sartorius

vastus intermedius

rectus femoris

vastus lateralis

tibialis anterior

gastrocnemius

FACT FILE

SANSKRIT
• Utkatasana

TARGETS
• Legs
• Back
• Arms

BENEFITS
• Strengthens thighs, ankles, spine, and arms
• Stretches shoulders and chest

CAUTIONS
• Knee issues

Twisting Chair Pose

Perform Twisting Chair Pose to improve digestion and elimination. Imagine wringing out your stomach as if it were a sponge, twisting a little deeper with each breath.

HOW TO DO IT

- Begin in Chair Pose (pages 54–55), with your arms parallel to each other above your head and your knees bent deeply.

- Inhale as you lengthen your spine and join your hands in a prayer position in front of your heart.

- Keep your hips square as you exhale and twist to the right, bringing your left elbow to the outside of your right thigh. Press your left elbow into your right knee and your knee into your elbow.

- Inhale to lengthen the spine, letting your abdomen move outward, and then exhale to twist as your navel draws strongly back toward your spine.

- Hold for the recommended breaths, and then inhale as you return to the center and reach your arms upward. Repeat on the other side.

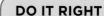

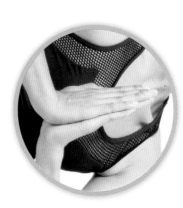

DO IT RIGHT

- Keep your hands in prayer position at the center of your chest, even though they will want to move toward one of your shoulders.
- Try to find a small bend in your upper back as you broaden across your collarbones.
- Twist from your torso, and keep your hips square; this will keep your knees in line with each other.
- Avoid rounding your shoulders as you twist.
- Avoid letting your left knee jut forward as you twist to the right, or vice versa.

FACT FILE

SANSKRIT
• Parivrtta Utkatasana

TARGETS
• Lower body
• Back
• Obliques

BENEFITS
• Strengthens thighs, ankles, spine, buttocks, and arms
• Stretches spine and obliques
• Tones abdomen
• Stimulates digestion

CAUTIONS
• Knee issues
• Back issues
• Pregnancy

Annotation Key

Bold text indicates target muscles
Light text indicates other working muscles
* indicates deep muscles

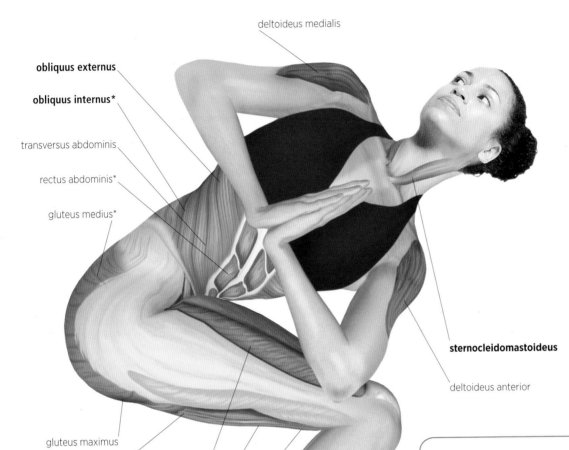

deltoideus medialis

obliquus externus

obliquus internus*

transversus abdominis

rectus abdominis*

gluteus medius*

sternocleidomastoideus

deltoideus anterior

gluteus maximus

biceps femoris

rectus femoris

semimembranosus

semitendinosus

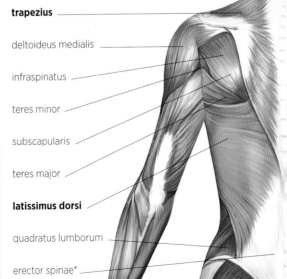

trapezius

deltoideus medialis

infraspinatus

teres minor

subscapularis

teres major

latissimus dorsi

quadratus lumborum

erector spinae*

Tree Pose

Tree Pose tests your balance. To perform it correctly, think of yourself as a tree, rooting your standing foot to the floor and reaching your head up toward the ceiling, so that you feel energy moving down and up at the same time.

HOW TO DO IT

• Stand in Mountain Pose (pages 32–33), with your feet together and arms by your sides.

• Bend your right knee, and bring your foot up to your left inner thigh, with toes pointing to the floor.

• Externally rotate your right thigh, allowing your right knee to point out to the right while keeping your hips level.

• Continue to open your right hip, rotating your inner thigh clockwise as you draw your tailbone down toward your left heel to neutralize your pelvis. Press your right foot into your left inner thigh as you draw your left outer hip in for stability.

• Find your balance, exhale, and draw your hands together into prayer position at the heart.

• Hold for the recommended breaths, and then inhale as you return to Mountain Pose. Repeat on the other side.

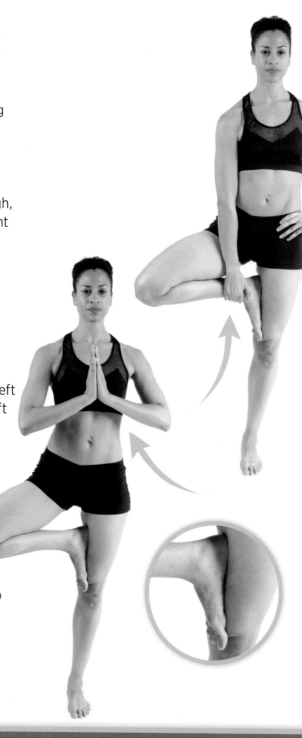
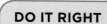

DO IT RIGHT

• Keep your standing leg in place with the foot facing straight ahead.
• If you need help placing your foot at your thigh, grasp your ankle with your hand; alternatively, you can rest your foot on the side of your shin instead.
• Ground down through all four corners of the raised foot to help you maintain balance.
• To assist in balancing, place your heel at your ankle with the ball of the foot on the floor, or lean against a wall.
• Avoid resting your foot on the sensitive kneecap area.

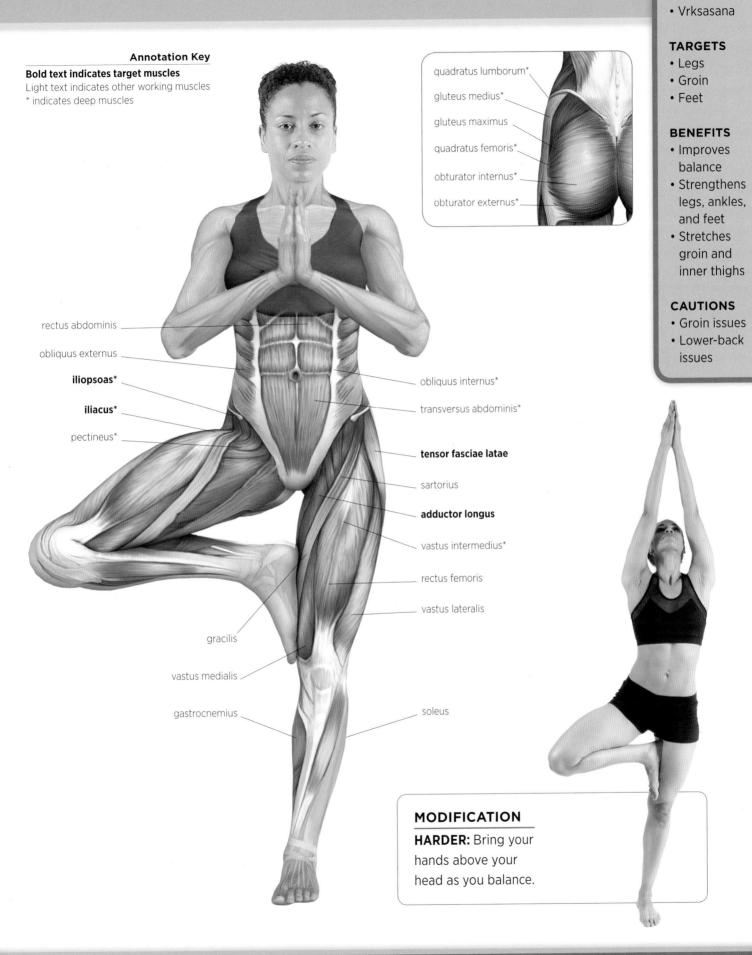

FACT FILE

SANSKRIT
• Vrksasana

TARGETS
• Legs
• Groin
• Feet

BENEFITS
• Improves balance
• Strengthens legs, ankles, and feet
• Stretches groin and inner thighs

CAUTIONS
• Groin issues
• Lower-back issues

Annotation Key

Bold text indicates target muscles
Light text indicates other working muscles
* indicates deep muscles

quadratus lumborum*
gluteus medius*
gluteus maximus
quadratus femoris*
obturator internus*
obturator externus*

rectus abdominis
obliquus externus
iliopsoas*
iliacus*
pectineus*

obliquus internus*
transversus abdominis*

tensor fasciae latae
sartorius
adductor longus
vastus intermedius*
rectus femoris
vastus lateralis

gracilis
vastus medialis
gastrocnemius
soleus

MODIFICATION

HARDER: Bring your hands above your head as you balance.

Eagle Pose

A standing pose with a lot to offer, Eagle Pose challenges your balance and demands focus, stamina, and endurance. It also opens your shoulders and lubricates your joints.

HOW TO DO IT

- Stand in Mountain Pose (pages 32–33), and then bend your knees and sit into Chair Pose (pages 54–55). Extend your arms out to your sides.

- Keep your right knee bent in the chair position as you shift your weight onto your right heel. Lift your left knee into your chest, and wrap your left thigh over your right thigh. If possible, wrap your left toes around the calf of your right leg.

- Bring your arms in front of you with your palms facing up, bend your elbows, and hook your right elbow underneath your left elbow. Wrap your right forearm around your left and bring your palms together with your fingers pointing toward the ceiling.

- Squeeze your arms together, and lift your elbows up as you bring your hands away from your face to broaden across your upper back.

- Hold for the recommended breaths, and then inhale as you return to Mountain Pose. Repeat on the other side.

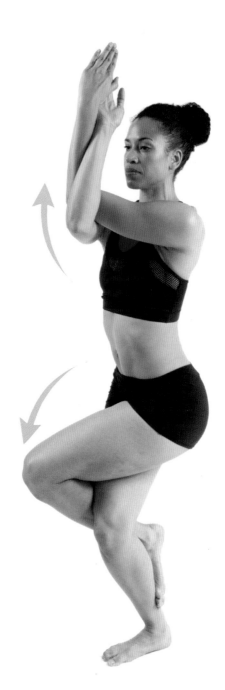

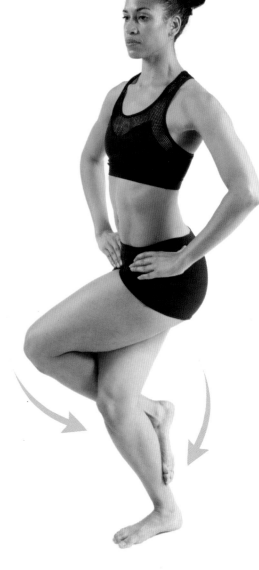

DO IT RIGHT

- If you have trouble balancing, bring your raised foot to the floor on the outside of the standing foot.
- Find a fixed gazing point, keeping your eyes soft.
- Avoid letting your hips twist to either side.

Annotation Key

Bold text indicates target muscles
Light text indicates other working muscles
* indicates deep muscles

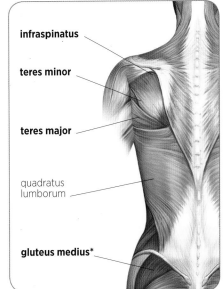

infraspinatus

teres minor

teres major

quadratus lumborum

gluteus medius*

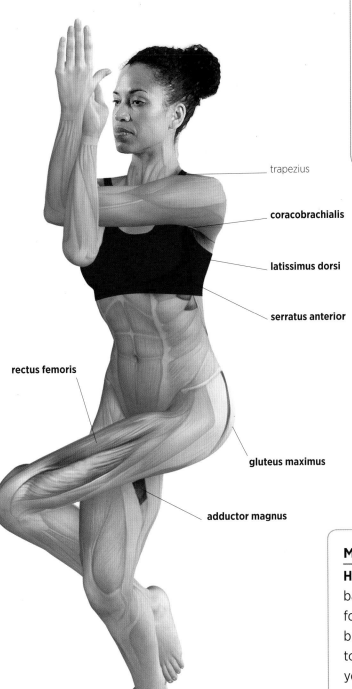

trapezius

coracobrachialis

latissimus dorsi

serratus anterior

rectus femoris

gluteus maximus

adductor magnus

FACT FILE

SANSKRIT
• Garudasana

TARGETS
• Back
• Hips
• Legs
• Buttocks

BENEFITS
• Releases tension in upper back
• Stretches hips and buttocks
• Strengthens thighs, ankles, and knees
• Builds stamina and endurance
• Improves concentration

CAUTIONS
• Groin issues
• Knee issues

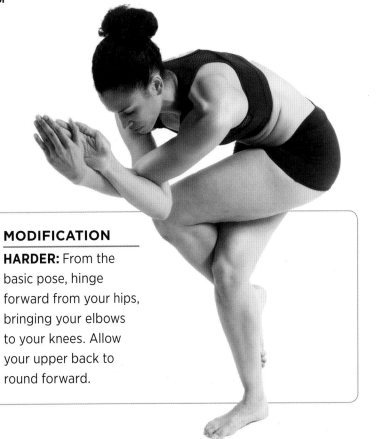

MODIFICATION

HARDER: From the basic pose, hinge forward from your hips, bringing your elbows to your knees. Allow your upper back to round forward.

Low Lunge

Also known as Crescent Moon Pose or simply as Lunge Pose, Low Lunge is found in many yoga flows. It offers a great lower-body stretch and also helps hone balance, coordination, and concentration.

HOW TO DO IT

• Begin in Downward-Facing Dog (pages 268–69). Exhale and step your right foot forward, planting it between your hands.

• Lower your left knee to the floor and, keeping your right knee fixed in place, slide your left back until you feel a comfortable stretch in the front of your left thigh and groin. Rest the top of your left foot on the floor.

• Inhale and lift your torso to an upright position. At the same time, sweep your arms out to the sides and up toward the ceiling. Draw your tailbone down toward the floor, and lift your pubis toward your navel.

• Tilt your head, and gaze upward while reaching your pinkies toward the ceiling. Hold for the recommended breaths.

• Exhale and fold your torso back down to your right thigh. Place your hands on the floor, and flip your toes so that the bottoms press against the floor. Exhale and lift your left knee off the floor, and step back to the Downward-Facing Dog Pose. Repeat on the other side.

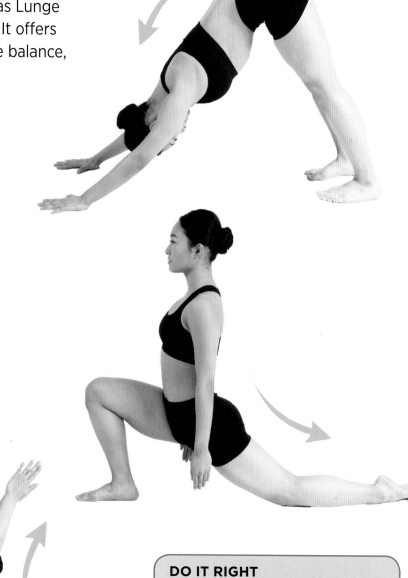

DO IT RIGHT

• Position your front knee and shin directly above your ankle, with the center of your knee aligned with your middle toes.
• Shift your pelvis forward to deepen the stretch.
• Place a blanket under your knees if they feel sensitive.
• Avoid sinking into your lower back.
• Avoid letting your front ribs pop forward.

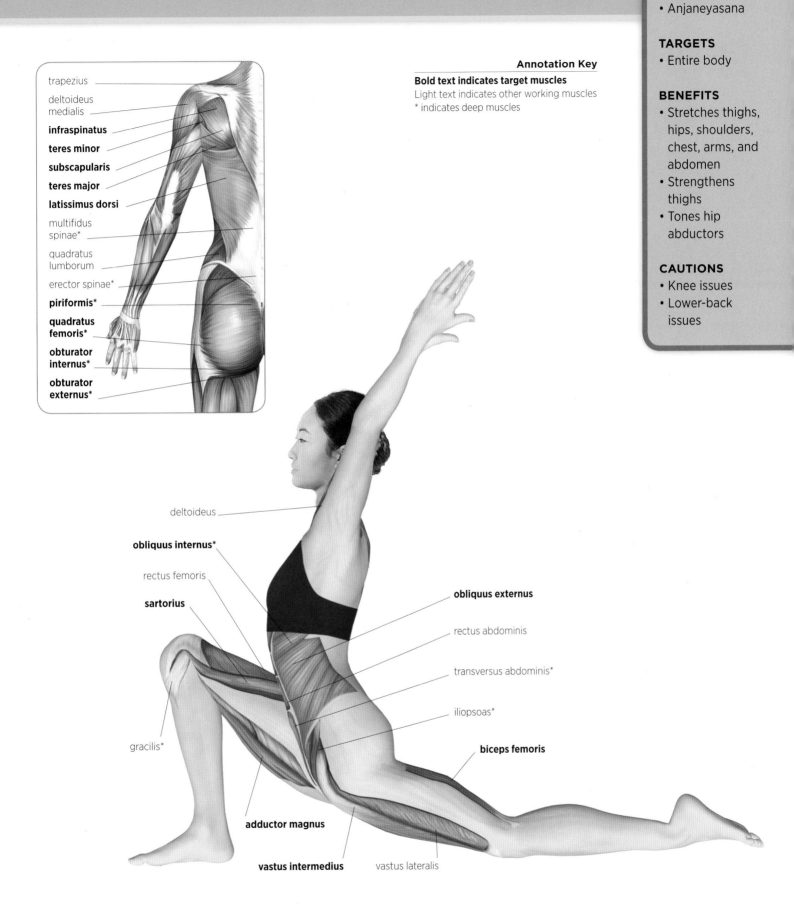

SANSKRIT
- Anjaneyasana

TARGETS
- Entire body

BENEFITS
- Stretches thighs, hips, shoulders, chest, arms, and abdomen
- Strengthens thighs
- Tones hip abductors

CAUTIONS
- Knee issues
- Lower-back issues

trapezius
deltoideus medialis
infraspinatus
teres minor
subscapularis
teres major
latissimus dorsi
multifidus spinae*
quadratus lumborum
erector spinae*
piriformis*
quadratus femoris*
obturator internus*
obturator externus*

Annotation Key

Bold text indicates target muscles
Light text indicates other working muscles
* indicates deep muscles

deltoideus
obliquus internus*
rectus femoris
sartorius
gracilis*
adductor magnus
vastus intermedius
vastus lateralis

obliquus externus
rectus abdominis
transversus abdominis*
iliopsoas*
biceps femoris

High Lunge

An integral component of many yoga flows, High Lunge provides a smooth transition to or from forward bends or arm supports, such as Downward-Facing Dog. Like other lunges, it strengthens the lower body, especially the thighs.

HOW TO DO IT

• Begin in Downward-Facing Dog (pages 268–69). Step your left foot forward in between your hands, with your left knee and shin lined up over your left ankle.

• With your fingertips resting on the floor, square your hips to the front of the mat, grounding your left heel into the floor and drawing your left hip crease back.

• Extend your right leg straight behind you, resting the ball of your foot on the mat. Lengthen all the way from the crown of your head to your right heel. Gaze slightly ahead, keeping the back of your neck long.

• Hold for the recommended breaths, and then repeat on the other side.

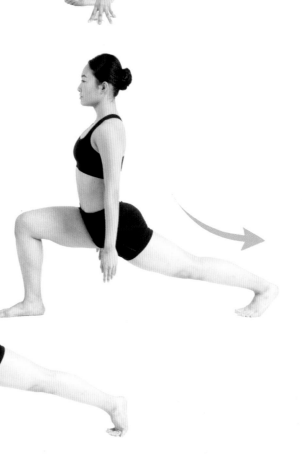

DO IT RIGHT

• Bring your abdomen in, away from your thigh.
• Keep your hips firm as you stretch.
• Roll the inner thigh of your straight leg toward the ceiling, finding its internal rotation.
• Place your hands on blocks to help elongate your spine if your back begins rounding when your fingertips touch the floor.
• Avoid positioning your knee past your ankle and over your toes, which can stress your knee joint.

SANSKRIT
• Prasarita
  Padottanasana

TARGETS
• Lower body

BENEFITS
• Strengthens
  thighs
• Stretches hip
  flexors, shoulders,
  and chest

CAUTIONS
• Knee issues

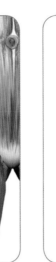

tensor fasciae latae

iliopsoas*

pectineus*

adductor longus

vastus intermedius*

rectus femoris

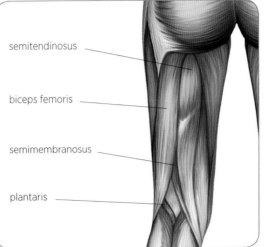

semitendinosus

biceps femoris

semimembranosus

plantaris

Annotation Key

Bold text indicates target muscles
Light text indicates other working muscles
* indicates deep muscles

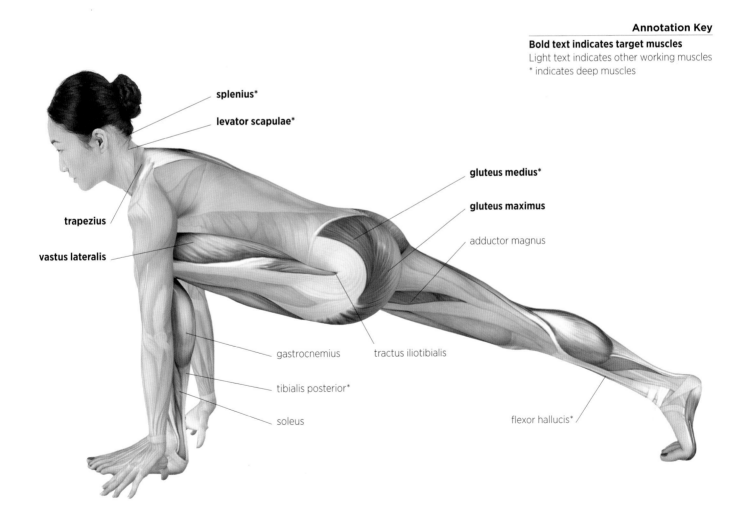

splenius*

levator scapulae*

gluteus medius*

gluteus maximus

adductor magnus

trapezius

vastus lateralis

gastrocnemius

tractus iliotibialis

tibialis posterior*

soleus

flexor hallucis*

Triangle Pose

The Triangle combines the core-strengthening benefits of the classical Pilates mat exercise with the flexibilty promotion of a yoga forward bend. It will help mobilize your spine, challenge your core muscles, flatten your abdominals, and strengthen your back. Let your breath guide you through the exercise, so that you use the same control rolling down as you do rolling up.

HOW TO DO IT

- Stand in Mountain Pose (pages 32–33), and then separate your feet slightly farther than shoulder-width apart.

- Inhale and raise both arms straight out to the side, keeping them parallel to the floor, with your palms facing down.

- Exhale slowly, and without bending your knees, pivot on your heels to turn your right foot all the way to the right and your left foot slightly toward the right, keeping your heels in line with each other.

- Drop your torso as far as is comfortable to the right side, keeping your arms parallel to the floor.

- Drop your right arm so that your right hand rests on your shin or on the front of your ankle. At the same time, extend your left arm straight up toward the ceiling.

- Gently twist your spine and torso counterclockwise, using your extended arm as a lever, while your spinal axis remains parallel to the ground. Extend your arms apart from each other in opposite directions. Turn your head to gaze at your left thumb, slightly intensifying the twist in your spine.

- Hold for the recommended breaths, and then inhale as you return to a standing position with your arms outstretched, strongly pressing the back heel into the floor. Reverse your foot position, and repeat on the other side.

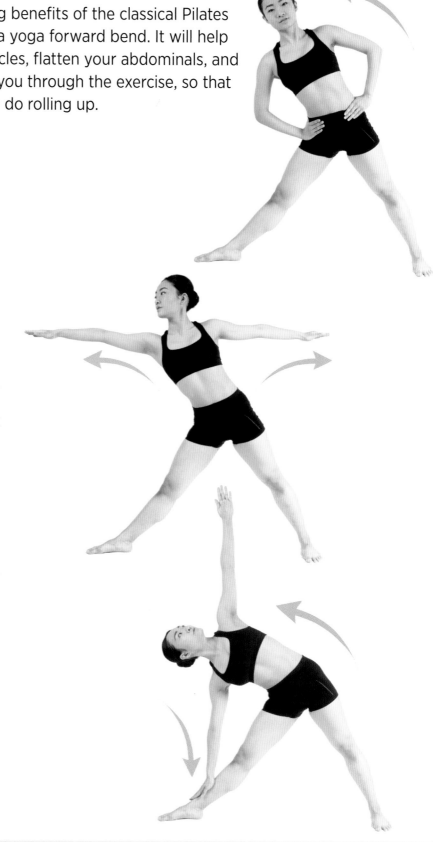

SANSKRIT
• Trikonasana

TARGETS
• Shoulders
• Chest
• Spine
• Legs

BENEFITS
• Stretches shoulders, chest, spine, and legs
• Relieves stress
• Stimulates digestion
• Relieves symptoms of menopause
• Relieves backache

CAUTIONS
• Diarrhea
• Headache
• High or low blood pressure
• Neck issues

DO IT RIGHT
• Keep your leading knee tight and aligned with the center of your foot, shin, and thigh.
• If you feel unsteady, brace your back heel against a wall.
• Avoid twisting your hips.

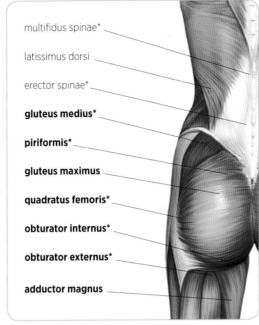

multifidus spinae*

latissimus dorsi

erector spinae*

gluteus medius*

piriformis*

gluteus maximus

quadratus femoris*

obturator internus*

obturator externus*

adductor magnus

latissimus dorsi

obliquus externus

rectus abdominis

transversus abdominis*

pectineus*

rectus femoris

vastus lateralis

adductor longus

tensor fasciae latae

sartorius

gracilis*

semitendinosus

Annotation Key
Bold text indicates target muscles
Light text indicates other working muscles
* indicates deep muscles

Warrior Pose I

The yoga Warrior poses are dramatic asanas that require a mix of fortitude and flexibility. Warrior I will build your strength and increase your confidence.

HOW TO DO IT

- Stand in the middle of your mat in Mountain Pose (pages 32–33), and place your hands on your hips. Step or jump your feet about 3 to 4 feet apart.

- Turn your left toes out about 45 degrees so that they face the upper-left corner of your mat, and walk your right foot to the right several inches until your feet are in heel-to-heel alignment.

- Keeping your left leg straight, bend your right knee as you inhale, lifting your torso and arms above your head so that your upper body and arms form a straight line. Externally rotate both arms with palms facing each other, and push energy up through your fingertips.

- Hold for the recommended breaths, and then repeat on the other side.

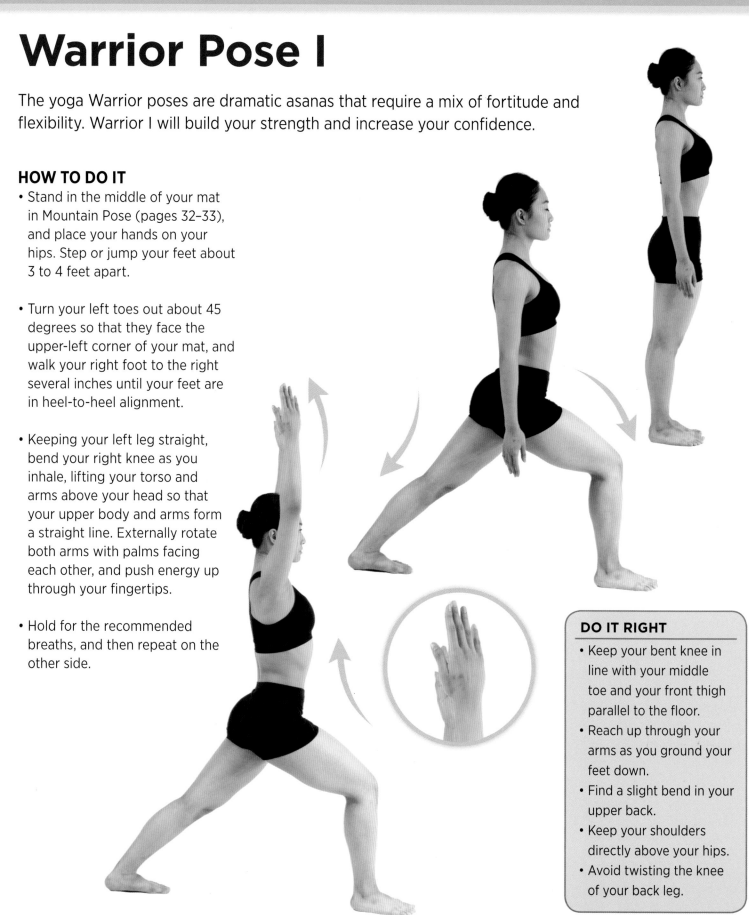

DO IT RIGHT

- Keep your bent knee in line with your middle toe and your front thigh parallel to the floor.
- Reach up through your arms as you ground your feet down.
- Find a slight bend in your upper back.
- Keep your shoulders directly above your hips.
- Avoid twisting the knee of your back leg.

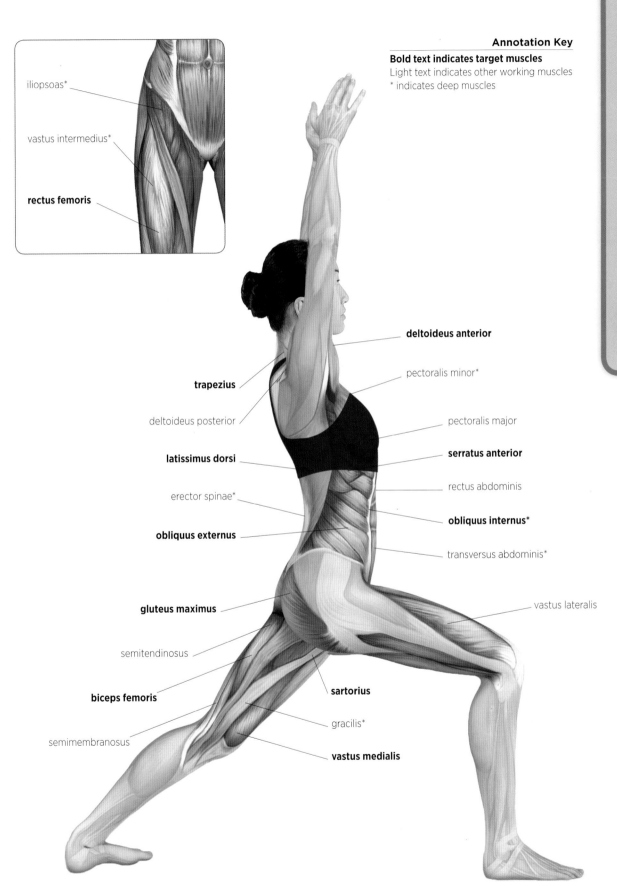

SANSKRIT
- Virabhadrasana I

TARGETS
- Hips
- Legs
- Shoulders

BENEFITS
- Increases stamina
- Strengthens shoulders, arms, thighs, ankles, and calves
- Stretches groin, abdomen, chest, and shoulders

CAUTIONS
- Knee issues
- Lower-back issues
- Shoulder issues

Annotation Key

Bold text indicates target muscles
Light text indicates other working muscles
* indicates deep muscles

iliopsoas*

vastus intermedius*

rectus femoris

deltoideus anterior

pectoralis minor*

trapezius

deltoideus posterior

pectoralis major

latissimus dorsi

serratus anterior

rectus abdominis

erector spinae*

obliquus internus*

obliquus externus

transversus abdominis*

gluteus maximus

vastus lateralis

semitendinosus

biceps femoris

sartorius

gracilis*

semimembranosus

vastus medialis

Crescent Lunge

Often confused with Warrior I (pages 68–69), Crescent Lunge is subtly different. It's all in the back leg—rather than turning your back foot to 45 degrees and keeping your heel on the floor as you would in Warrior I, in Crescent, you raise your heel as you square your hips.

HOW TO DO IT

• Stand in the middle of your mat in Mountain Pose (pages 32–33). Place your hands on your hips.

• Step or jump your feet about 3 to 4 feet apart with your right foot so that it faces the front of your mat, allowing your left foot to rise on your toes.

• Keeping your left leg straight, bend your right knee as you inhale, lifting your torso and arms above your head so that your upper body and arms form a straight line. Externally rotate both arms with palms facing each other, and push energy up through your fingertips.

• Hold for the recommended breaths, and then repeat on the other side.

DO IT RIGHT

• Find a slight bend in your upper back.
• Keep your shoulders directly above your hips.
• Draw your navel toward your spine.
• Bend your back leg slightly as you build the strength and balance to maintain the full pose.
• Avoid twisting the knee of your back leg.

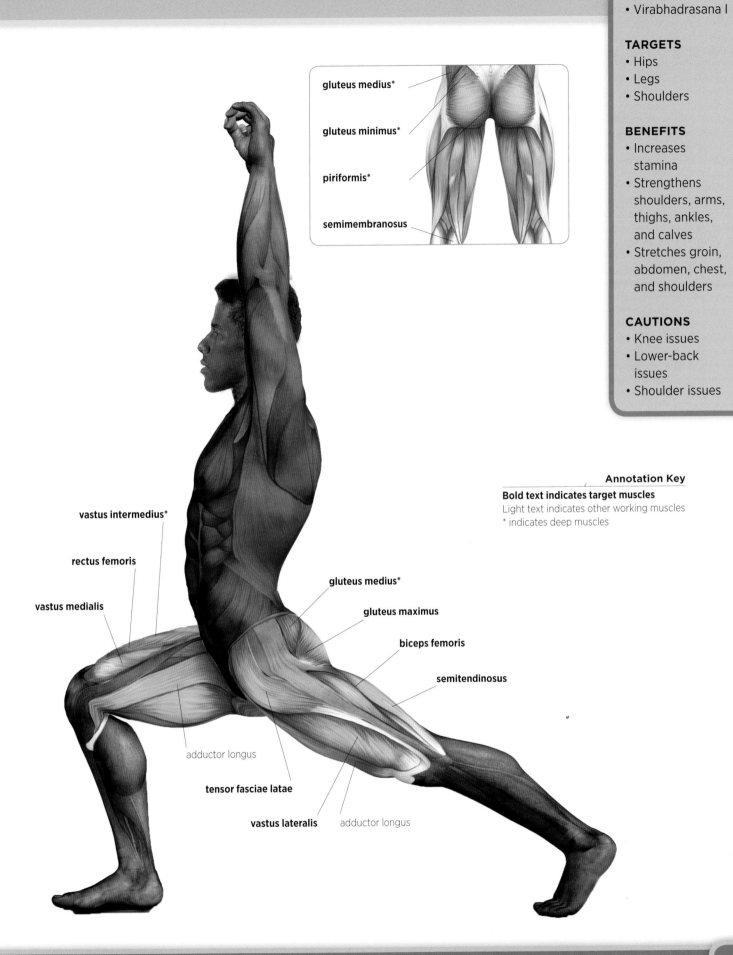

SANSKRIT
• Virabhadrasana I

TARGETS
• Hips
• Legs
• Shoulders

BENEFITS
• Increases stamina
• Strengthens shoulders, arms, thighs, ankles, and calves
• Stretches groin, abdomen, chest, and shoulders

CAUTIONS
• Knee issues
• Lower-back issues
• Shoulder issues

gluteus medius*

gluteus minimus*

piriformis*

semimembranosus

Annotation Key
Bold text indicates target muscles
Light text indicates other working muscles
* indicates deep muscles

vastus intermedius*

rectus femoris

vastus medialis

gluteus medius*

gluteus maximus

biceps femoris

semitendinosus

adductor longus

tensor fasciae latae

vastus lateralis

adductor longus

Warrior Pose II

Despite its name, Warrior II often comes earlier in a sequence than Warrior I. Like all of the Warrior poses, this version tones your lower body and helps you increase your confidence.

HOW TO DO IT

- Stand in the middle of your mat in Mountain Pose (pages 32–33), and place your hands on your hips. Step or jump your feet about 3 to 4 feet apart.

- Turn your left toes so they face the upper-left corner of your mat, and walk your right foot to the right several inches until your feet are in heel-to-heel alignment. Walk your left foot to the right several inches so that your left heel aligns with the inner arch of your right foot.

- Keeping your left knee bent, lift your torso so that your shoulders line up over your hips. Keep a slight internal rotation to the back leg to keep your leg neutral. Extend both arms out to the sides, parallel to the floor, with palms facing downward.

- Continue to bend your left knee, externally rotating your left hip to open your thigh as you find a neutral pelvis. Turn your head toward the left, and gaze past your fingers.

- Hold for the recommended breaths, and then repeat on the other side.

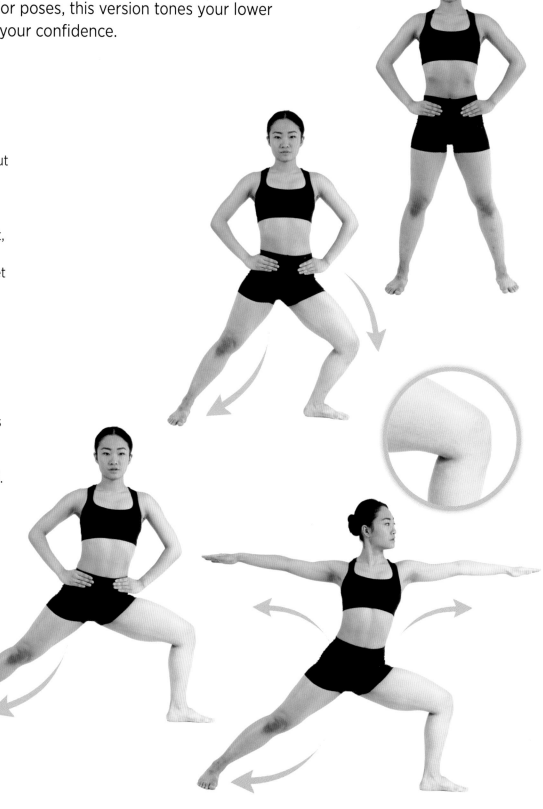

SANSKRIT
• Virabhadrasana II

TARGETS
• Hips
• Legs
• Shoulders

BENEFITS
• Strengthens thighs and arms
• Stretches shoulders, chest, and groin
• Increases stamina

CAUTIONS
• Knee issues
• Lower-back issues
• Shoulder issues

Annotation Key

Bold text indicates target muscles
Light text indicates other working muscles
* indicates deep muscles

DO IT RIGHT

• Press your heels into the floor, using your inner-thigh muscles.
• Keep your shoulders directly above your hips.
• Keep your front knee in line with your middle toe.
• Avoid arching your lower back.
• Avoid leaning over your bent leg.

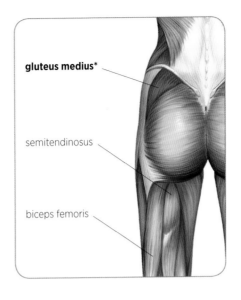

gluteus medius*

semitendinosus

biceps femoris

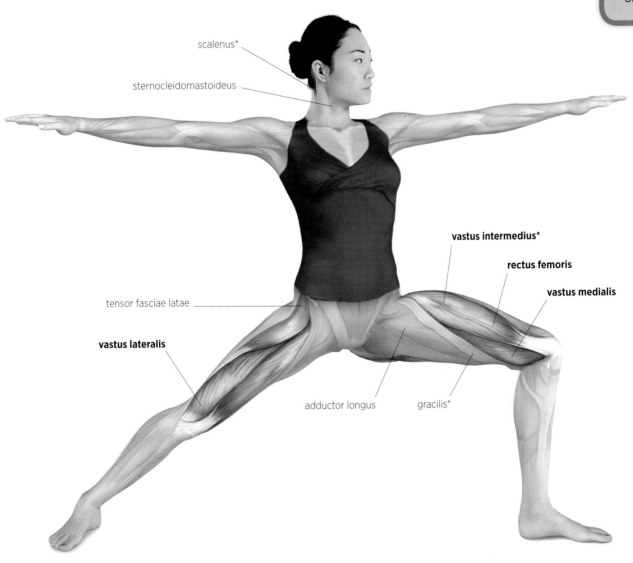

scalenus*

sternocleidomastoideus

vastus intermedius*

rectus femoris

vastus medialis

tensor fasciae latae

vastus lateralis

adductor longus

gracilis*

Side Angle Pose

Mastering Side Angle Pose is the first step in achieving the strength and flexibility necessary to move on to the more difficult standing postures. On its own, it's a great side stretch and core strengthener.

HOW TO DO IT

- Leading with your right foot, begin in Warrior II (pages 72–73).

- Bend your torso toward your right knee, reaching your fingers to the floor as you raise your left arm straight toward the ceiling.

- Hold for the recommended breaths, and then repeat on the other side.

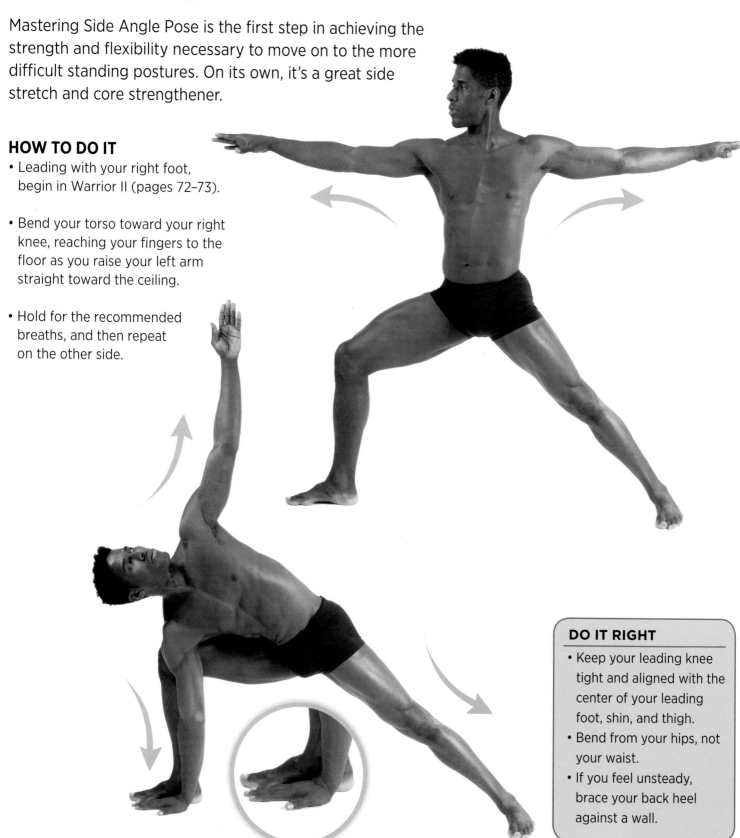

DO IT RIGHT
- Keep your leading knee tight and aligned with the center of your leading foot, shin, and thigh.
- Bend from your hips, not your waist.
- If you feel unsteady, brace your back heel against a wall.

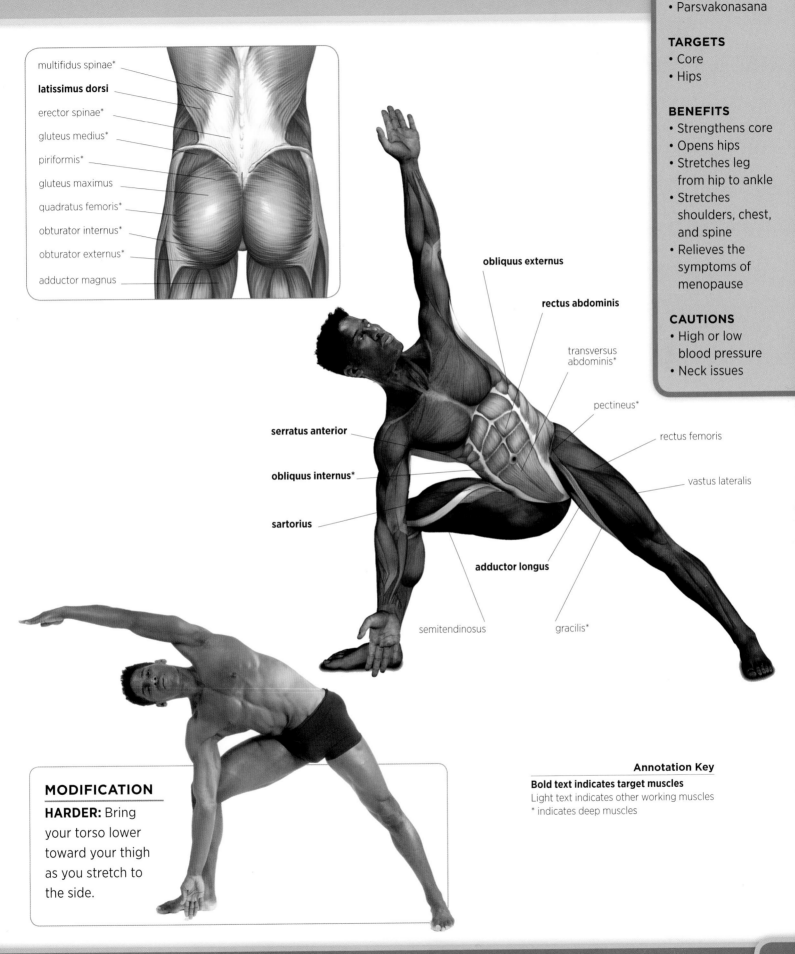

SANSKRIT
• Parsvakonasana

TARGETS
• Core
• Hips

BENEFITS
• Strengthens core
• Opens hips
• Stretches leg from hip to ankle
• Stretches shoulders, chest, and spine
• Relieves the symptoms of menopause

CAUTIONS
• High or low blood pressure
• Neck issues

multifidus spinae*
latissimus dorsi
erector spinae*
gluteus medius*
piriformis*
gluteus maximus
quadratus femoris*
obturator internus*
obturator externus*
adductor magnus

obliquus externus

rectus abdominis

transversus abdominis*

pectineus*

rectus femoris

vastus lateralis

serratus anterior

obliquus internus*

sartorius

adductor longus

semitendinosus

gracilis*

MODIFICATION

HARDER: Bring your torso lower toward your thigh as you stretch to the side.

Annotation Key

Bold text indicates target muscles
Light text indicates other working muscles
* indicates deep muscles

Extended Triangle Pose

A pose with multiple benefits, Extended Triangle works your entire body. It functions as a hip opener, core strengthener, side bend, twist, and heart opener.

HOW TO DO IT

• Stand in the middle of your mat in Mountain Pose (pages 32–33). Step or jump your feet about 3 to 4 feet apart. Turn your left foot out 90 degrees and your right foot in slightly.

• Walk your left foot to the right several inches so that your left heel aligns with the inner arch of your right foot.

• Keeping both legs straight with firm thighs and your arms extended out to your sides parallel to the floor, exhale, and reach your left arm and torso down to the left as you shift your hips to the right, deepening the crease in your left hip.

• Place your left hand on the floor on the outside of your left leg. Extend your right arm straight up. Inhale as you find length across your collarbones.

• Exhale and turn the left side of your torso toward the ceiling.

• Hold for the recommended breaths, and then repeat on the other side.

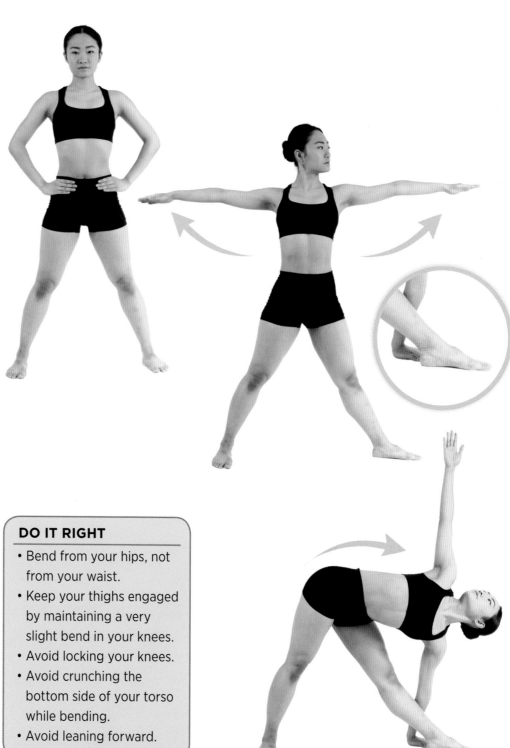

DO IT RIGHT

• Bend from your hips, not from your waist.
• Keep your thighs engaged by maintaining a very slight bend in your knees.
• Avoid locking your knees.
• Avoid crunching the bottom side of your torso while bending.
• Avoid leaning forward.

SANSKRIT
- Utthita Trikonasana

TARGETS
- Obliques
- Hips
- Buttocks

BENEFITS
- Alleviates sciatica
- Stretches shoulders, chest, hips, thighs, and groin
- Strengthens ankles, knees, and core

CAUTIONS
- Diarrhea
- Headache
- High or low blood pressure
- Neck issues

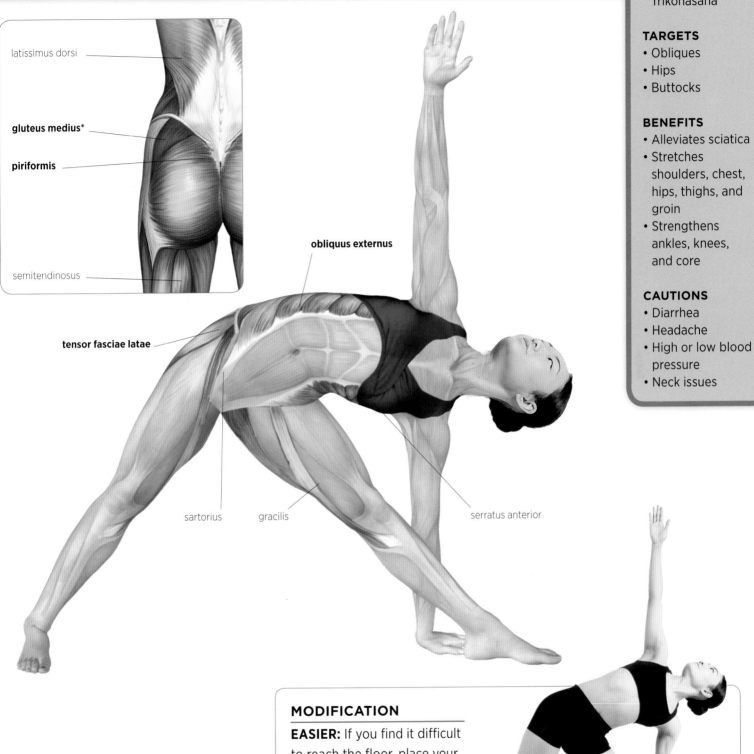

latissimus dorsi

gluteus medius*

piriformis

semitendinosus

obliquus externus

tensor fasciae latae

sartorius

gracilis

serratus anterior

Annotation Key
Bold text indicates target muscles
Light text indicates other working muscles
* indicates deep muscles

MODIFICATION
EASIER: If you find it difficult to reach the floor, place your hand on a block, positioning it on the floor directly under your shoulder. Using a block means less stress on tight hamstrings or hips.

Revolved Triangle Pose

This pose takes the Triangle Pose to a new level. Revolved Triangle Pose challenges your hamstring and spine flexibility while strengthening and stabilizing your legs and hips.

HOW TO DO IT

- Stand in the middle of your mat in Mountain Pose (pages 32–33), and place your hands on your hips. Step or jump your feet about 3 to 4 feet apart.

- Turn your right toes about 45 degrees so that they face the upper-right corner of your mat, and walk your left foot to the left several inches, coming into heel-to-heel alignment.

- Inhale and raise both arms over your head into Upward Salute (pages 36–37). Exhale and bring your left hand to your left hip.

- Inhale and extend your right arm as high as possible, finding length along the right side of your body, and hinge forward with a flat back as you twist to the left.

- Place your right hand onto the floor on the outside of your left foot. Reach your left arm up to the ceiling, broadening across your collarbones.

- Exhale and twist the right side of your torso to the left, and gaze toward the thumb of your upper hand.

- Hold for the recommended breaths, and then repeat on the other side.

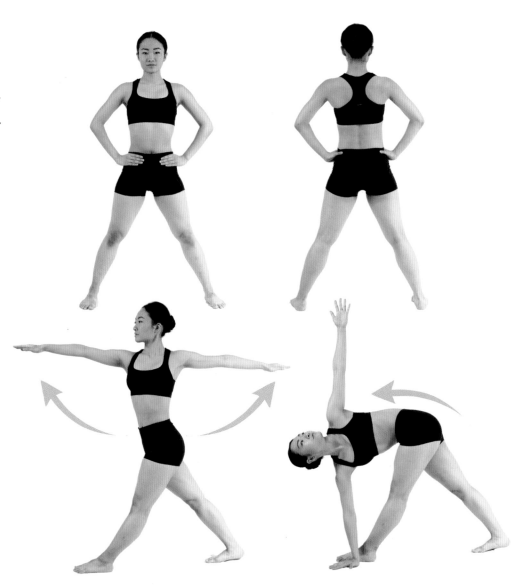

DO IT RIGHT

- Keep your arms and legs straight.
- Use the inhalation to lengthen your spine, and the exhalation to twist.
- If you have tight hamstrings, widen your feet by walking your front foot closer to the edge of the mat, making sure your feet are not lined up as if you were on a tightrope.
- Avoid rounding your spine.

TARGETS
- Hamstrings
- Spine
- Obliques

BENEFITS
- Detoxifies
- Aids digestion
- Stretches hamstrings, hips, shoulders, and arms
- Strengthens thighs and core
- Improves balance

CAUTIONS
- Diarrhea
- Headache
- High or low blood pressure
- Neck issues
- Pregnancy

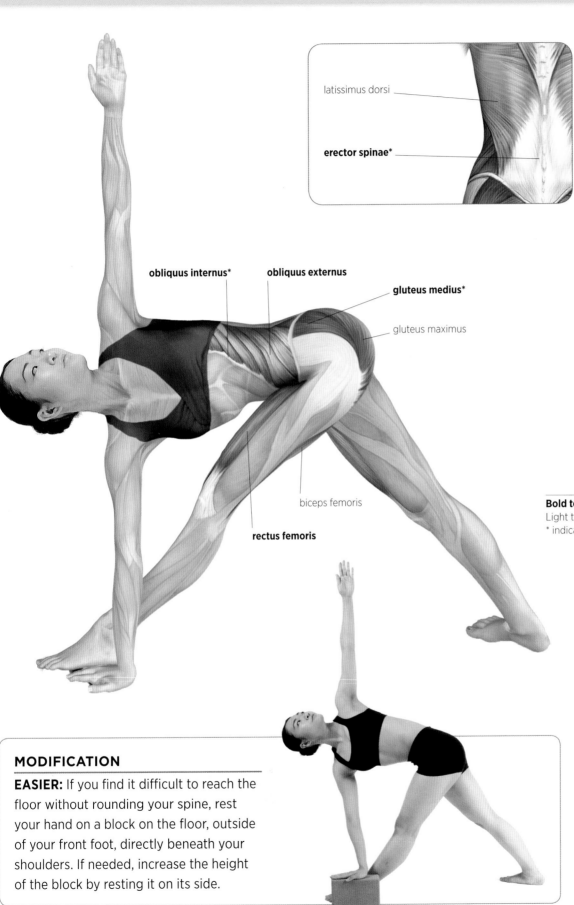

latissimus dorsi

erector spinae*

obliquus internus*   **obliquus externus**

gluteus medius*

gluteus maximus

biceps femoris

rectus femoris

Annotation Key
Bold text indicates target muscles
Light text indicates other working muscles
* indicates deep muscles

MODIFICATION
EASIER: If you find it difficult to reach the floor without rounding your spine, rest your hand on a block on the floor, outside of your front foot, directly beneath your shoulders. If needed, increase the height of the block by resting it on its side.

Revolved Crescent Lunge

Yoga poses that call for you to revolve at the torso aid digestion and relieve lower-back pain. Revolved Crescent Lunge also strengthens your lower body and provides a full-body stretch.

HOW TO DO IT

- Begin in High Lunge (pages 64–65), with your right leg forward and your hands on the floor on either side of your right foot.

- Balance your weight on your left hand, and carefully and slowly guide your right arm up toward the ceiling, twisting your torso to the right. Gaze upward toward your fingers.

- Hold for the recommended breaths, return to the center, and repeat on the other side.

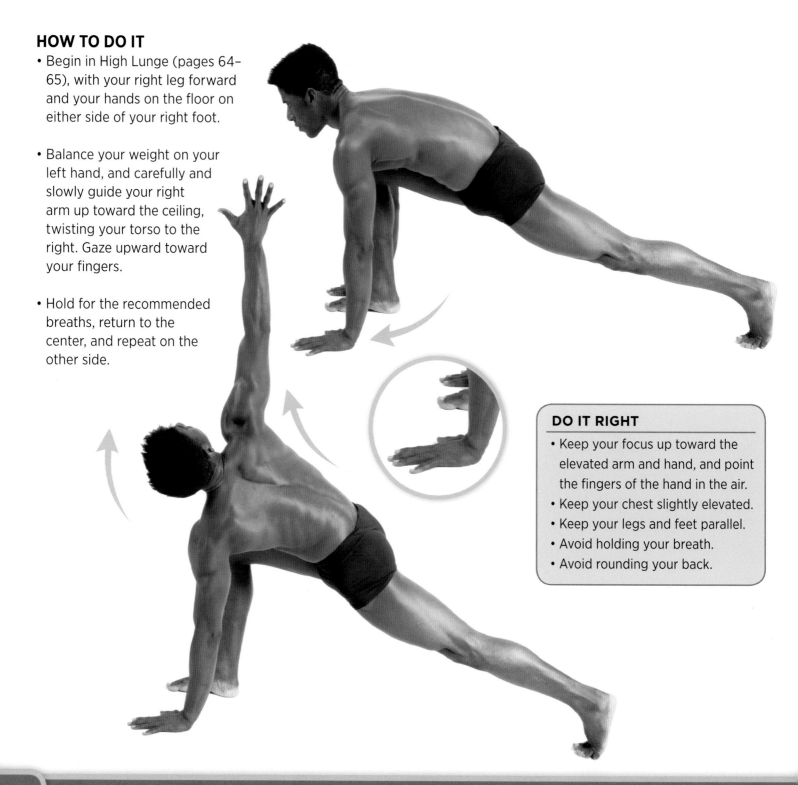

DO IT RIGHT

- Keep your focus up toward the elevated arm and hand, and point the fingers of the hand in the air.
- Keep your chest slightly elevated.
- Keep your legs and feet parallel.
- Avoid holding your breath.
- Avoid rounding your back.

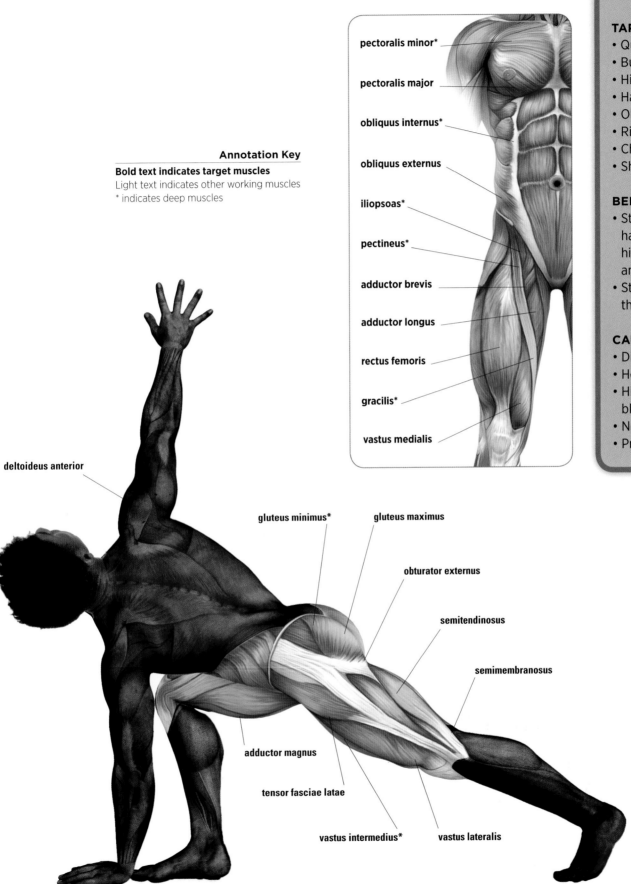

SANSKRIT
• Parivrtta
  Anjaneyasana

TARGETS
• Quadriceps
• Buttocks
• Hip adductors
• Hamstrings
• Obliques
• Rib cage
• Chest
• Shoulders

BENEFITS
• Stretches
  hamstrings,
  hips, shoulders,
  and arms
• Strengthens
  thighs and core

CAUTIONS
• Diarrhea
• Headache
• High or low
  blood pressure
• Neck issues
• Pregnancy

pectoralis minor*

pectoralis major

obliquus internus*

obliquus externus

iliopsoas*

pectineus*

adductor brevis

adductor longus

rectus femoris

gracilis*

vastus medialis

Annotation Key

Bold text indicates target muscles
Light text indicates other working muscles
* indicates deep muscles

deltoideus anterior

gluteus minimus*

gluteus maximus

obturator externus

semitendinosus

semimembranosus

adductor magnus

tensor fasciae latae

vastus intermedius*

vastus lateralis

Extended Side Angle Pose

An excellent stretch for the sides of your torso, Extended Side Angle Pose demands focus on form. When performed correctly, your upper arm, spine, and back leg should form a graceful diagonal line.

HOW TO DO IT

- Stand in the middle of your mat in Mountain Pose (pages 32–33). Step or jump your feet about 3 to 4 feet apart. Turn your left foot out 90 degrees and your right foot in slightly.

- Walk your left foot to the right several inches so that your left heel aligns with the inner arch of your right foot. Extend your arms out to your sides, parallel to the floor.

- Keeping your right leg straight with the thigh slightly internally rotated, press your weight into the pinkie-toe edge of your right foot. Exhale as you extend your torso to the left, reaching your left hand to the floor on the outside of your foot.

- Inhale and extend your right arm straight up toward the ceiling. Turn your right hand to face the floor, externally rotating your entire arm as you exhale and reach over your ear.

- Inhale and lengthen your torso. Exhale and pivot the left side of your body clockwise toward the ceiling.

- Turn your gaze underneath your right arm up toward the ceiling. Hold for the recommended breaths, and then repeat on the other side.

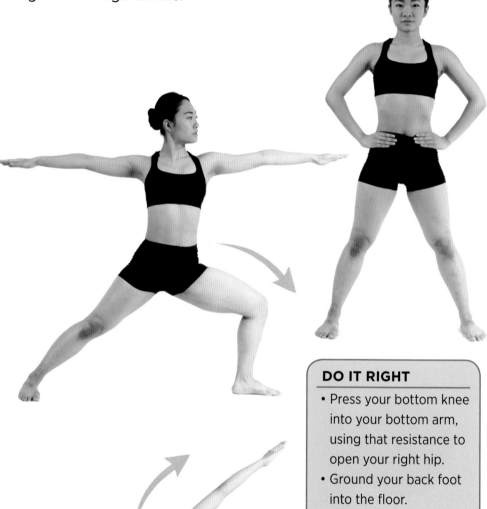

DO IT RIGHT

- Press your bottom knee into your bottom arm, using that resistance to open your right hip.
- Ground your back foot into the floor.
- Keep your upper arm extended and your back leg straight.
- Keep the knee of your bottom foot in line with your toes, pointing forward.
- Avoid crunching your bottom ribs.
- Avoid allowing your shoulders to round forward.

TARGET
- Quadriceps
- Buttocks
- Hip adductors
- Hamstrings
- Obliques
- Rib cage
- Chest
- Shoulders

BENEFITS
- Stretches hips, groin, sides, and spine
- Strengthens and stretches thighs, knees, and ankles
- Strengthens core

CAUTIONS
- Knee issues
- Shoulder issues
- Diarrhea
- Headache
- High or low blood pressure
- Neck issues

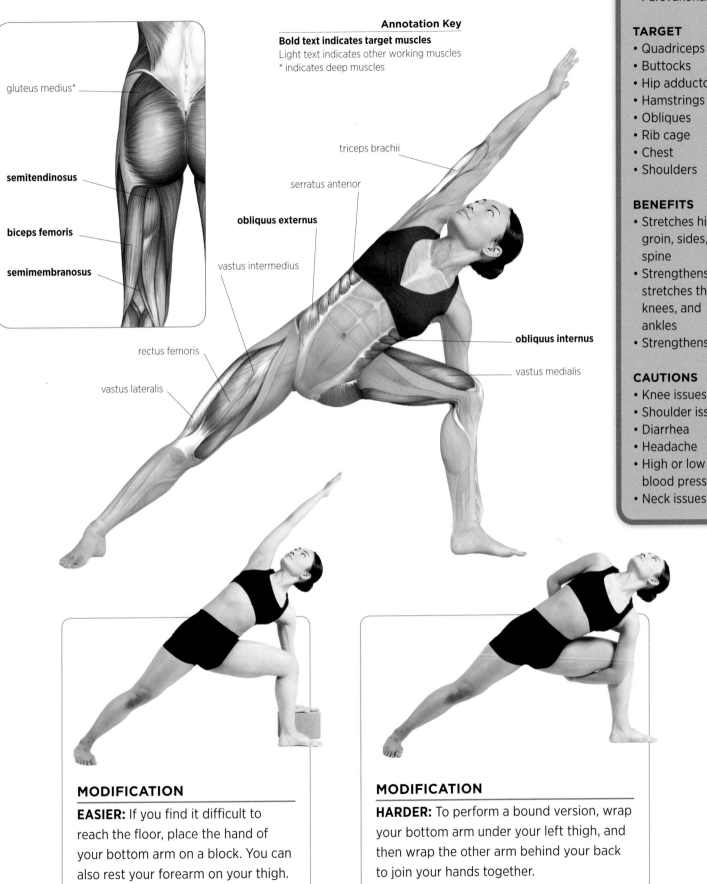

Annotation Key

Bold text indicates target muscles
Light text indicates other working muscles
* indicates deep muscles

gluteus medius*

semitendinosus

biceps femoris

semimembranosus

triceps brachii

serratus anterior

obliquus externus

vastus intermedius

rectus femoris

vastus lateralis

obliquus internus

vastus medialis

MODIFICATION

EASIER: If you find it difficult to reach the floor, place the hand of your bottom arm on a block. You can also rest your forearm on your thigh.

MODIFICATION

HARDER: To perform a bound version, wrap your bottom arm under your left thigh, and then wrap the other arm behind your back to join your hands together.

Revolved Extended Side Angle Pose

This deep twist calls for excellent balance, along with thigh and core strength. Like other revolved asanas, Revolved Extended Side Angle Pose aids digestion and relieves lower-back pain.

HOW TO DO IT

- Stand in the middle of your mat in Mountain Pose (pages 32–33). Bring your hands to your hips, and then step or jump your feet about 3 to 4 feet apart.

- Turn your left toes 45 degrees inward, and walk your right foot to the right several inches, until your feet are in heel-to-heel alignment.

- Bring your hands together in a prayer position in front of your heart. Bend your right knee so that your thigh is parallel to the floor. Firm your left thigh, keeping your leg straight.

- Twist your torso to the right, positioning your left elbow on the outside of your right thigh. Keep your hips square, drawing your right hip crease back.

- Turn your gaze upward and to the back right-hand corner of the room. Hold for the recommended breaths, and then repeat on the other side.

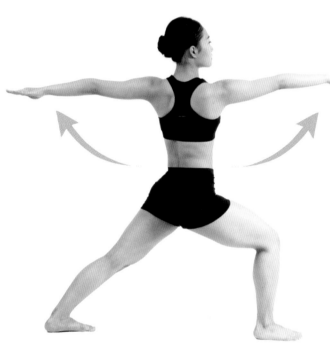

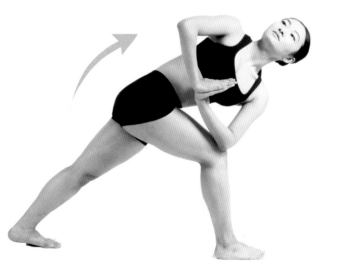

DO IT RIGHT

- Keep your hands and arms in the prayer position as you twist.
- Your front foot should form a 90-degree angle with the front of your mat.
- Keep your front knee facing forward, in line with your middle toes.
- Press the pinkie-toe edge of your back foot firmly downward, and use the grounding of your back leg to help you twist.
- Push your elbow into your thigh, and vice versa, to deepen the twist as you hold.

TARGETS
- Spine
- Obliques
- Hip adductors
- Hamstrings
- Rib cage
- Chest
- Shoulders

BENEFITS
- Stretches hips, groin, torso, arms, and spine
- Strengthens thighs and ankles
- Stimulates digestion and elimination
- Improves balance

CAUTIONS
- Knee issues
- Shoulder issues
- Diarrhea
- Headache
- High or low blood pressure
- Neck issues

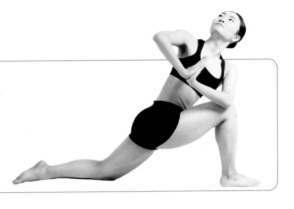

MODIFICATION

EASIER: Instead of keeping your back leg extended, bend your back knee to lower your leg to the floor, making it easier to balance.

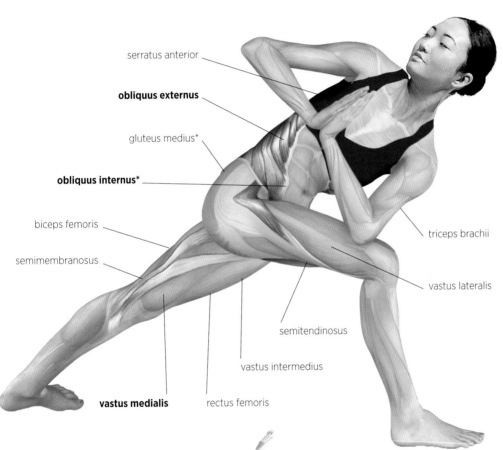

serratus anterior

obliquus externus

gluteus medius*

obliquus internus*

biceps femoris

semimembranosus

triceps brachii

vastus lateralis

semitendinosus

vastus intermedius

vastus medialis

rectus femoris

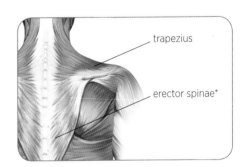

trapezius

erector spinae*

Annotation Key

Bold text indicates target muscles
Light text indicates other working muscles
* indicates deep muscles

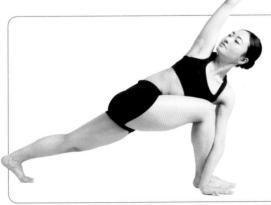

MODIFICATION

SIMILAR DIFFICULTY: Instead of keeping your hands and arms in the prayer position, place the hand of the arm opposite your front leg on the floor, and extend the other arm in line with your body, feeling a stretch along the side of your body.

Half Moon Pose

Open your hips and hone your balance and coordination with Half Moon Pose.
This posture will also strengthen your entire core.

HOW TO DO IT

- Stand in Extended Triangle Pose (pages 76–77) with your left palm or fingertips resting on your shin or on the floor. Gaze down toward your left foot, and bring your right hand onto your hip.

- Bend your left knee slightly, keeping it extended over your middle toe. At the same time, shift more weight onto your left leg, and step your right foot in about 12 inches.

- Straighten your left leg, opening the thigh while lifting your right leg to hip height. Keep your right leg in a neutral position, and flex your ankle.

- Once you have found your balance, extend your right arm straight up toward the ceiling, opening up across the front of your chest.

- Hold for the recommended breaths, and then repeat on the other side.

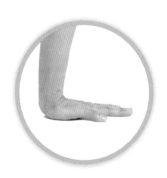

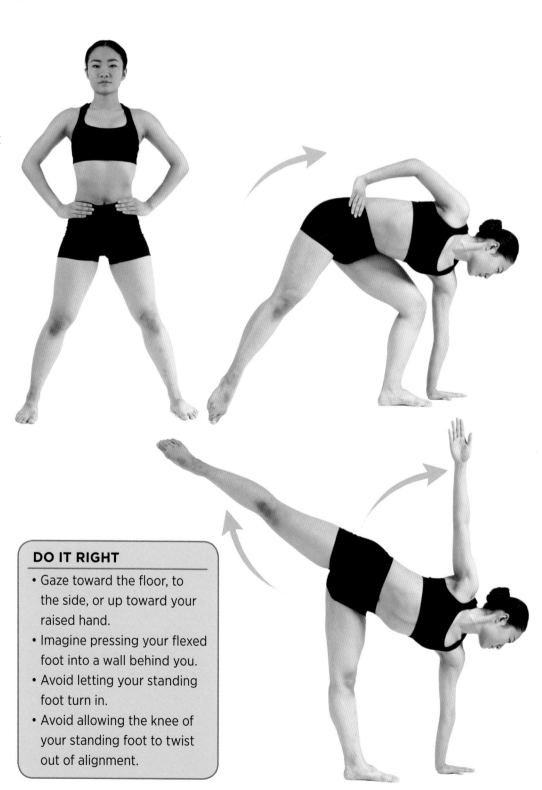

DO IT RIGHT

- Gaze toward the floor, to the side, or up toward your raised hand.
- Imagine pressing your flexed foot into a wall behind you.
- Avoid letting your standing foot turn in.
- Avoid allowing the knee of your standing foot to twist out of alignment.

TARGET
- Spine
- Hip adductors
- Hamstrings
- Rib cage
- Chest
- Shoulders

BENEFITS
- Stretches hip, groin, torso, arms, and spine
- Strengthens thighs and ankles
- Stimulates digestion and elimination
- Improves balance

CAUTIONS
- Knee issues
- Shoulder issues
- Diarrhea
- Headache
- High or low blood pressure
- Neck issues

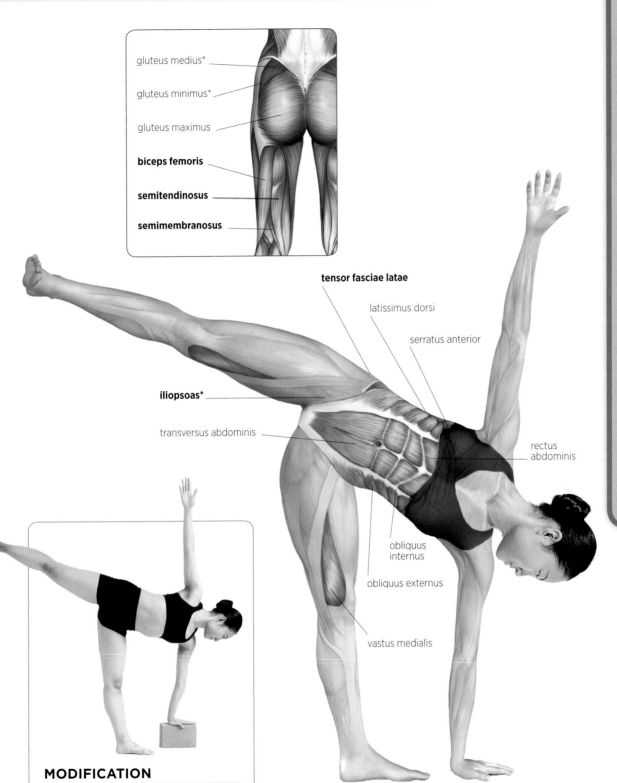

gluteus medius*
gluteus minimus*
gluteus maximus
biceps femoris
semitendinosus
semimembranosus

tensor fasciae latae
latissimus dorsi
serratus anterior
iliopsoas*
transversus abdominis
rectus abdominis
obliquus internus
obliquus externus
vastus medialis

MODIFICATION

EASIER: Rest your hand on a block if it is challenging for you to straighten your standing leg. If needed, increase the height of the block by resting it on its side.

Annotation Key
Bold text indicates target muscles
Light text indicates other working muscles
* indicates deep muscles

Extended Hand-to-Big-Toe Pose

The revitalizing Extended Hand-to-Big-Toe Pose provides your hamstrings with a deep stretch while challenging your sense of balance. Focus on grounding your standing leg, allowing yourself enough time to find your equilibrium.

HOW TO DO IT

- Stand in Mountain Pose (pages 32–33). Shift some of your weight onto your left foot as you bend your right knee into your chest, placing your left hand on your hip.

- Grab your right toe in a yogi toe lock, with your index finger and middle finger wrapped around the inside of your big toe and your thumb wrapped around the outside of the toe.

- Slightly internally rotate your left thigh, and firm the whole leg. Exhaling, extend your right leg forward, aiming to straighten it.

- Hold for the recommended breaths, and then repeat on the other side.

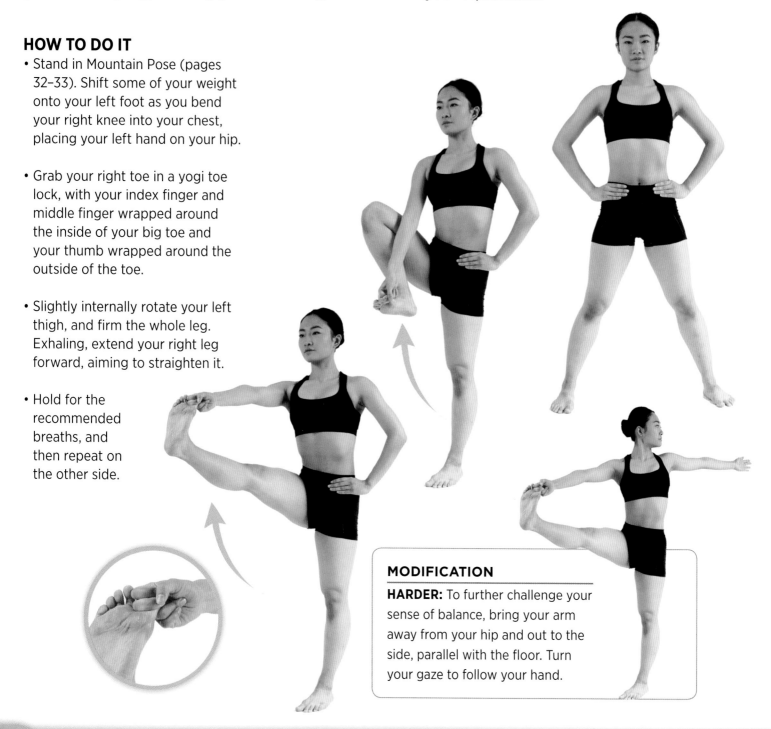

MODIFICATION

HARDER: To further challenge your sense of balance, bring your arm away from your hip and out to the side, parallel with the floor. Turn your gaze to follow your hand.

TARGETS
- Hamstrings

BENEFITS
- Stretches hamstrings and shoulders
- Strengthens spine, legs, and ankles
- Improves balance

CAUTIONS
- Ankle issues
- Foot issues
- Lower-back issues

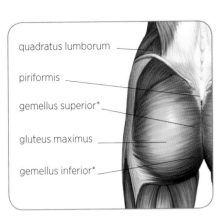

quadratus lumborum

piriformis

gemellus superior*

gluteus maximus

gemellus inferior*

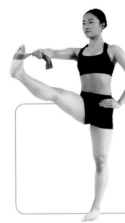

MODIFICATION

EASIER: Place a strap around the ball of your foot to help extend your leg.

DO IT RIGHT

- If you find yourself leaning your torso forward and rounding your back to straighten your leg, then keep it bent; it is more important to elongate your spine than to straighten your extended leg.
- On the side of your lifted leg, draw your hip crease back to keep your hips square.
- Keep your spine upright with your shoulders in line over your hips.
- Ground the heel of your standing leg into the floor to maintain your balance.
- Keep your standing leg straight.
- Avoid letting your hip lift upward in an attempt to raise your leg.
- Avoid locking the knee of your standing leg.
- Avoid allowing your shoulder to protract forward as you hold your toe.
- Avoid twisting your hips.

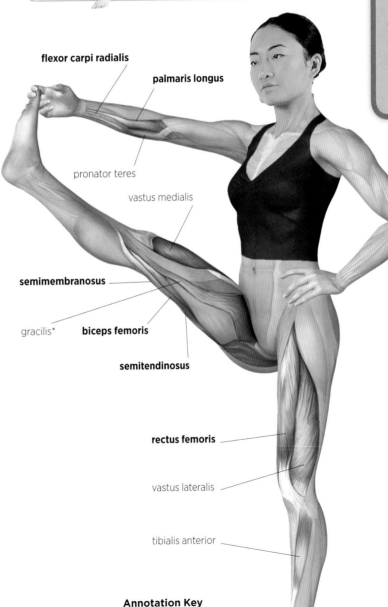

flexor carpi radialis

palmaris longus

pronator teres

vastus medialis

semimembranosus

gracilis*

biceps femoris

semitendinosus

rectus femoris

vastus lateralis

tibialis anterior

Annotation Key

Bold text indicates target muscles
Light text indicates other working muscles
* indicates deep muscles

Revolved Half Moon Pose

The Revolved Half Moon is a balancing pose and a twist. An ideal counterpose to Half Moon Pose (pages 86–87), this asana relies on your core strength.

HOW TO DO IT

• Begin in Revolved Triangle Pose (pages 78–79), with your left hand on the floor on the outside of your right foot and your right arm reaching straight up.

• Bring your right hand onto your right hip. Staying in the twist, turn your gaze toward the floor, and bend your right knee slightly as you step your left foot about 12 inches in toward your right, shortening the stance. Lift your left leg up to hip height as you straighten your right leg.

• Keep your hips squared to the floor as you twist your left ribs to the right. Once you have found your balance, extend your right arm up to the ceiling. Externally rotate your arm and reach up through the fingertips.

• Hold for the recommended breaths, as you continue to square your hips, drawing your right hip crease back and your left down toward the floor.

DO IT RIGHT
• Imagine pressing your lifted foot into a wall behind you.
• Find a comfortable gazing point, either at the floor or to the side, before eventually turning your gaze up to your thumb.
• Avoid allowing the hip on the side of your lifted leg to drop toward the floor.

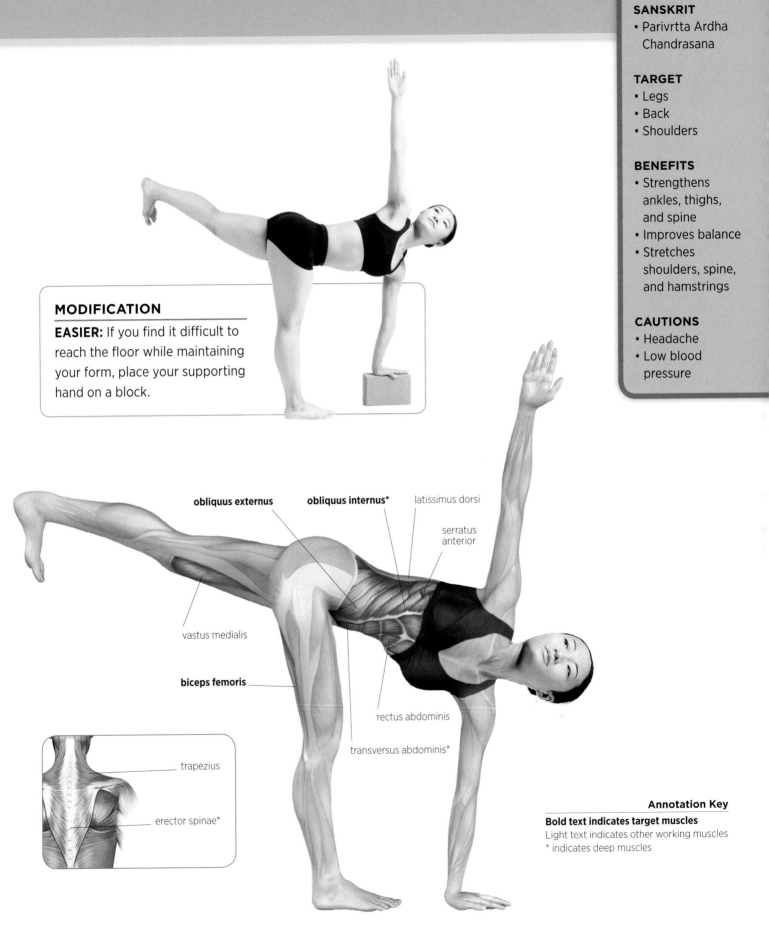

FACT FILE

SANSKRIT
• Parivrtta Ardha Chandrasana

TARGET
• Legs
• Back
• Shoulders

BENEFITS
• Strengthens ankles, thighs, and spine
• Improves balance
• Stretches shoulders, spine, and hamstrings

CAUTIONS
• Headache
• Low blood pressure

MODIFICATION

EASIER: If you find it difficult to reach the floor while maintaining your form, place your supporting hand on a block.

obliquus externus

obliquus internus*

latissimus dorsi

serratus anterior

vastus medialis

biceps femoris

rectus abdominis

transversus abdominis*

trapezius

erector spinae*

Annotation Key

Bold text indicates target muscles
Light text indicates other working muscles
* indicates deep muscles

Warrior Pose III

Appearing in many yoga flows, Warrior III is a versatile asana. You can come into it in several ways, such as from Mountain Pose, as described here. It will challenge your balance while providing an effective arm, shoulder, and upper-back stretch. It also tones your abdominals.

HOW TO DO IT

• Stand in the middle of a mat in Mountain Pose (pages 32–33), with your feet together and arms at your sides. Step your right foot forward about 12 inches.

• Extend your arms over your head, keeping them parallel to each other. Lift your left heel upward, shifting your weight onto the ball of your right foot.

• Square your hips to the front of the mat, drawing your right hip back and your left hip forward. Keeping your arms extended over your head, hinge your torso forward over your right thigh.

• Continue to shift your weight onto your right leg as you lift your left leg to hip height, foot flexed. Your arms and left leg should be parallel to the floor.

• Hold for the recommended breaths, and then repeat on the other side.

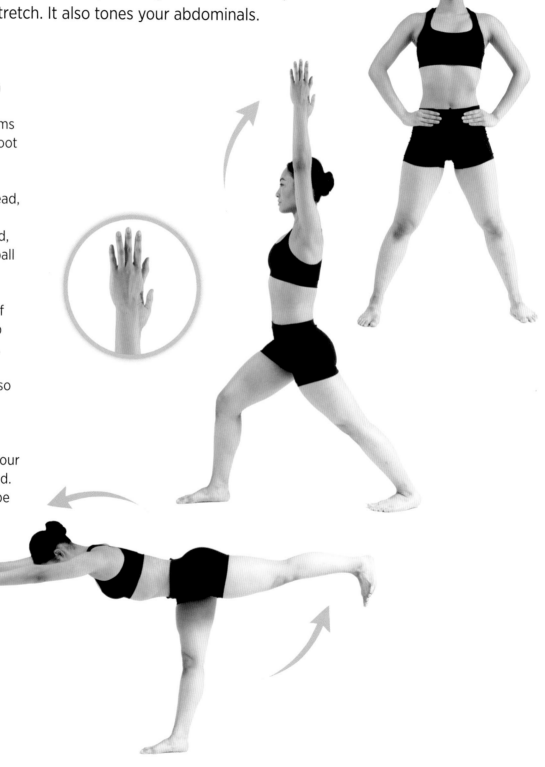

TARGET
• Legs
• Back
• Shoulders

BENEFITS
• Stretches shoulders, spine, and hamstrings
• Strengthens ankles, thighs, and spine
• Improves balance

CAUTIONS
• Headache
• Low blood pressure

DO IT RIGHT

• Keep your hips squared.
• Keep length in your spine as you extend from your fingertips to your lifted heel.
• Energize your lifted leg to help you find balance.
• Ground down with the heel of your standing foot.
• Avoid allowing your lifted leg to bend or hang without control.

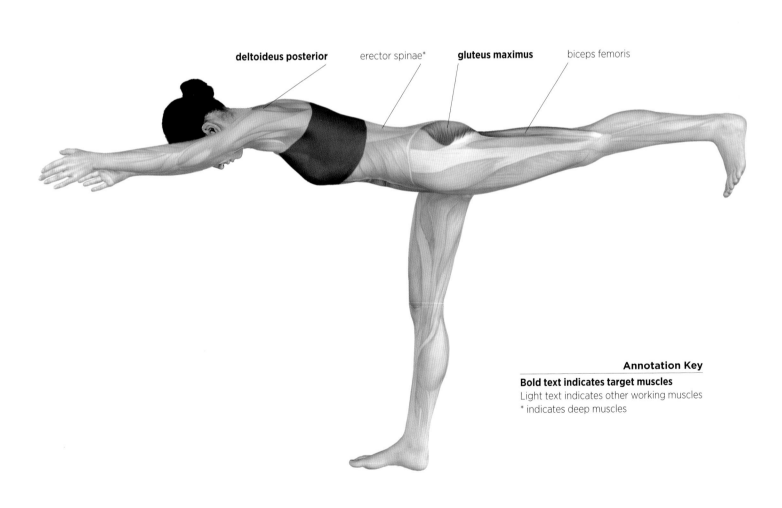

rectus abdominis

obliquus internus*

transversus abdominis*

deltoideus posterior

erector spinae*

gluteus maximus

biceps femoris

Annotation Key

Bold text indicates target muscles
Light text indicates other working muscles
* indicates deep muscles

Bowing with Respect Pose

This advanced pose takes Warrior III to a new level, calling for strength, balance, and flexibility. Include it in a yoga flow designed to work your hamstrings. This pose will also provide a deep hip-opening stretch.

HOW TO DO IT

• Begin in Warrior III (pages 92–93), balancing on your right leg, and then bend your raised left leg into your chest.

• Grab your left toe with your left hand, and extend your left arm and leg out to your side. Keep your right arm extended to the right side.

• Hold for the recommended breaths, and then release back into Warrior III.

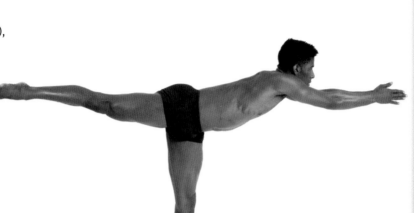

FACT FILE

SANSKRIT
• None

TARGET
• Legs
• Glutes
• Core
• Back
• Shoulders

BENEFITS
• Stretches shoulders, spine, and hamstrings
• Strengthens ankles, thighs, and spine
• Opens hips
• Improves balance
• Engages core

CAUTION
• Hip issues
• Shoulder issues
• Knee issues
• Headache
• Low blood pressure

DO IT RIGHT

• Keep your free arm extended throughout for balance.
• Point your supporting foot forward, keeping your toes spread and grounded.
• Keep your knee over your ankle.

Annotation Key

Bold text indicates target muscles
Light text indicates other working muscles
* indicates deep muscles

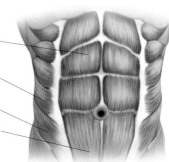

rectus abdominis

obliquus externus*

obliquus internus*

transversus abdominis*

Bowing Bird of Paradise Prep

Another advanced balance, this pose prepares you for the extreme challenge of the full Bowing Bird of Paradise. On its own, it has much to offer—as a hip opener, it can help remedy hip muscle imbalances that manifest as lower-back pain, muscle stiffness, and an inability to walk distances.

HOW TO DO IT

- Begin in Warrior III (pages 92–93), balancing on your right leg, and then bend your raised left leg into your chest.

- Extend your left leg out to the side, and extend your left arm, weaving it under your raised knee and out alongside your leg. Keep your right arm extended to the right side, bending the knee over the arm.

- Hold for the recommended breaths, and then release back into Warrior III.

DO IT RIGHT

- Keep your free arm extended throughout for balance.
- Point your supporting foot forward, keeping your toes spread and grounded.
- Keep your knee over your ankle.

FACT FILE

SANSKRIT
- Namitum Svarga Dvijasana prep

TARGET
- Legs
- Glutes
- Core
- Back
- Shoulders

BENEFITS
- Stretches shoulders, spine, and hamstrings
- Strengthens ankles, thighs, and spine
- Opens hips
- Improves balance
- Engages core

CAUTIONS
- Hip issues
- Shoulder issues
- Knee issues
- Headache
- Low blood pressure

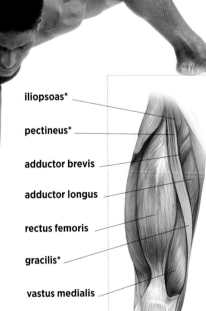

iliopsoas*
pectineus*
adductor brevis
adductor longus
rectus femoris
gracilis*
vastus medialis

Annotation Key
Bold text indicates target muscles
Light text indicates other working muscles
* indicates deep muscles

Bowing Bird of Paradise

This advanced strengthening stretch combines a forward bend, a twist, and a balance. Be sure to master the intermediate-level balancing poses before attempting this demanding asana.

HOW TO DO IT

- Begin in Warrior III (pages 92–93), balancing on your right leg, and then bend your raised left leg into your chest.

- Extend your left leg out to the side, and extend your left arm, weaving it under your raised knee and out alongside your leg.

- Reach your right arm behind your back, and bind your hands together behind your hips.

- Hold for the recommended breaths, and then release back into Warrior III.

DO IT RIGHT

- Point your supporting foot forward, keeping your toes spread and grounded.
- Keep your knee over your ankle.

FACT FILE

SANSKRIT
- Namitum Svarga Dvijasana

TARGET
- Legs
- Glutes
- Core
- Back
- Shoulders

BENEFITS
- Stretches shoulders, spine, and hamstrings
- Strengthens ankles, thighs, and spine
- Opens hips
- Improves balance
- Engages core

CAUTION
- Hip issues
- Shoulder issues
- Knee issues
- Headache
- Low blood pressure

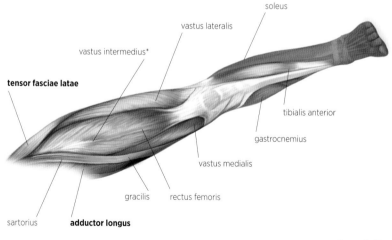

vastus lateralis

soleus

vastus intermedius*

tensor fasciae latae

tibialis anterior

gastrocnemius

vastus medialis

gracilis

rectus femoris

sartorius

adductor longus

Annotation Key
Bold text indicates target muscles
Light text indicates other working muscles
* indicates deep muscles

Bird of Paradise Pose

Known as Bird of Paradise, this pose takes on the asymmetrical shape of its namesake, a tropical flower with petals that resemble a bird taking flight. It challenges your shoulder and hip flexibility, and it also demands keen balance and a great deal of strength.

HOW TO DO IT

• Begin in Extended Side Angle Pose (pages 82–83), with your right leg bent.

• Exhale and reach your left arm behind your back, and then reach your right arm underneath your left leg to join your hands near the outermost part of your left thigh.

• Exhale and turn your gaze down toward your right toes, and then bring your left foot to the top of your mat, planting your feet hip-width apart.

• Straighten both legs, and twist your torso to the right, keeping your hands bound around your left leg.

• Shift your weight onto your right leg, and slowly make your way up to standing.

• Gaze straight ahead to steady yourself, and gradually straighten your left leg to fully extend it.

• Hold for the recommended breaths, and then lower your left leg back to the floor. Carefully release your bound hands, and assume a Standing Forward Bend. Repeat on the other side.

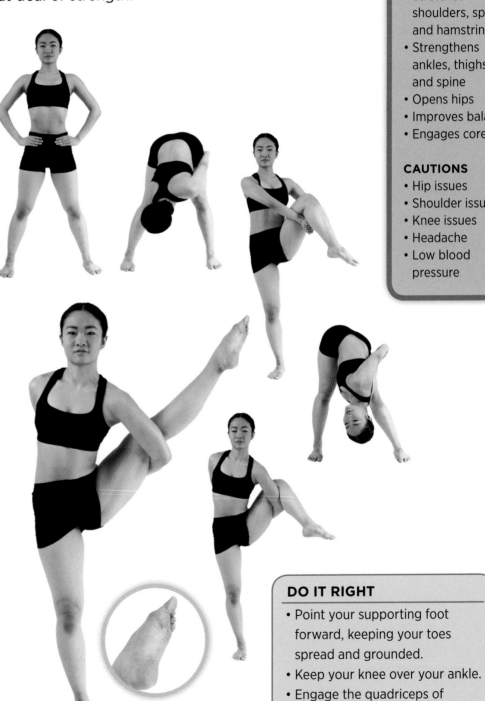

DO IT RIGHT

• Point your supporting foot forward, keeping your toes spread and grounded.
• Keep your knee over your ankle.
• Engage the quadriceps of both legs.

Extended Standing Split Pose

Extended Standing Split Pose is an extremely advanced asana that calls for maximum flexibility and superb balance. A standing pose, it also involves a twist and builds strength.

HOW TO DO IT

• Stand with your legs and feet parallel and shoulder-width apart. Bend your right leg, grasping your ankle with your right hand and your toes with your left.

• Keeping hold of your ankle and toes, hinge your right leg upward from the hip.

• Continue stretching your leg upward until your right leg is fully extended perpendicular to the floor.

• To assume the full pose, point the toes of your right foot, allowing your hand to slide downward to grasp the bottom of your foot.

• Bring your right arm in front of your raised leg, extending parallel to the floor at shoulder height.

• Hold for the recommended breaths, carefully release the stretch, and then repeat on the opposite side.

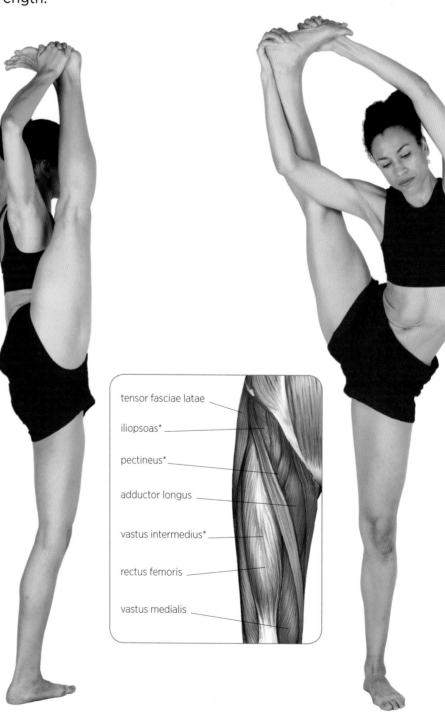

tensor fasciae latae

iliopsoas*

pectineus*

adductor longus

vastus intermedius*

rectus femoris

vastus medialis

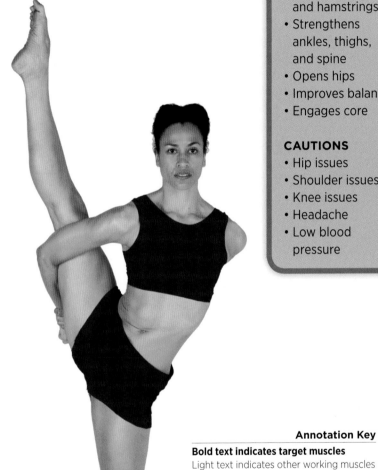

TARGETS
- Hip adductors
- Hamstrings
- Inner thighs
- Glutes

BENEFITS
- Stretches shoulders, spine, and hamstrings
- Strengthens ankles, thighs, and spine
- Opens hips
- Improves balance
- Engages core

CAUTIONS
- Hip issues
- Shoulder issues
- Knee issues
- Headache
- Low blood pressure

DO IT RIGHT
- Keep your back straight.
- Keep your chest open.
- Pull your leg upward only as high as you can without hurting your hips.
- Avoid holding your breath.

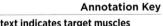

Annotation Key

Bold text indicates target muscles
Light text indicates other working muscles
* indicates deep muscles

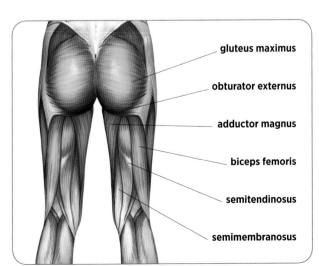

- gluteus maximus
- obturator externus
- adductor magnus
- biceps femoris
- semitendinosus
- semimembranosus

CHAPTER TWO

STANDING FORWARD AND SIDE BENDS

Standing forward bends offer numerous benefits. Because they are weight-bearing, they strengthen your legs, stabilize your hips, and are great for stretching your hamstrings, calves, ankles, and lower back. As you release your head downward into each pose, the tension in your upper back, shoulders, and neck dissipates. These bends can also help to calm your nerves, alleviate symptoms of mild depression, and ease headaches.

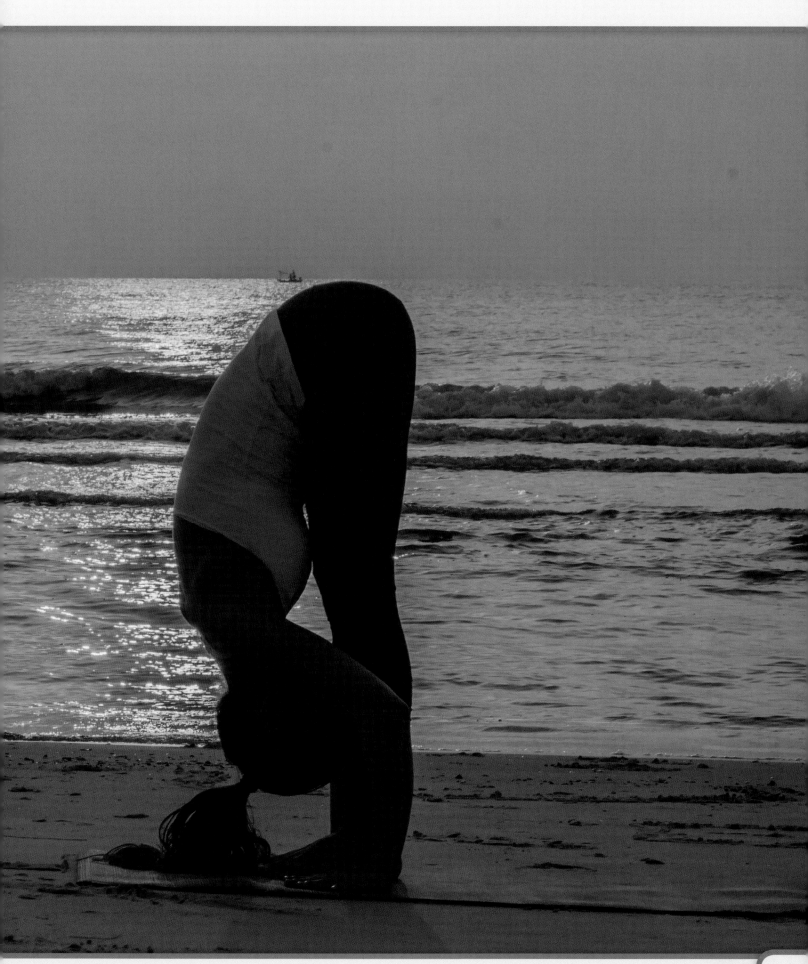

Cat Pose

Cat Pose is an essential yoga move that helps keep your spine mobile. Often paired with Cow Pose (pages 166–67), it teaches beginners how to move with articulation, meaning one vertebra at a time.

HOW TO DO IT

- Begin on all fours, with your hands planted directly below your shoulders and your knees aligned beneath your hips. Your hips should be in a neutral position and the tops of your feet on the floor.

- Spread your fingers wide, grounding down through your thumb and index fingers. Externally rotate your arms, thinking of opening your right upper arm clockwise and your left upper arm counterclockwise.

- Drop your head as you round your upper back, and draw your belly into your spine. Gazing down at the floor or toward your navel, hold for the recommended breaths, and then exhale to release the stretch.

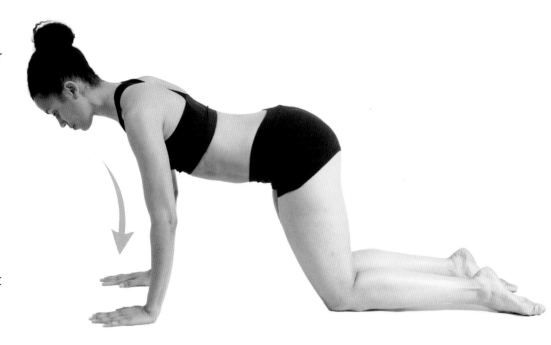

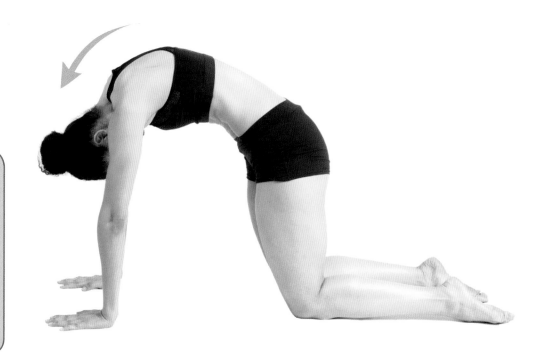

DO IT RIGHT

- Allow your shoulder blades to separate, and breathe more space into your upper spine.
- Keep your shoulders over your wrists as you round your back.
- Avoid bringing your weight back toward your knees as you round your spine.

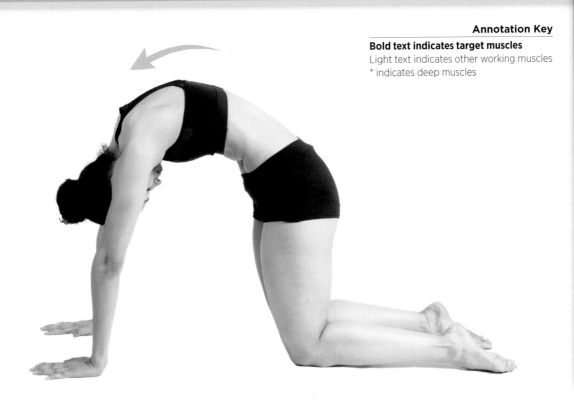

FACT FILE

SANSKRIT
• Marjaryasana

TARGETS
• Spine
• Chest
• Neck

BENEFITS
• Stretches upper body and back
• Strengthens the muscles in the hands and wrists
• Massages spine
• Increases mobility

CAUTIONS
• Neck issues
• Wrist issues

Annotation Key

Bold text indicates target muscles
Light text indicates other working muscles
* indicates deep muscles

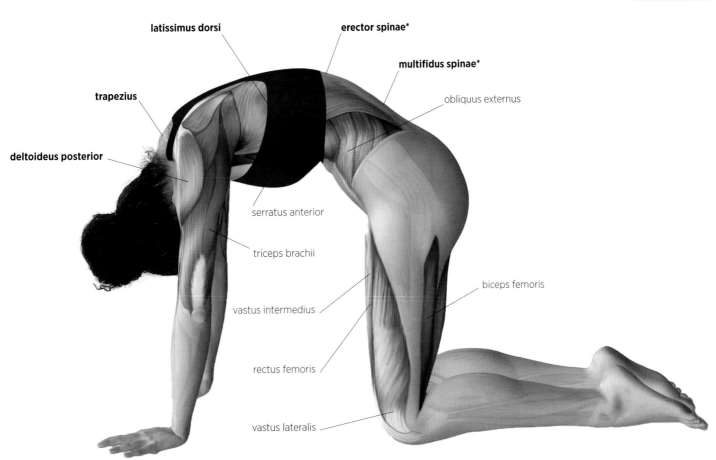

latissimus dorsi

erector spinae*

multifidus spinae*

trapezius

obliquus externus

deltoideus posterior

serratus anterior

triceps brachii

biceps femoris

vastus intermedius

rectus femoris

vastus lateralis

Straight-Leg Lunge Pose

This stretching pose helps improve core stability and balance while strengthening your legs and buttocks. It also benefits hip mobility and spinal health.

HOW TO DO IT

• Stand with your legs and feet parallel and shoulder-width apart. Bend your knees slightly and tuck your pelvis forward. Lift your chest and press your shoulders downward and back.

• Step forward with your right foot.

• Keep your legs straight as you lean your torso forward as far as possible over your right leg. Place your hands on your right thigh to help with balance. Allow the weight of your upper body to intensify the stretch.

• Hold for the recommended breaths, return to the standing position, and repeat on the other side.

DO IT RIGHT

• Flex your front foot by lifting the ball of your foot off the floor to maximize the intensity of the stretch.
• Keep the heel of your rear leg on the floor throughout the stretch.
• Keep your chest elevated, and focus your gaze toward your front foot; this will help elongate your torso and intensify the stretch in both your lower back and hamstrings.
• Avoid retaining unnecessary tension in your upper body—relax and breathe in and out naturally.

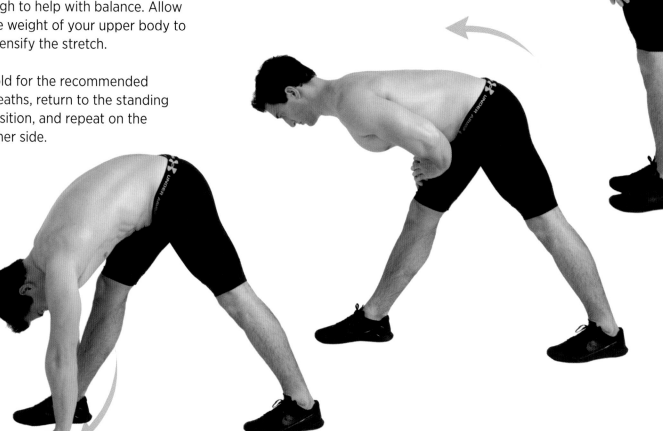

FACT FILE

SANSKRIT
• None

TARGETS
• Hamstrings
• Lower back
• Calves

BENEFITS
• Improves mid- and lower-body balance
• Strengthens legs and buttocks

CAUTIONS
• Neck issues

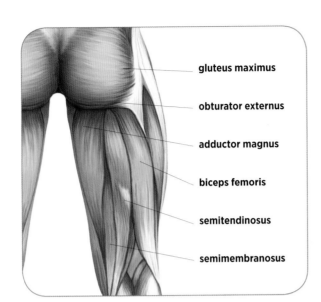

gluteus maximus

obturator externus

adductor magnus

biceps femoris

semitendinosus

semimembranosus

Annotation Key

Bold text indicates target muscles
Light text indicates other working muscles
* indicates deep muscles

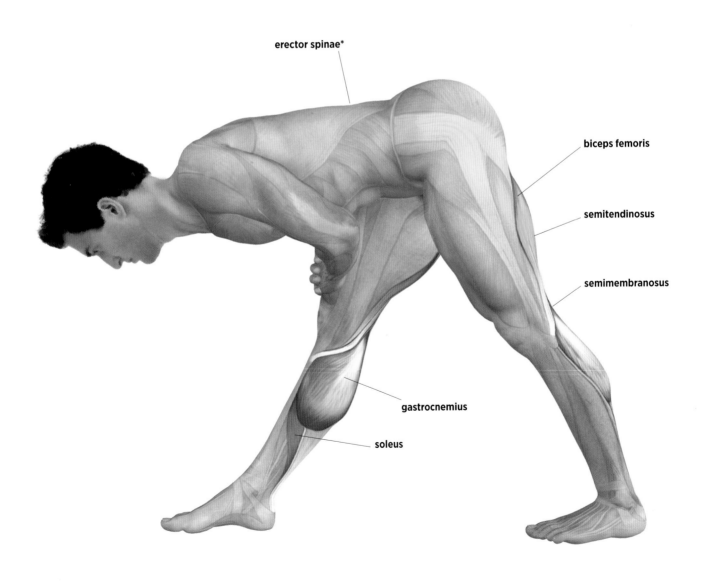

erector spinae*

biceps femoris

semitendinosus

semimembranosus

gastrocnemius

soleus

Standing Half Forward Bend to Forward Bend

Often repeated throughout yoga classes, Standing Half Forward Bend and Standing Forward Bend form part of the well-known Sun Salutation sequences. Each time you perform these two poses, you will be able to fold a little deeper into the forward bend.

HOW TO DO IT

• Begin in Mountain Pose (pages 32–33). Inhale and raise your arms toward the ceiling. Exhale as you hinge at the hips to fold forward, bringing your arms down until your fingertips reach the floor. Spread out your toes and press down evenly through all four corners of your feet. Plant your fingertips in line with your toes and look forward.

• Straighten your legs and arms as you lift your chest up away from your legs. Broaden across the front of your chest, finding a slight backward bend in your upper back as you draw in your stomach.

• Press your heels into the floor as you lift your tailbone up toward the ceiling, keeping your hips in line with your heels. Gaze forward and hold this pose, Standing Half Forward Bend, for the recommended breaths.

• Next, inhale to lengthen your spine and transition to Standing Forward Bend. Exhale as you fold further from your hips and rest your palms on the floor.

• Lengthen your torso as you bring your belly closer to your thighs. Ground your heels into the floor, and lift your tailbone toward the ceiling.

• Hold for the recommended breaths, inhaling to lengthen your spine and exhaling to fold deeper.

DO IT RIGHT

• Keep a slight bend in your knees if your lower back or hamstrings are tight.
• If you cannot reach your fingertips to the floor during Standing Half Forward Bend, place your hands on your shins.
• If you cannot reach your palms to the floor during Standing Forward Bend, place your hands on blocks or cross your arms and hold your elbows.
• Avoid shifting your weight backward and positioning your hips behind your heels.
• Avoid compressing your neck as you look forward.
• Avoid rolling your spine into or out of the pose.

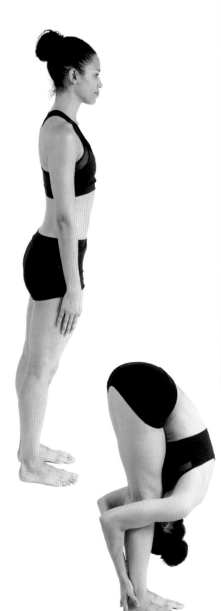

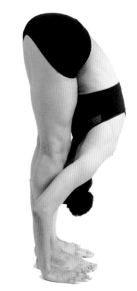

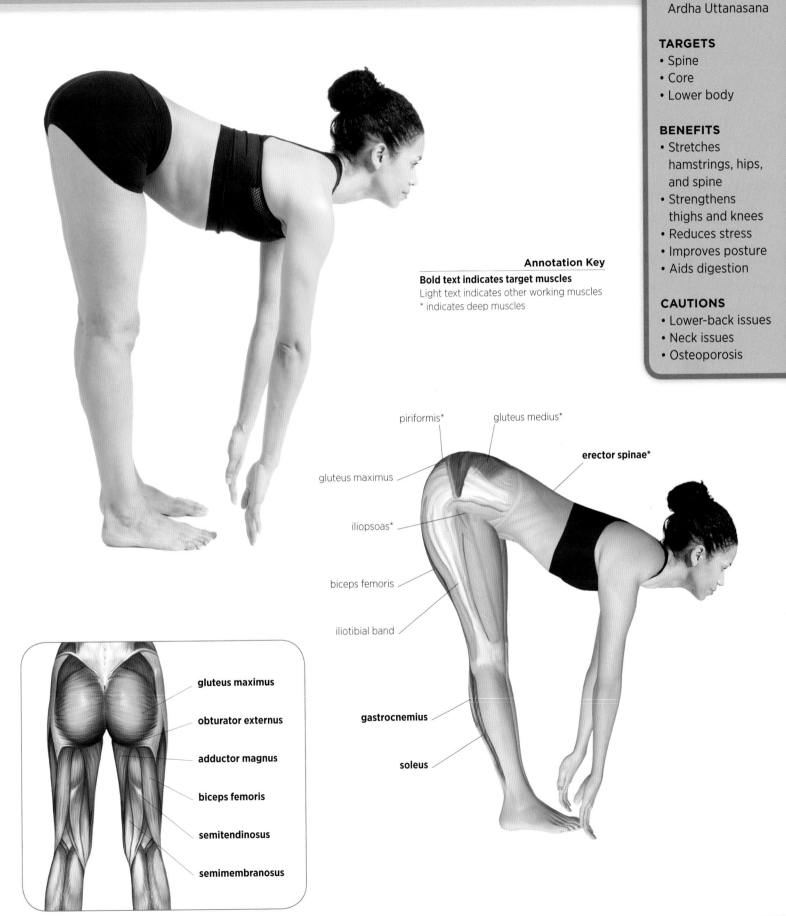

FACT FILE

SANSKRIT
- Uttanasana to Ardha Uttanasana

TARGETS
- Spine
- Core
- Lower body

BENEFITS
- Stretches hamstrings, hips, and spine
- Strengthens thighs and knees
- Reduces stress
- Improves posture
- Aids digestion

CAUTIONS
- Lower-back issues
- Neck issues
- Osteoporosis

Annotation Key

Bold text indicates target muscles
Light text indicates other working muscles
* indicates deep muscles

piriformis*

gluteus medius*

erector spinae*

gluteus maximus

iliopsoas*

biceps femoris

iliotibial band

gastrocnemius

soleus

gluteus maximus

obturator externus

adductor magnus

biceps femoris

semitendinosus

semimembranosus

Side Bend to Half Forward Bend Circle

This pose is great for toning your core muscles and those of your shoulders and upper body. It also increases overall flexibility.

HOW TO DO IT

• Stand in Mountain Pose (pages 32–33), with your arms relaxed at your sides, and feet together.

• Raise both arms above your head, and lace your fingers together, palms facing upward.

• Keep your elbows straight as you reach to the left side, and begin to trace a circle pattern with your torso.

• Lean forward and then to your right as you continue to trace a circle pattern.

• Repeat for the recommended repetitions. Return to Mountain Pose, and repeat on the other side.

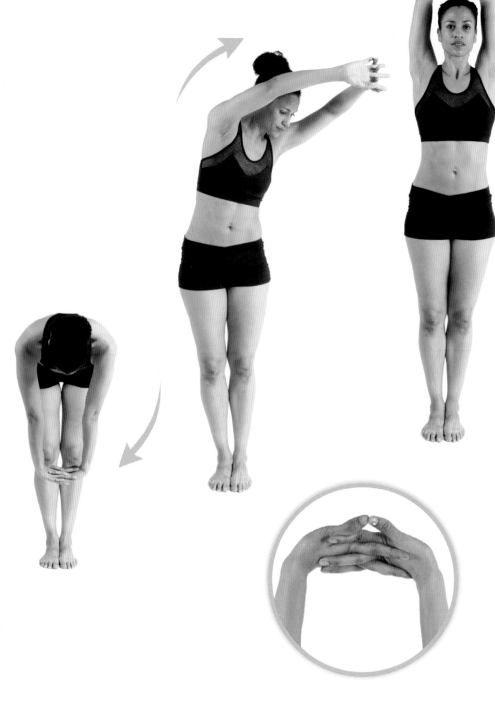

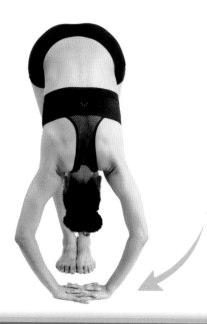

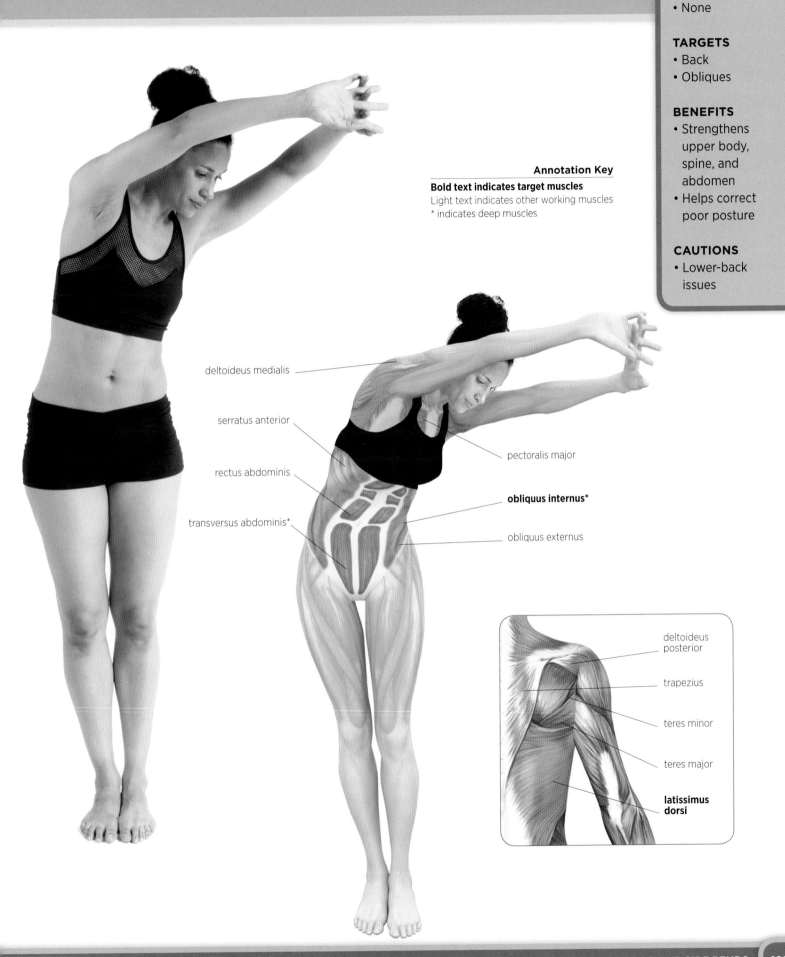

FACT FILE

SANSKRIT
• None

TARGETS
• Back
• Obliques

BENEFITS
• Strengthens upper body, spine, and abdomen
• Helps correct poor posture

CAUTIONS
• Lower-back issues

Annotation Key

Bold text indicates target muscles
Light text indicates other working muscles
* indicates deep muscles

deltoideus medialis

serratus anterior

rectus abdominis

transversus abdominis*

pectoralis major

obliquus internus*

obliquus externus

deltoideus posterior

trapezius

teres minor

teres major

latissimus dorsi

Standing Toe Touch

This forward-bending pose lengthens the entire back of your body, providing a deep stretch from the back of your neck and the top of your spine down to your toes.

HOW TO DO IT

- Stand with your legs and feet parallel and shoulder-width apart. Bend your knees slightly.

- Slowly round your spine downward, from your neck through your lower back, and lower your arms down along the sides of your legs as you reach for your toes.

- Continue to lower your torso downward as you bend at your waist, and let the weight of your body draw your head toward the floor as you stretch.

- Hold for the recommended breaths.

DO IT RIGHT

- Relax your neck and jaw.
- Breathe naturally and steadily throughout the stretch.
- Avoid letting your knees touch—keep your thighs slightly apart to help engage and stretch your gluteal muscles.

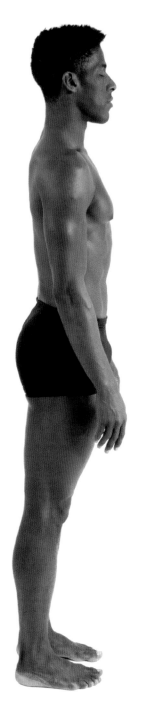

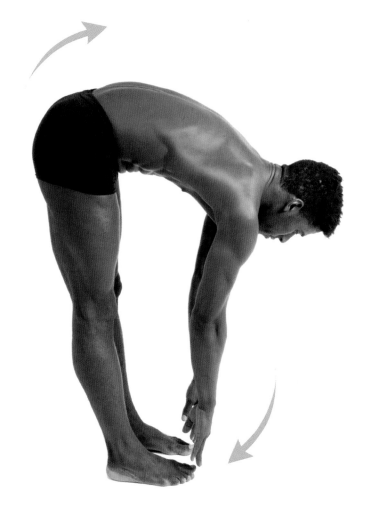

SANSKRIT
• None

TARGETS
• Hamstrings
• Upper back
• Lower back
• Calves

BENEFITS
• Stretches spine
• Eases tight leg muscles and glutes
• Aids in relaxation

CAUTIONS
• Back issues

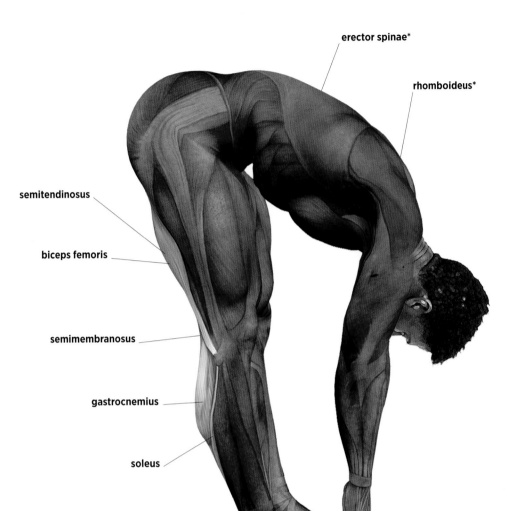

erector spinae*

rhomboideus*

semitendinosus

biceps femoris

semimembranosus

gastrocnemius

soleus

Annotation Key
Bold text indicates target muscles
Light text indicates other working muscles
* indicates deep muscles

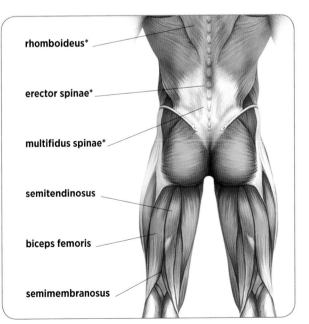

rhomboideus*

erector spinae*

multifidus spinae*

semitendinosus

biceps femoris

semimembranosus

MODIFICATION

HARDER: Place your palms on the floor and bring your face as close to your knees as possible to gain the ultimate benefits of this stretching pose.

Crossed-Foot Forward Bend

This Crossed-Foot Forward Bend improves flexibility and loosens tight leg muscles and glutes. The foot position also engages your iliotibial band, the fibrous tissue that runs along your outer thigh and stabilizes your hip and knee joints.

HOW TO DO IT

• Stand with your arms relaxed at your sides. Cross one foot over the other so that the outer edges of your soles are aligned.

• Bend at your waist, and gradually reach toward the floor with your hands.

• Press your palms to the floor, and hold for the recommended breaths. Release, slowly roll up, and repeat on the other side.

DO IT RIGHT

• Keep your knees straight, yet soft, throughout the exercise.
• Let your head drop.
• Avoid bending or locking your knees.
• Avoid twisting your neck, shoulders, or torso to either side.

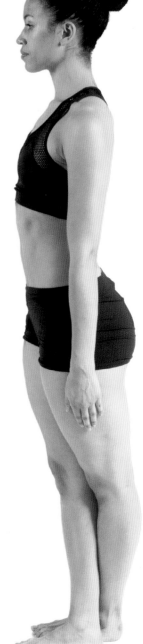

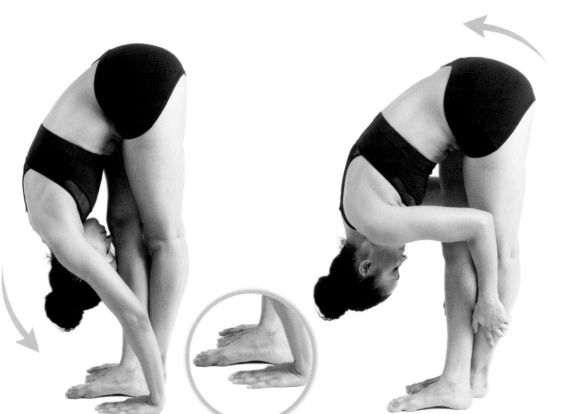

MODIFICATION

EASIER: If you find it difficult to reach your hands to the floor while maintaining your form, reach only to the point where you are comfortable. Try to extend your hands slightly lower each time you stretch.

FACT FILE

SANSKRIT
• None

TARGETS
• Hamstrings
• Upper back
• Lower back
• Calves
• Iliotibial band

BENEFITS
• Stretches iliotibial band
• Counteracts effects of wearing high heels

CAUTIONS
• Hip injury

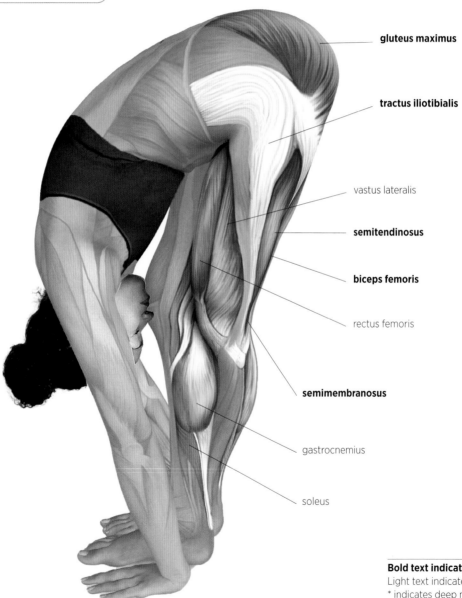

gluteus maximus

tractus iliotibialis

vastus lateralis

semitendinosus

biceps femoris

rectus femoris

semimembranosus

gastrocnemius

soleus

Annotation Key

Bold text indicates target muscles
Light text indicates other working muscles
* indicates deep muscles

Wide-Legged Forward Bend

Wide-Legged Forward Bend is one of the most effective ways to stretch your hamstrings and spine. Dancers frequently use it to relieve stress before a performance. This forward bend is also technically an inversion pose because your head is positioned below your heart.

HOW TO DO IT

- Stand with your legs and feet parallel and generously more than shoulder-width apart. Bend your knees slightly, and tuck your pelvis forward. Press your shoulder blades together and downward.

- Inhale and lengthen your spine. Lift your chest, and find a slight bend in your upper back, bringing your gaze up to the ceiling.

- Exhale and hinge forward from your hips with your back flat. Reach your palms to the floor, with your fingers facing forward. Bring the crown of your head toward the floor, lifting your shoulders toward your ears to make space for your neck.

- Firm your thighs, and lift your kneecaps. Let your sit bones move toward the ceiling as your tailbone draws down toward the floor.

- Hold for the recommended breaths.

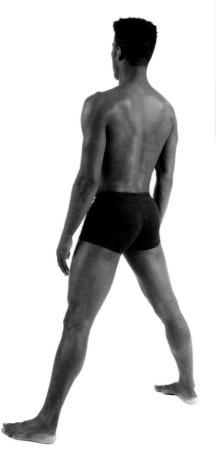

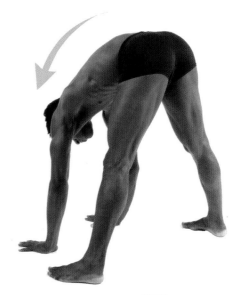

DO IT RIGHT

- Keep your knees soft.
- Hinge forward with your chest open and your back flat.
- Bend only as far forward as you can go while keeping your back flat.
- Keep your hips lined up above your heels.
- Avoid rounding your back to cheat your hands to the floor.
- Avoid locking your knees.

MODIFICATION

EASIER: If you find it difficult to reach the floor with your hands, place some blocks on the floor and reach for them instead.

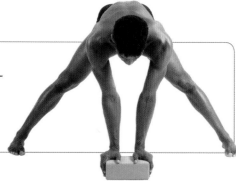

SANSKRIT
• Prasarita
  Padottanasana

TARGETS
• Hamstrings
• Lower back
• Glutes
• Calves

BENEFITS
• Strengthens
  spine
• Stretches inner
  and outer hips
• Releases groin
• Calms mind and
  body

CAUTIONS
• Back issues
• Hamstring issues

MODIFICATION

ADVANCED: Walk your hands in between your legs, bend your elbows, and gently rest your forehead on the floor. Your hands should be available, if necessary, to keep your balance.

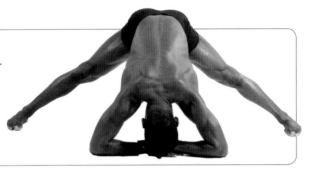

erector spinae*

gluteus medius*

gluteus minimus*

transversus abdominis*

gluteus maximus

obliquus externus

obliquus internus*

biceps femoris

rectus abdominis

semitendinosus

semimembranosus

gastrocnemius

soleus

Annotation Key

Bold text indicates target muscles
Light text indicates other working muscles
* indicates deep muscles

Intense Side Stretch Pose I

This forward bend is known for its calming properties. It also provides a very effective stretch for your hamstrings.

HOW TO DO IT

- Begin in Mountain Pose (pages 32–33), and step your left foot back about 3 feet. Turn your toes in about 45 degrees so that they face the upper-left corner of your mat. Come into heel-to-heel alignment, squaring your hips to the front of your mat.

- Bring your arms into reverse prayer position by reaching your arms behind you, with your fingers pointing downward and your palms together. Rotate your hands so that your fingers point up to the sky.

- Inhale, broadening the space across your collarbones, drawing your shoulder blades together and lifting your chest while keeping your hips squared.

- Ground through the pinkie toe of your left foot. Press your left thigh back as you exhale and fold forward over your right leg. Lead with your heart, and keep your spine elongated.

- Hold the pose for the recommended breaths. Inhale, draw your shoulders back, and lift your sternum, leading with your heart to come up to standing position. Step your left foot forward to meet your right foot in Mountain Pose, and repeat on the other side.

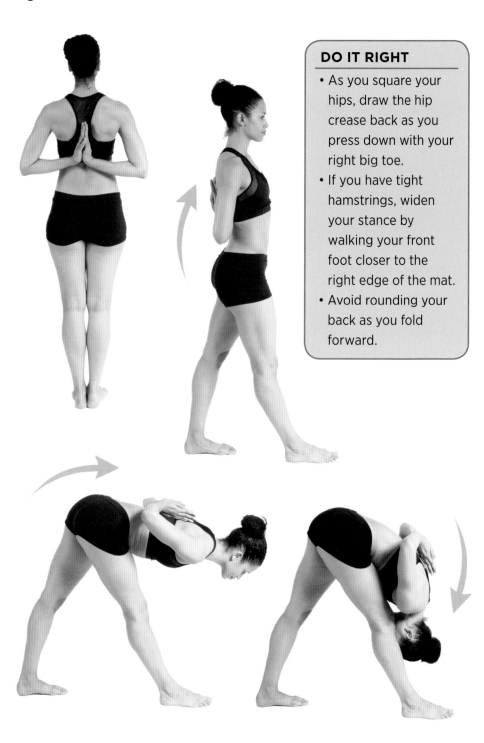

DO IT RIGHT

- As you square your hips, draw the hip crease back as you press down with your right big toe.
- If you have tight hamstrings, widen your stance by walking your front foot closer to the right edge of the mat.
- Avoid rounding your back as you fold forward.

FACT FILE

SANSKRIT
• Parsvottanasana

TARGETS
• Back
• Shoulders
• Arms
• Lower body

BENEFITS
• Strengthens legs and spine
• Stretches legs, spine, shoulders, and wrists
• Improves posture
• Calms mind and body

CAUTIONS
• Hamstring issues
• Spine issues

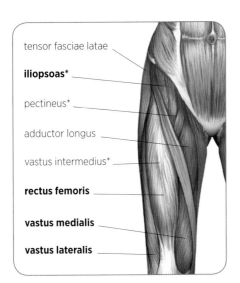

tensor fasciae latae

iliopsoas*

pectineus*

adductor longus

vastus intermedius*

rectus femoris

vastus medialis

vastus lateralis

Annotation Key

Bold text indicates target muscles
Light text indicates other working muscles
* indicates deep muscles

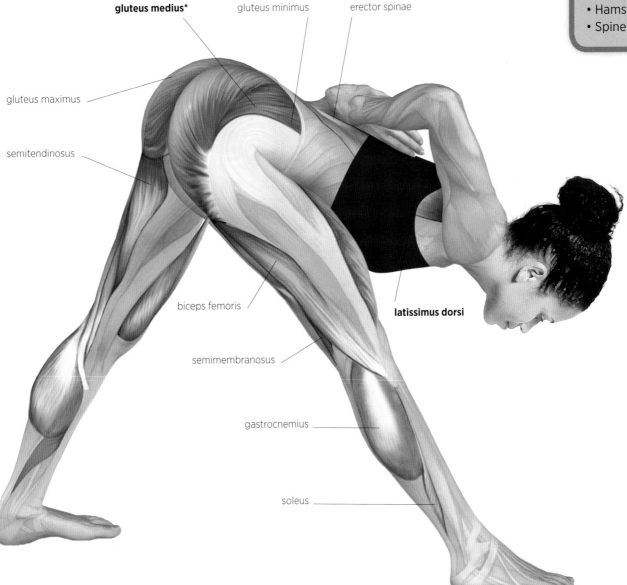

gluteus medius*

gluteus minimus

erector spinae

gluteus maximus

semitendinosus

biceps femoris

latissimus dorsi

semimembranosus

gastrocnemius

soleus

Tiptoe Intense Pose I

This advanced stretching pose is a forward bend that qualifies as an inversion because your heart is positioned above your head.

HOW TO DO IT

- Begin in Standing Half Forward Bend (pages 106–07), and then position your feet shoulder-width apart.

- As you rise onto your tiptoes, reach your hands back between your legs. Keeping your arms straight, touch the floor with your fingertips, with your palms apart and facing forward. Gaze down at the floor.

- Lower your head so that you are now looking back between your lowered arms. Hold for the recommended breaths, and ease yourself upright.

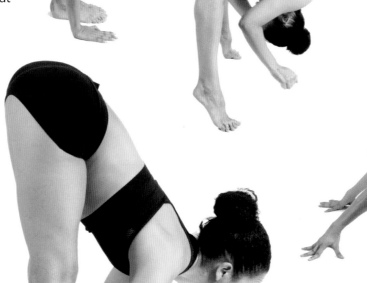

FACT FILE

SANSKRIT
- Prapada Uttanasana

TARGETS
- Spine
- Glutes
- Legs
- Abdominals

BENEFITS
- Stretches spine and glutes
- Loosens tight hamstrings
- Improves balance

CAUTION
- Balance issues

DO IT RIGHT

- Keep your legs straight and your fingers outspread on the mat to create a balancing platform.
- Bring your torso as close to your thighs as possible.
- Avoid tension in your neck.

Tiptoe Intense Pose II

This advanced forward bend—an inversion because your head is below your heart—is an excellent pose for improving balance. It also stretches your spine and strengthens your core and shoulders.

HOW TO DO IT

• Begin in Standing Half Forward Bend (pages 106–07). Reach your hands out in front of you, and place them flat on the floor, palms down and shoulder-width apart.

• At the same time, raise your torso by standing on tiptoe, with your knees straight and your toes curled away from you. Your head should be facing your legs.

• Hold for the recommended breaths.

DO IT RIGHT
• Keep your elbows soft.
• Keep your neck in a neutral position.
• Avoid rounding your back excessively.

FACT FILE

SANSKRIT
• Uttana Kulpa
  Uttanasana I

TARGETS
• Spine
• Abdominals
• Wrists
• Ankles

BENEFITS
• Stretches
  lower back and
  hamstrings
• Strengthens
  shoulders and
  abdomen
• Improves balance
  and stability

CAUTIONS
• Balance issues
• Wrist or ankle
  pain

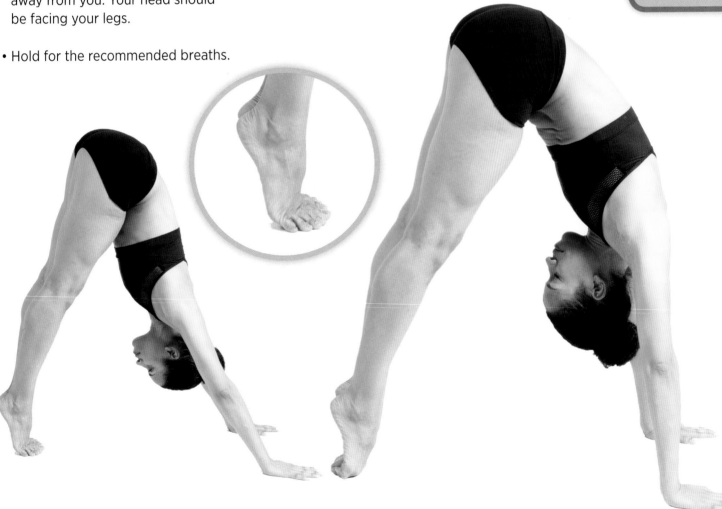

Intense Side Stretch Pose II

This pose improves your flexibility and balance while stretching and strengthening the muscles of your shoulders, sides, abdomen, and lower back. It can also stimulate your abdominal organs and aid in digestion.

HOW TO DO IT

• Begin in Standing Half Forward Bend (pages 106–07), with your palms on the floor.

• With your left hand, grasp the outer edge of your right foot.

• Draw your right foot off the floor while keeping your knee straight.

• Hold the pose for the recommended breaths, and repeat on the other side.

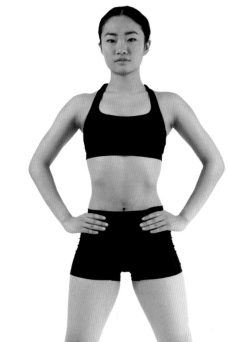

FACT FILE

SANSKRIT
• Parsvottanasana

TARGETS
• Hamstrings
• Shoulders
• Lower back

BENEFITS
• Opens hips and spine
• Stretches hamstrings
• Improves balance
• Stimulates digestion

CAUTION
• Wrist issues
• Ankle pain
• Elbow pain
• Balance issues

DO IT RIGHT

• Relax your head and neck.
• Keep your torso elongated and your back slightly rounded.
• Avoid bending your raised leg.

Sideways Intense Stretch Pose

This twisting pose works well for stretching and strengthening the muscles of your shoulders, sides, abdomen, and lower back.

HOW TO DO IT

- From Standing Half Forward Bend (pages 106–07), position your feet more than shoulder-width apart.

- Bend your torso down to the left with your right side facing up toward the ceiling.

- Reach down with your left hand and clasp the front of your right ankle.

- Drape your right arm over your head and reach with your right hand to grasp the side of your left ankle.

- Hold the pose for the recommended breaths, and repeat on the other side.

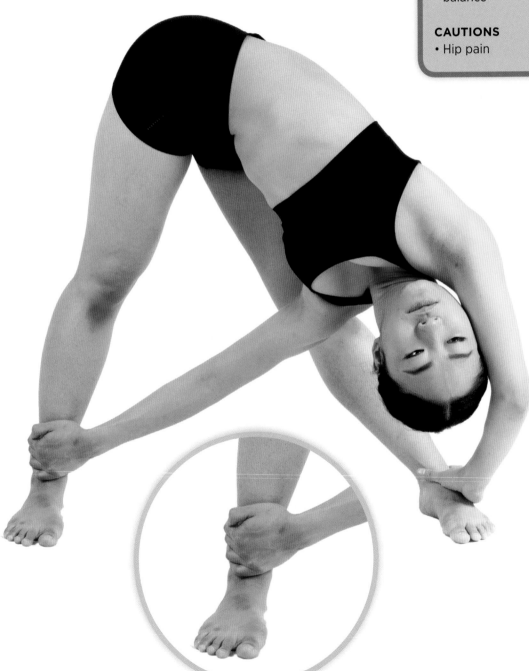

Standing Split Pose Prep

If you haven't had any dance training, you've probably never performed a standing split. Do not be intimidated if you start out less than perfect—the purpose of this pose is simply to stretch the legs.

HOW TO DO IT

- Begin in Mountain Pose (pages 32–33).

- Lift your arms above your head, and hinge from your hips to bend forward, bringing your hands to the floor.

- Walk your hands about 12 inches forward and shift your weight onto your right leg.

- Lift your left leg, keeping your hips square with the front of your mat.

- Hold for the recommended breaths, and repeat on the other side.

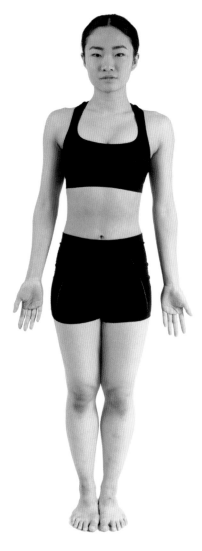

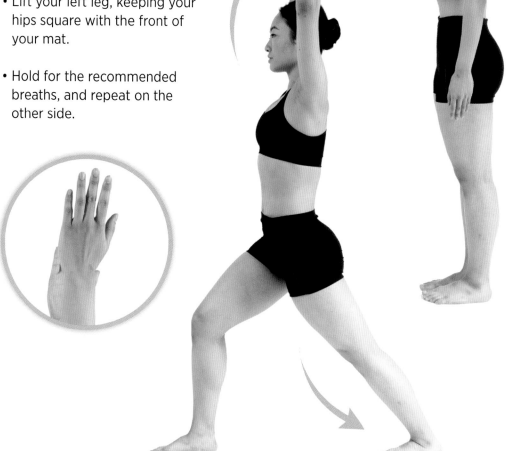

DO IT RIGHT

- Contract your leg muscles, and ground your standing foot throughout the pose.
- If you have trouble reaching the floor with your hands, place blocks on the floor for support.
- Avoid compressing the back of your neck while holding the pose.

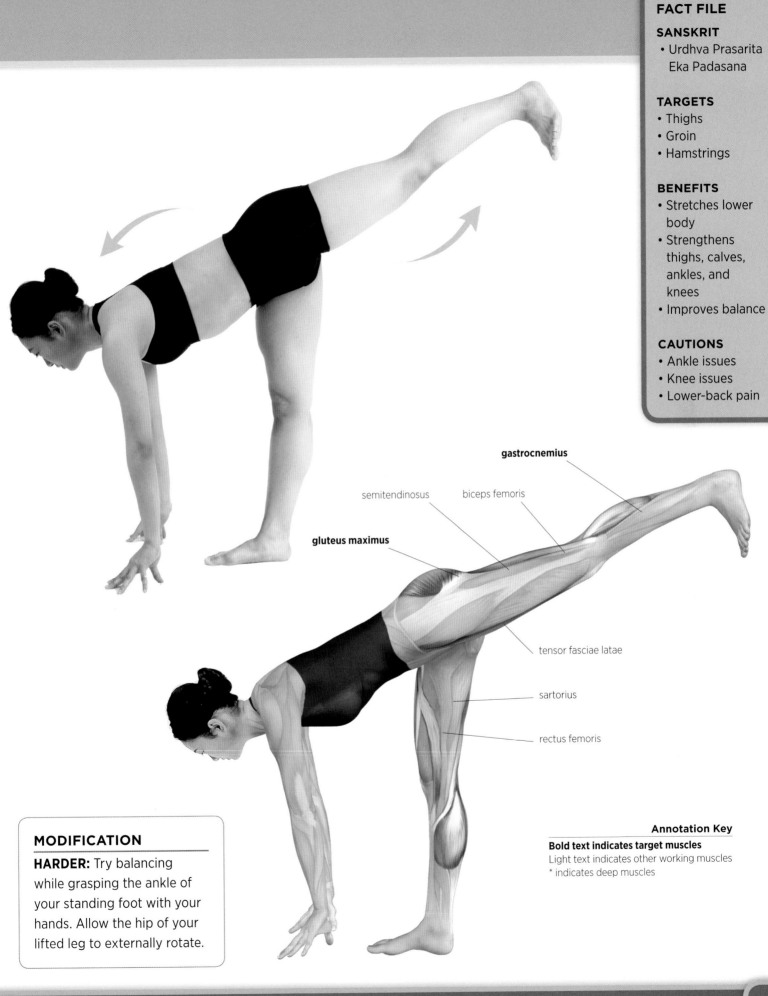

SANSKRIT
• Urdhva Prasarita Eka Padasana

TARGETS
• Thighs
• Groin
• Hamstrings

BENEFITS
• Stretches lower body
• Strengthens thighs, calves, ankles, and knees
• Improves balance

CAUTIONS
• Ankle issues
• Knee issues
• Lower-back pain

gastrocnemius

semitendinosus

biceps femoris

gluteus maximus

tensor fasciae latae

sartorius

rectus femoris

MODIFICATION

HARDER: Try balancing while grasping the ankle of your standing foot with your hands. Allow the hip of your lifted leg to externally rotate.

Annotation Key
Bold text indicates target muscles
Light text indicates other working muscles
* indicates deep muscles

Standing Split Pose

This inversion pose is an excellent way to stretch the muscles of your lower body while improving your balance and stability.

HOW TO DO IT

- Begin in Mountain Pose (pages 32–33), and then shift your weight onto your left foot.

- Bend forward with your back flat, simultaneously raising your right leg behind you. Square your shoulders and your hips. Reach your fingertips toward the floor.

- Exhale and contract your leg muscles as you fold your torso onto your left thigh. Lift your right heel toward the ceiling, extending your legs in opposite directions.

- Relax your shoulders down toward the floor. In this position, your left knee is pointed forward and your right knee is pointed straight behind you with your leg straight. If possible, grasp the back of your left ankle with both hands. Maintain balance with your left palm on the floor.

- Hold the pose for the recommended breaths, and repeat on the other side.

DO IT RIGHT

- Lower your torso and lift your back leg simultaneously.
- Tuck in your chin and elongate the back of your neck.
- Avoid rotating your standing knee inward, rounding your spine, or bending forward from your waist.

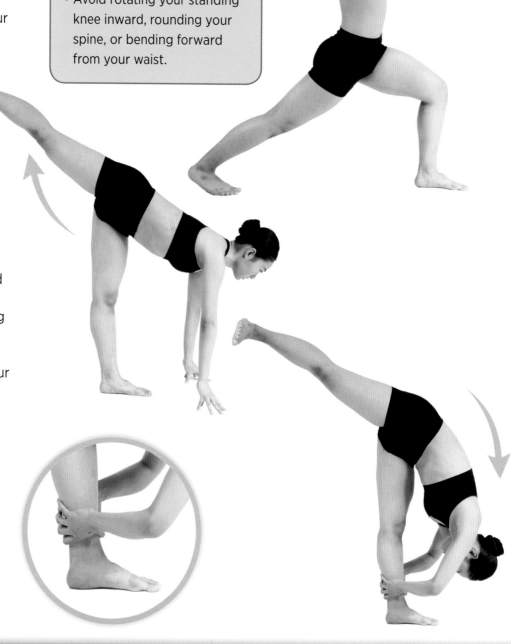

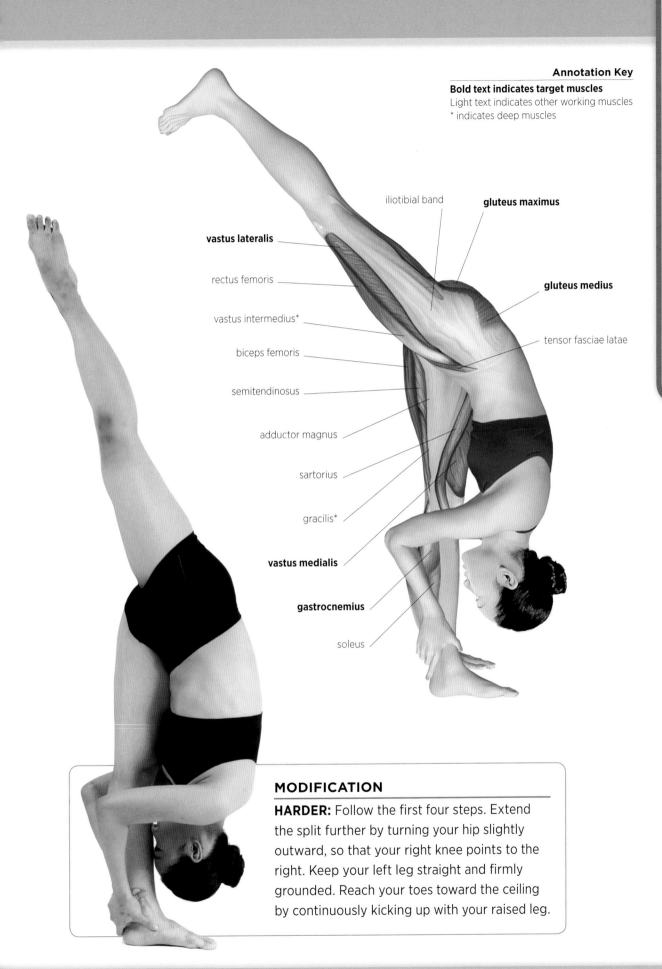

SANSKRIT
- Urdhva Prasarita Eka Padasana

TARGETS
- Thighs
- Calves
- Glutes

BENEFITS
- Stretches groin, thighs, and calves
- Strengthens thighs, knees, and ankles
- Improves balance

CAUTIONS
- Lower-back pain
- Ankle issues
- Knee pain

Annotation Key

Bold text indicates target muscles
Light text indicates other working muscles
* indicates deep muscles

iliotibial band

gluteus maximus

vastus lateralis

rectus femoris

gluteus medius

vastus intermedius*

tensor fasciae latae

biceps femoris

semitendinosus

adductor magnus

sartorius

gracilis*

vastus medialis

gastrocnemius

soleus

MODIFICATION

HARDER: Follow the first four steps. Extend the split further by turning your hip slightly outward, so that your right knee points to the right. Keep your left leg straight and firmly grounded. Reach your toes toward the ceiling by continuously kicking up with your raised leg.

CHAPTER THREE

SEATED
FORWARD BENDS

Seated forward bends provide a healthy stretch for the back of your body, from your neck to your heels, especially your hamstrings. Forward folds calm the nervous system and reduce fatigue, as well as allow the student to refocus a distracted mind and gain serenity. These poses should be avoided, however, in cases of recent or chronic injury to your arms, hips, ankles, or shoulders.

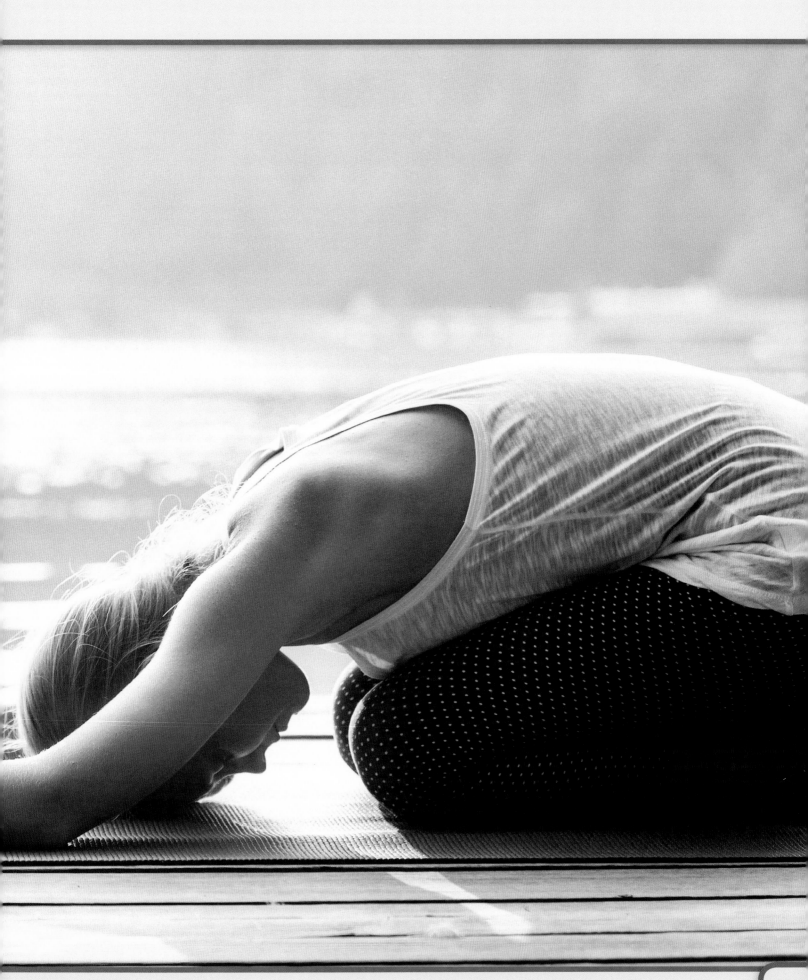

Seated Forward Bend Prep

This pose prepares you for the Seated Forward Bend. It loosens your lower back, hamstrings, and calves. It also improves digestion and calms the mind.

HOW TO DO IT

- Sit on the floor, sitting up as straight as possible with your legs extended in front of you in a parallel position. Your feet should be relaxed and flexed slightly.

- Lean forward, lowering your abdominals over your thighs, with your forearms resting above your kneecaps as you stretch.

- Hold for the recommended breaths, then slowly roll up to sitting position, and repeat as recommended.

DO IT RIGHT

- Be sure to bend at your hips and keep your spine fairly straight as you stretch.
- Extend your torso as far forward over your legs as possible.
- Avoid holding your breath during the stretch.

MODIFICATION

ADVANCED: To achieve a deeper stretch in your hamstrings, place an elastic exercise band around the balls of your feet, and use both hands to draw the band upward.

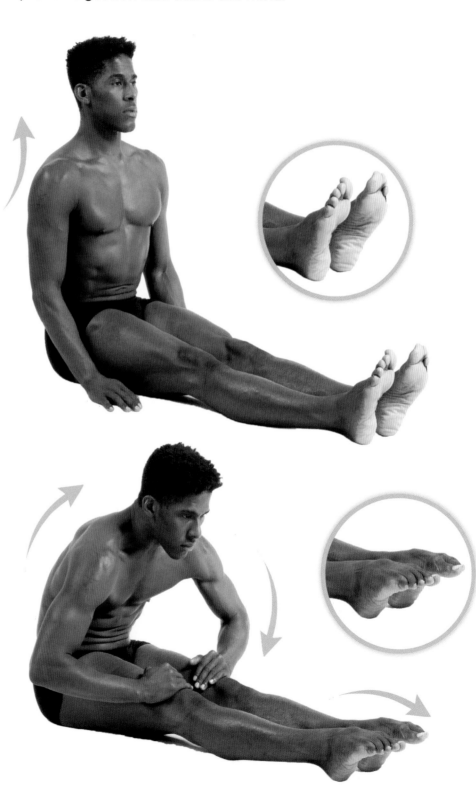

SANSKRIT
• Paschimottanasana

TARGETS
• Hamstrings
• Calves

BENEFITS
• Stretches spine
  and hamstrings
• Improves
  digestion

CAUTIONS
• Lower-back
  issues

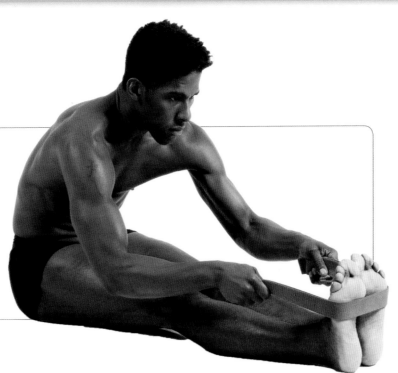

MODIFICATION

EASIER: If your hamstrings or lower back feel tight, place a yoga strap around the balls of your feet and pull the ends toward your hips to help you reach forward.

Annotation Key

Bold text indicates target muscles
Light text indicates other working muscles
* indicates deep muscles

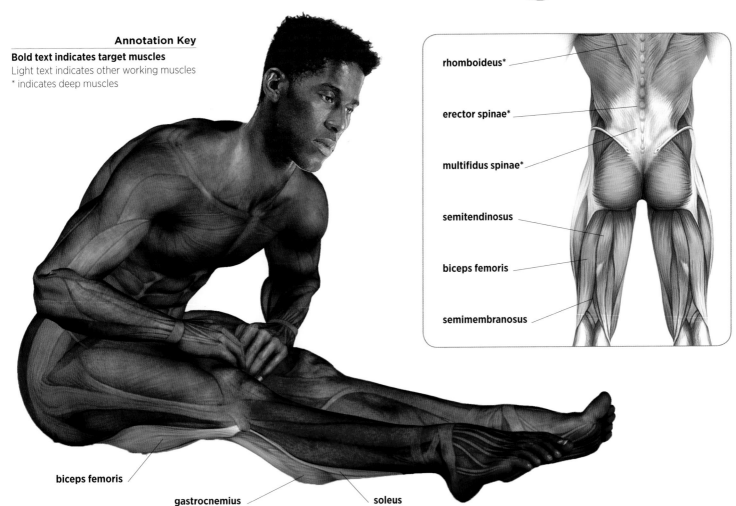

rhomboideus*

erector spinae*

multifidus spinae*

semitendinosus

biceps femoris

semimembranosus

biceps femoris

gastrocnemius   **soleus**

Head-to-Knee Forward Bend Prep

This pose helps prepare you for the intermediate Head-to-Knee Forward Bend. It can help loosen tight hamstrings and calf muscles as well as aid in digestion.

HOW TO DO IT

- Sit on the floor, as straight as possible, with your legs extended in front of you in a parallel position.

- Bend your left leg. Lower your knee out to the side, resting the bottom of your left foot against your right inner thigh, just above your kneecap. Rest your clasped hands on your right knee.

- Bend from your waist, and lean forward over your right leg. Place your forearms above your right kneecap.

- Hold for the recommended breaths, then switch legs, and repeat on the opposite side.

DO IT RIGHT

- For a more intense overall stretch, drop your head to benefit your rhomboids.
- Avoid straining your back if it feels tight. Try performing this stretch with a sofa behind you. Be sure to position your lower back as close to the sofa as possible.

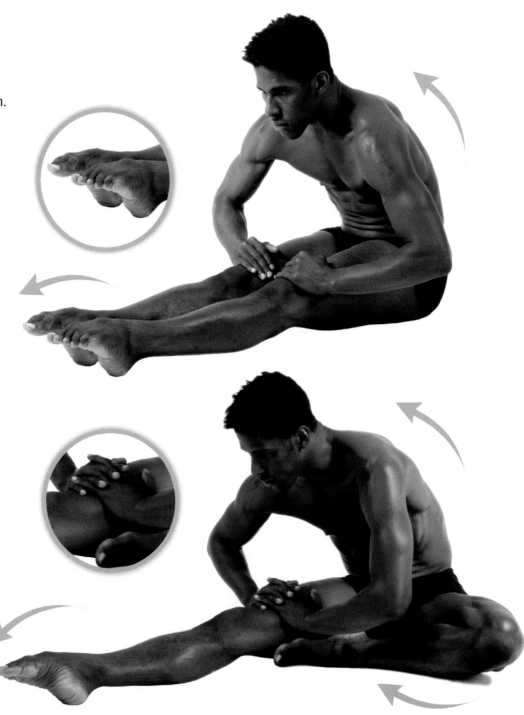

SANSKRIT
- Janu Sirsasana

TARGETS
- Upper hamstrings
- Calves

BENEFITS
- Stretches spine and legs
- Eases digestion

CAUTIONS
- Lower-back issues

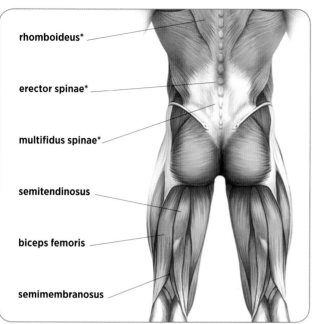

rhomboideus*

erector spinae*

multifidus spinae*

semitendinosus

biceps femoris

semimembranosus

Annotation Key
Bold text indicates target muscles
Light text indicates other working muscles
* indicates deep muscles

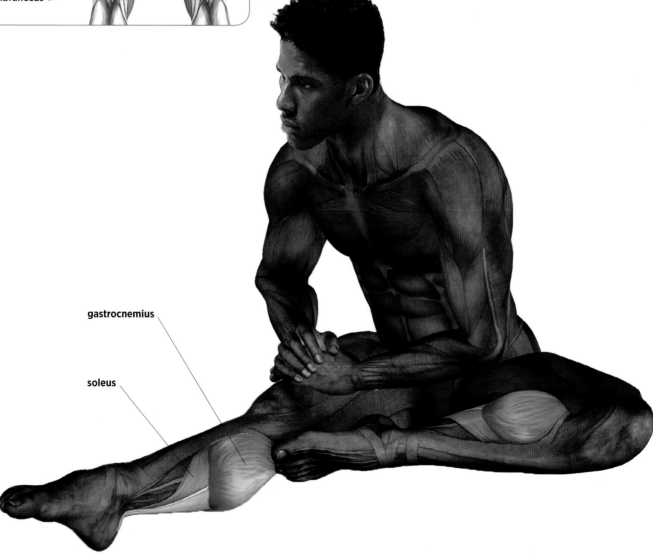

gastrocnemius

soleus

Child's Pose

Child's Pose not only gently stretches the back and hips, it is also relaxing and restorative. You will find it makes a perfect resting position, one that you can assume at any point during your session.

HOW TO DO IT

- Kneel on your hands and knees, hands planted shoulder-width apart.

- Bring your big toes together, and place your knees about hip-width apart.

- Shift your hips back toward your heels as you extend your torso forward, lowering your stomach onto your thighs. Let your shoulders round forward, allowing your forehead to rest gently on the floor.

- Slide your arms back along your thighs, with the palms of your hands facing upward. Breathe into the back of your body. Hold for the recommended breaths.

DO IT RIGHT

- Relax any tension you may be retaining in your jaw and face muscles.
- Place your forehead on a folded towel or low cushion if desired.
- Expand the space between your shoulder blades as you breathe.
- Avoid bringing your knees too far apart.

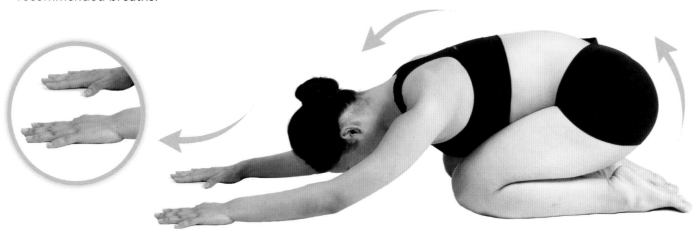

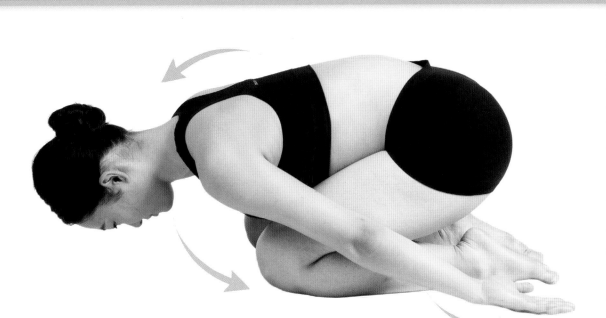

FACT FILE

SANSKRIT
• Balasana

TARGETS
• Back
• Hips
• Ankles

BENEFITS
• Relaxes anterior muscles
• Passively stretches posterior muscles
• Reduces stress and anxiety
• Relieves back pain

CAUTIONS
• Knee issues

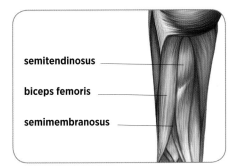

semitendinosus

biceps femoris

semimembranosus

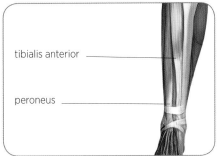

tibialis anterior

peroneus

Annotation Key

Bold text indicates target muscles
Light text indicates other working muscles
* indicates deep muscles

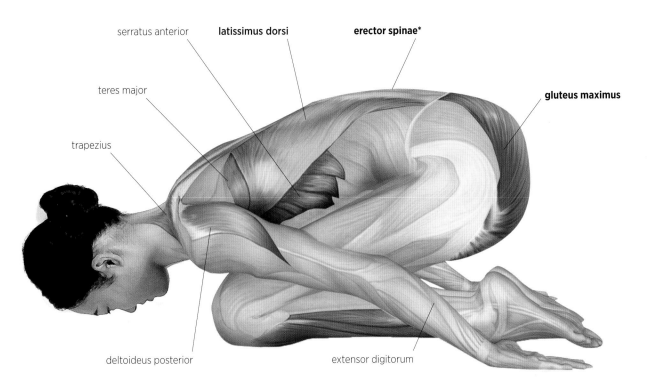

serratus anterior

latissimus dorsi

erector spinae*

teres major

gluteus maximus

trapezius

deltoideus posterior

extensor digitorum

Child's Pose with Arms Extended

This pose offers the same benefits as Child's Pose—gently stretching the back of your torso while relaxing the abdominal muscles—with an additional extension of your arms.

HOW TO DO IT

- Kneel on your hands and knees, hands planted shoulder-width apart.

- Bring your big toes together and place your knees about hip-width apart.

- Drop your torso down onto your thighs, and extend your arms on the floor above your head so that your forehead comes to rest on the floor. Hold for the recommended breaths.

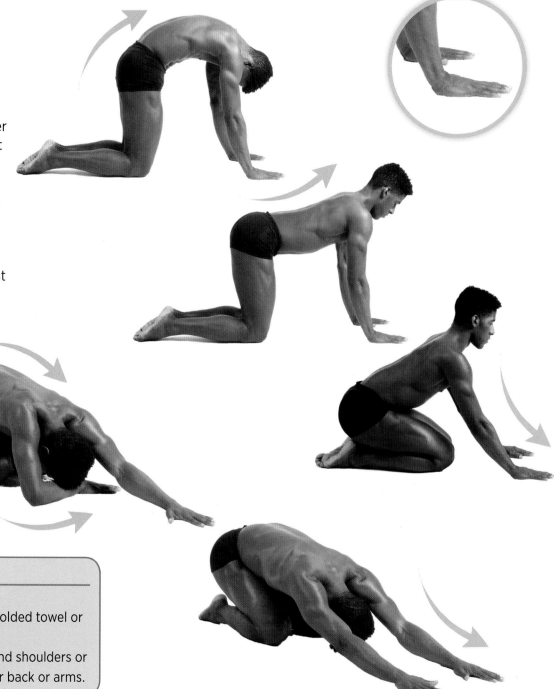

DO IT RIGHT

- Don't forget to breathe.
- Place your forehead on a folded towel or low cushion if desired.
- Avoid tensing your neck and shoulders or hyperextending your lower back or arms.

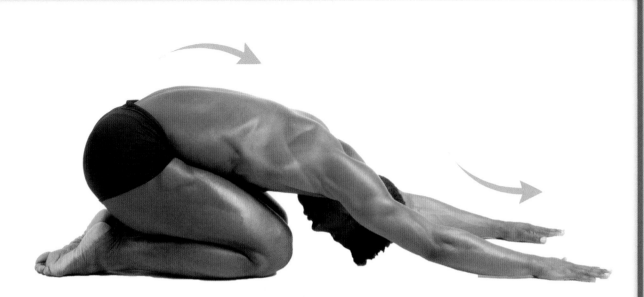

FACT FILE

SANSKRIT
• Utthita Balasana

TARGETS
• Back
• Quadriceps
• Ankles

BENEFITS
• Stretches posterior muscles
• Relaxes anterior muscles
• Eases stress and improves digestion
• Relieves lower-back pain

CAUTIONS
• Knee issues

Annotation Key

Bold text indicates target muscles
Light text indicates other working muscles
* indicates deep muscles

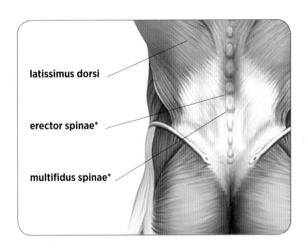

latissimus dorsi

erector spinae*

multifidus spinae*

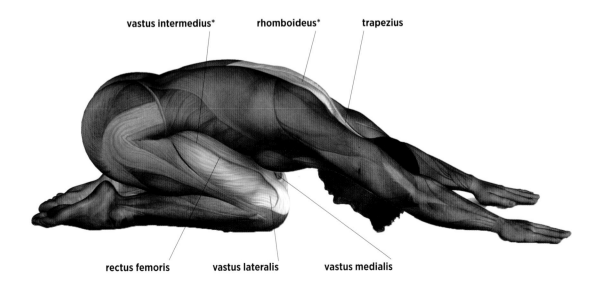

vastus intermedius*

rhomboideus*

trapezius

rectus femoris

vastus lateralis

vastus medialis

Extended Puppy Pose

This versatile resting pose offers the shoulder- and arm-stretching benefits of Downward-Facing Dog along with the restorative qualities of Child's Pose.

HOW TO DO IT

• Begin on all fours with your hands beneath your shoulders and your knees directly below your hips.

• Keep your knees in place as you walk your hands forward and stretch your arms straight out. Externally rotate your outer upper arms toward your ears. Keep your arms active.

• Adopt a Downward-Facing Dog (pages 268–69) position with your upper body. Place your hands shoulder-width apart, fingers widely spread, and hands pressed down to lengthen your spine. Keep your forearms off the floor and your elbows lifted.

• Bring your abdominal muscles into play to support your lower back as you stretch.

• Let your forehead rest on the floor, and allow your neck to soften. Close your eyes, and hold for the recommended breaths.

DO IT RIGHT

• Be sure to keep your neck and shoulders soft.
• Avoid sinking into your lower back or letting your ribcage jut forward.

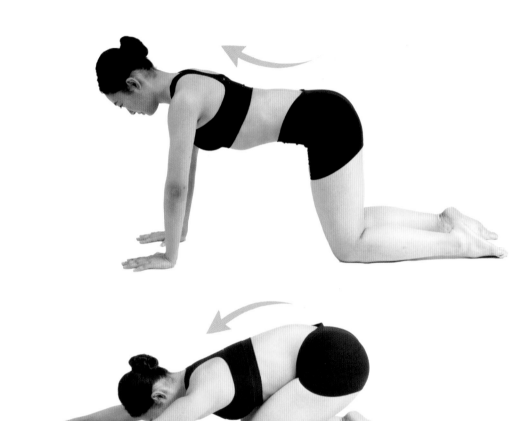

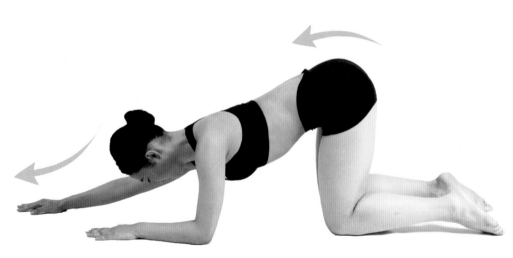

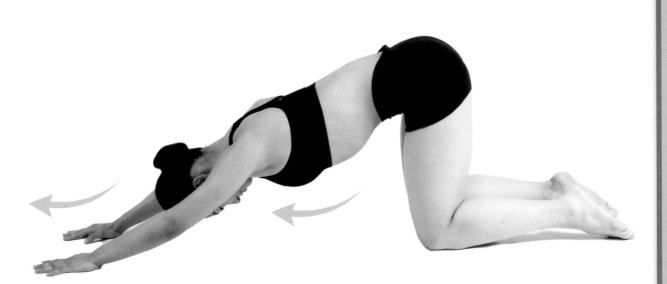

FACT FILE

SANSKRIT
- Uttana Shishosana

TARGETS
- Upper back
- Glutes
- Hamstrings

BENEFITS
- Lengthens spine
- Stretches shoulders and lower torso
- Relaxes mind and body

CAUTIONS
- Knee issues
- Lower-back issues

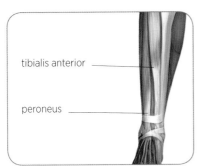

tibialis anterior

peroneus

Annotation Key

Bold text indicates target muscles
Light text indicates other working muscles
* indicates deep muscles

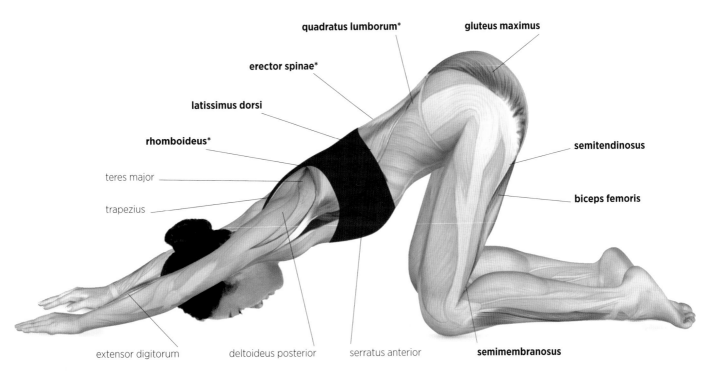

quadratus lumborum*

gluteus maximus

erector spinae*

latissimus dorsi

rhomboideus*

teres major

trapezius

semitendinosus

biceps femoris

extensor digitorum

deltoideus posterior

serratus anterior

semimembranosus

Bound Angle Pose with Forward Bend

Bound Angle poses are excellent hip openers that also improve overall flexibility. They stimulate many internal organs and can relieve mild depression. The forward bend deepens the benefits of this pose.

HOW TO DO IT

- Sit up tall on your mat, with the soles of your feet pressed together.

- Place your forearms or elbows on your inner thighs, and grab your feet and toes with your hands.

- Draw your heels closer, keeping your heels a comfortable distance from your core.

- Fold your upper body forward until you feel a stretch in your groin.

- Hold for the recommended breaths, and then slowly roll up.

DO IT RIGHT

- Make sure you exhale as you drop your chest toward the floor.
- Avoid slouching or rocking backward off your hip bones; instead, you should feel them anchored on the floor.
- Avoid holding your breath.

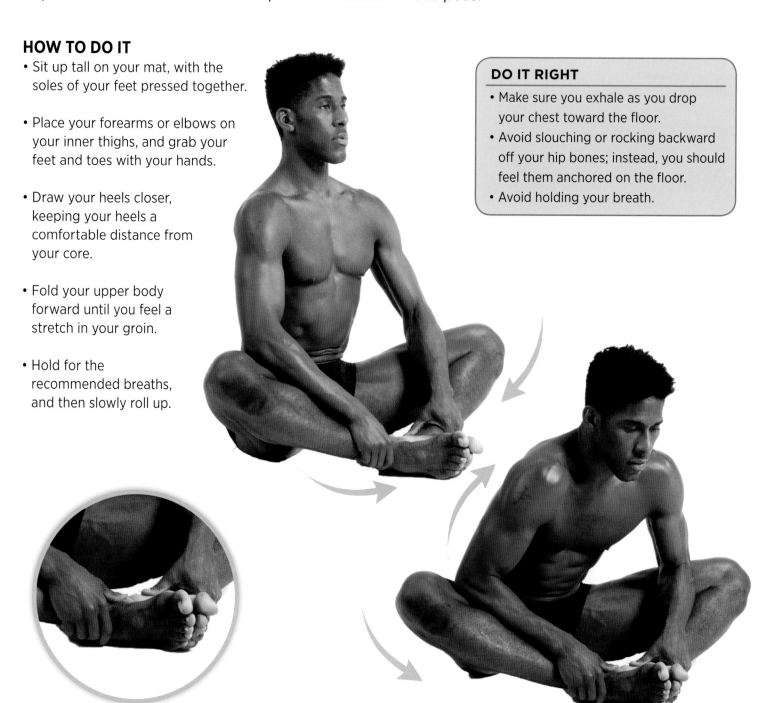

SANSKRIT
- Baddha
  Konasana
  Uttanasana

TARGETS
- Lower torso
- Spine
- Thighs

BENEFITS
- Opens hips
- Stretches glutes
  and thighs

CAUTIONS
- Lower-back
  issues
- Hip injuries

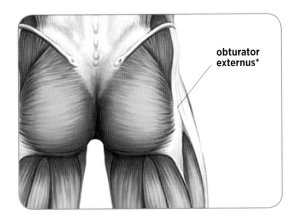

obturator externus*

Annotation Key

Bold text indicates target muscles
Light text indicates other working muscles
* indicates deep muscles

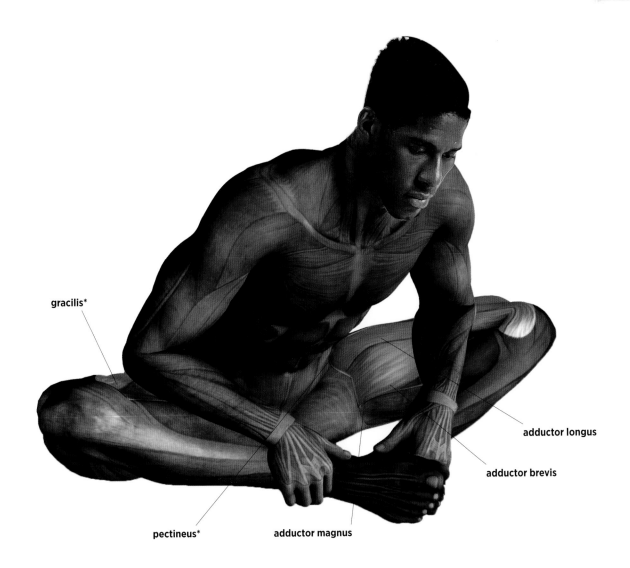

gracilis*

pectineus*

adductor magnus

adductor longus

adductor brevis

Seated Forward Bend

This pose stretches your spine, shoulders, and hamstrings. It also improves digestion and stimulates internal organs such as the liver, kidneys, ovaries, and uterus. Seated Forward Bend can also ease headaches. An introspective posture, its gesture of surrender helps to reduce stress and calm your mind.

HOW TO DO IT

- Sit in Staff Pose (pages 218–19), with your legs extended in front of you and your feet flexed.

- Inhale and lift your arms above your head, parallel to each other. Sit up tall to lengthen your spine.

- Exhale and fold forward. Grasp the outside of your right foot with your right hand, and the outside of your left foot with your left hand.

- Hinge at your hips, easing your abdomen down toward your thighs. Allow your head to release downward, and hold for the recommended breaths.

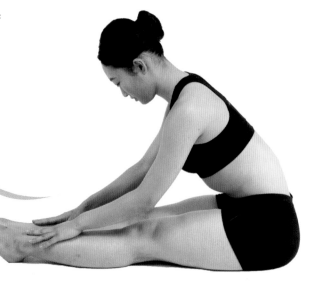

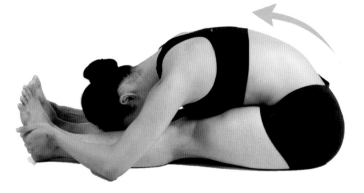

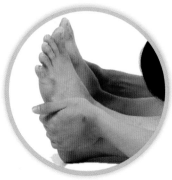

DO IT RIGHT
- Keep your feet flexed.
- Try sitting on a folded blanket if desired.
- To help you fold deeper onto your thighs, think of having a slight arch in your lower back as you root your thighs into the floor.
- Close your eyes if you feel comfortable doing so.
- Try to lengthen your exhalations so that they are longer than your inhalations.
- Avoid letting your big toes move closer to you than the other toes; as you flex, your feet should be straight, as if you were standing on the floor.

SANSKRIT
- Paschimottanasana

TARGETS
- Shoulders
- Hamstrings
- Back

BENEFITS
- Stretches spine, shoulders, and hamstrings
- Calms mind
- Relieves headaches and depression

CAUTIONS
- Hamstring issues
- Lower-back issues

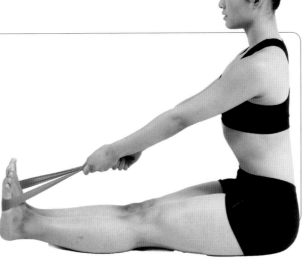

MODIFICATION

EASIER: If your hamstrings and/or lower back feel tight, try placing a yoga strap around the balls of your feet instead of reaching all the way to your feet.

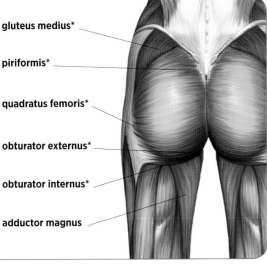

gluteus medius*

piriformis*

quadratus femoris*

obturator externus*

obturator internus*

adductor magnus

Annotation Key
Bold text indicates target muscles
Light text indicates other working muscles
* indicates deep muscles

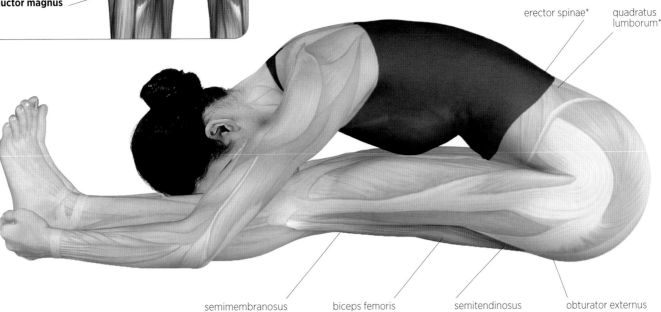

erector spinae*

quadratus lumborum*

semimembranosus

biceps femoris

semitendinosus

obturator externus

Head-to-Knee Forward Bend

This versatile bending pose stretches your spine and lower body and eases an anxious mind. Use it to relieve the symptoms of fatigue, headache, or painful menstruation.

HOW TO DO IT

- Sit in Staff Pose (pages 218–19), with your legs extended in front of you and your feet flexed.

- Bend your right knee, and draw your right heel in toward your groin, placing the sole of your foot on your left inner thigh. Your right shin should be at a right angle to your left shin. Draw both sit bones to the floor.

- Inhale and lift up through your spine. As you exhale, turn your torso slightly to your left so that it aligns with your left leg. Flex your foot, and contract the muscles in your left thigh to push the back of your leg toward the floor.

- Exhale and stretch your sternum forward to fold your torso over your left leg. Grasp the inside of your left foot with your left hand. Use your right hand to guide your torso to the left.

- Extend your right arm forward toward your left foot. You may either grasp your left foot with both hands or place your hands on the floor on either side of your left foot, with your elbows bent. Place your forehead on your left shin. With each inhalation, lengthen your spine. With each exhalation, deepen the stretch.

- Hold for the recommended breaths, return to the starting position, and then repeat on the opposite side.

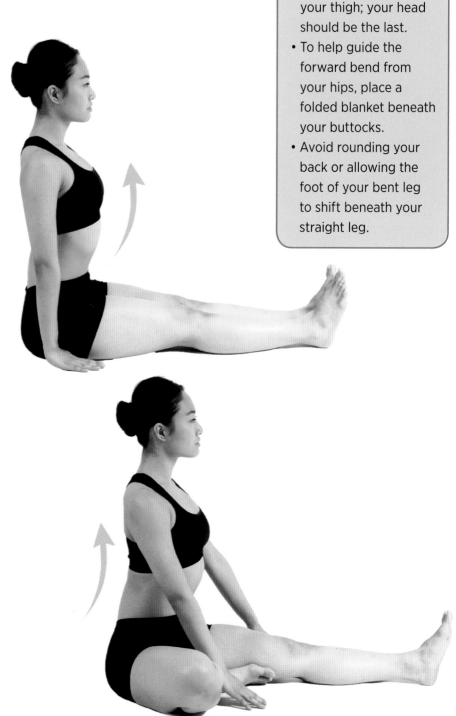

DO IT RIGHT

- Your abdominals should be the first part of your body to touch your thigh; your head should be the last.
- To help guide the forward bend from your hips, place a folded blanket beneath your buttocks.
- Avoid rounding your back or allowing the foot of your bent leg to shift beneath your straight leg.

FACT FILE

SANSKRIT
• Janu Sirsasana

TARGETS
• Hamstrings
• Groin
• Spine

BENEFITS
• Stretches back, core, and thighs
• Stimulates digestion
• Eases stress and mild depression

CAUTIONS
• Knee issues
• Lower-back issues
• Diarrhea

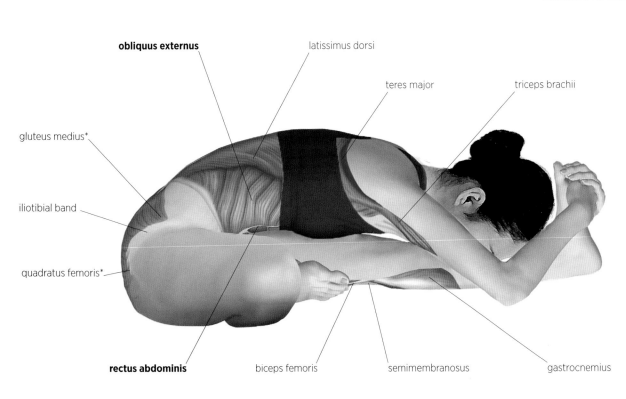

Annotation Key

Bold text indicates target muscles
Light text indicates other working muscles
* indicates deep muscles

obliquus externus

latissimus dorsi

teres major

triceps brachii

gluteus medius*

iliotibial band

quadratus femoris*

rectus abdominis

biceps femoris

semimembranosus

gastrocnemius

Heron Pose Prep

This pose tones your abdominal muscles and stretches your hamstrings and calf muscles in preparation for performing the challenging Heron Pose.

HOW TO DO IT

• Lie on your back with your legs extended in front of you, toes pointed.

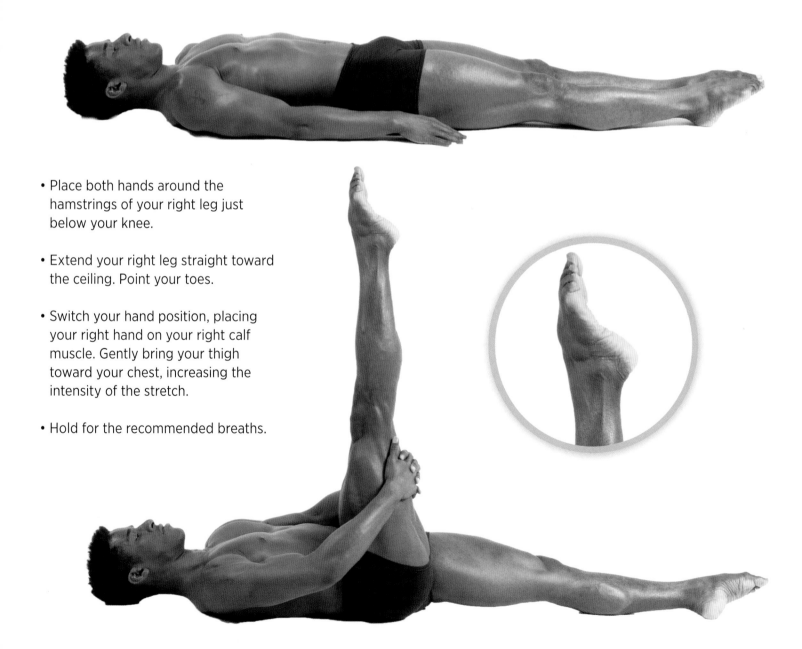

• Place both hands around the hamstrings of your right leg just below your knee.

• Extend your right leg straight toward the ceiling. Point your toes.

• Switch your hand position, placing your right hand on your right calf muscle. Gently bring your thigh toward your chest, increasing the intensity of the stretch.

• Hold for the recommended breaths.

FACT FILE

SANSKRIT
• Krounchasana

TARGETS
• Hamstrings
• Abdominals

BENEFITS
• Stretches
  thighs and
  lower legs
• Extends spine
• Stimulates
  abdominal
  organs

CAUTIONS
• Back issues
• Groin issues

semimembranosus

semitendinosus

biceps femoris

gluteus maximus

erector spinae*   gluteus medius*   gluteus minimus*   gastrocnemius   soleus

DO IT RIGHT
• Keep the toes of both feet pointed
  throughout the pose.
• Avoid jerking your raised leg
  toward your chest; ease it forward.

Annotation Key
Bold text indicates target muscles
Light text indicates other working muscles
* indicates deep muscles

Heron Pose

This intense pose stretches the hamstrings and glutes of your extended leg, and lengthens the quadriceps of your bent leg. It also stimulates your abdominal organs and can actually be therapeutic for flat feet and for combating flatulence. Heron Pose is usually performed as part of a longer seated forward bend sequence.

HOW TO DO IT

• Sit in Staff Pose (pages 218–19), with your legs extended in front of you and your feet flexed.

• Bring your left leg into Hero Pose (pages 224–25), so that your calf is next to your left thigh. The sole of your left foot should be facing up.

• Bend your right knee, and place your foot on the floor, just in front of your right sit bone. Place your right arm against the inside of the right leg so that your shoulder is pressed against your inner knee. Cross your right hand in front of your right ankle, and grasp the outside of your right foot. With your left hand, grasp the inside of your right foot.

• Keeping your torso long, lean back slightly. Firm your shoulder blades against your back to help maintain the lift of your chest. Inhale and raise your right leg diagonally to the floor so that your foot is as high as, or slightly higher than, your head.

• Hold for the recommended breaths, and then exhale as you release your raised leg. Carefully unbend, and then repeat on the opposite side.

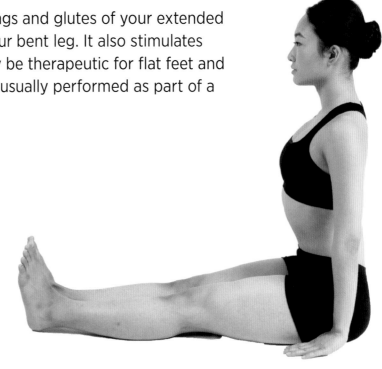

DO IT RIGHT

• Make sure that your bent leg is beside your thigh, not under it.
• If you cannot lift your foot to head height, continue with the Heron Pose prep to increase flexibility.
• Avoid leaning back and using your torso weight to lift the raised leg.

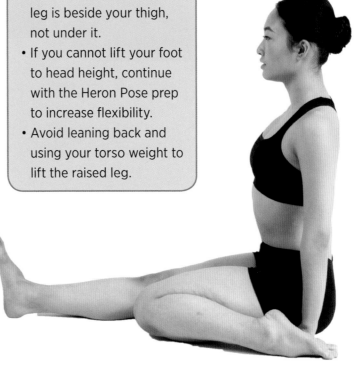

FACT FILE

SANSKRIT
• Krounchasana

TARGETS
• Hamstrings
• Hips
• Glutes

BENEFITS
• Stretches hamstrings and calves
• Strengthens abdominals
• Increases hip flexibility

CAUTIONS
• Hip injuries
• Groin issues

gluteus maximus

obturator externus

adductor magnus

biceps femoris

semitendinosus

semimembranosus

Annotation Key

Bold text indicates target muscles
Light text indicates other working muscles
* indicates deep muscles

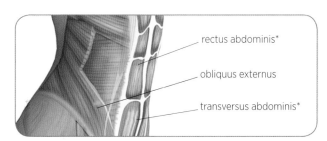

rectus abdominis*

obliquus externus

transversus abdominis*

Revolved Head-to-Knee Pose

This pose, the counterpose to Head-to-Knee Forward Bend, creates a deep toning of your core muscles as it stretches your shoulders, spine, lower back, hamstrings, and the sides of your abdomen.

HOW TO DO IT

- Sit in Staff Pose (pages 218–19), with your legs extended in front of you and your feet flexed.

- Bend your left leg out to the left, externally rotating your hip, as you place the sole of your left foot on the inner thigh of your right leg.

- Bring your right foot slightly to your right, externally rotate your hip, and open your left leg out to the left to widen the foundation.

- Place your right forearm on the inside of your right shin, and use your right hand to grasp the inside of your right foot.

- Reach your left arm toward the ceiling and outwardly rotate your arm, bringing it over your left ear. Bend to your right, reaching for the outside of your right foot with your left hand.

- Nestle your right shoulder toward the inside of your right leg. Slightly bend both elbows away from each other, and lean back. Use this resistance to twist your right ribs and torso toward the ceiling.

- Hold for the recommended breaths, release the stretch, and repeat on the opposite side.

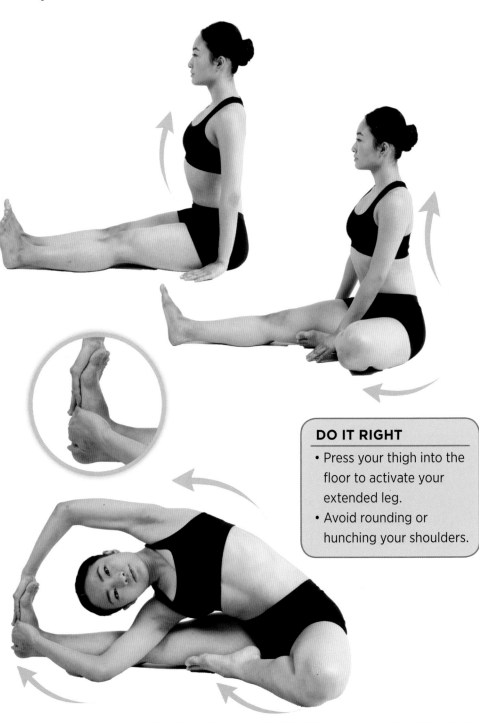

DO IT RIGHT

- Press your thigh into the floor to activate your extended leg.
- Avoid rounding or hunching your shoulders.

SANSKRIT
• Parivrtta Janu Sirsasana

TARGETS
• Shoulders
• Back
• Lower torso
• Hamstrings

BENEFITS
• Stretches shoulders and hamstrings
• Offers deep side stretch
• Stimulates digestive organs

CAUTIONS
• Knee issues
• Lower-back issues

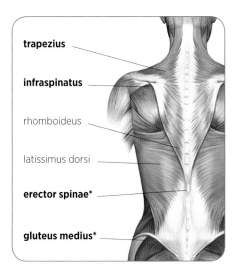

- trapezius
- infraspinatus
- rhomboideus
- latissimus dorsi
- erector spinae*
- gluteus medius*

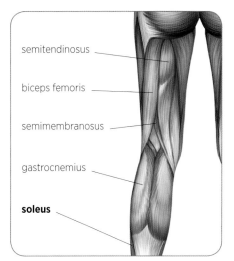

- semitendinosus
- biceps femoris
- semimembranosus
- gastrocnemius
- soleus

MODIFICATION

EASIER: Instead of leaning all the way to the side, place one hand on your shin, and extend the other arm over your ear as you bend slightly to the side.

Annotation Key
Bold text indicates target muscles
Light text indicates other working muscles
* indicates deep muscles

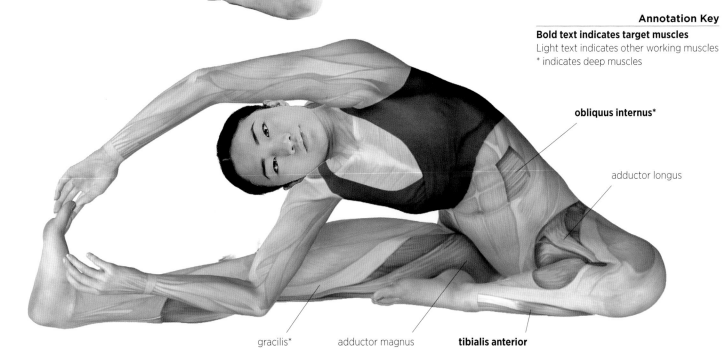

- obliquus internus*
- adductor longus
- gracilis*
- adductor magnus
- tibialis anterior

Seated Leg Cradle

This pose offers a great stretch to your gluteal muscles, while targeting your hips and hamstrings. It also helps to relieve the tension in your lower back and hips after long hours sitting at a desk or computer.

HOW TO DO IT

• Sit in Staff Pose (pages 218–19), with your legs extended in front of you and your feet flexed.

• Bend your right knee, and grasp your calf with your right hand. With your left hand, support your raised foot as you hug it into your chest, as if you were cradling a baby. Keep your heel roughly 12 inches away from your chest.

• Hold for the recommended breaths, release the stretch, and then repeat on the opposite side.

DO IT RIGHT

• Keep your chest lifted and open.
• Contract your glutes as you raise your leg.
• Avoid holding your breath.

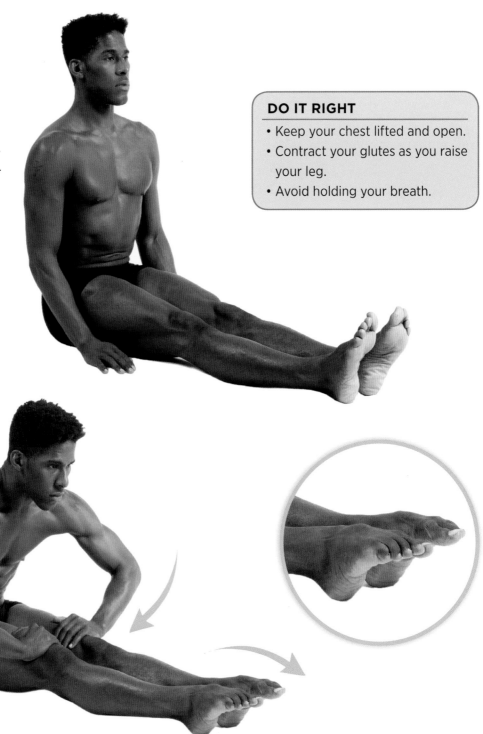

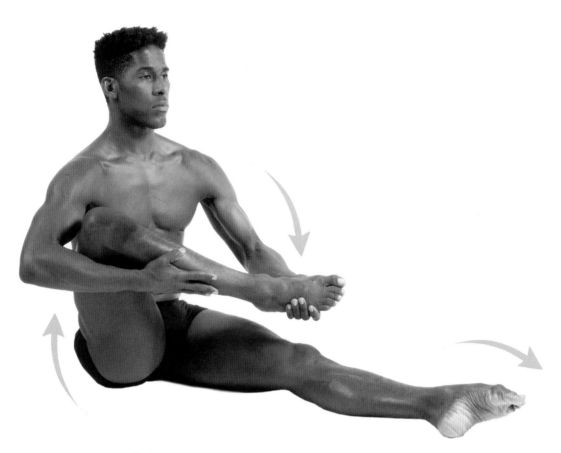

FACT FILE

SANSKRIT
- Hindolasana

TARGETS
- Upper hamstrings
- Glutes

BENEFITS
- Opens hips
- Stretches hamstrings, pelvic floor, and glutes
- Relieves tension in lower back

CAUTIONS
- Groin injury
- Hip issues

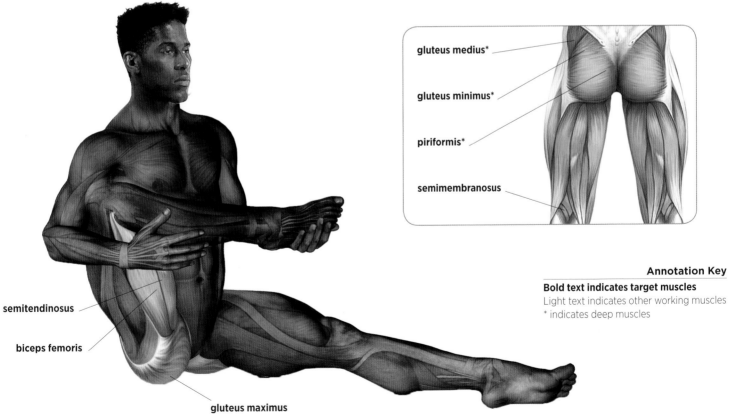

gluteus medius*

gluteus minimus*

piriformis*

semimembranosus

semitendinosus

biceps femoris

gluteus maximus

Annotation Key

Bold text indicates target muscles
Light text indicates other working muscles
* indicates deep muscles

Half Straddle Pose

This pose is beneficial to your lower torso and legs, providing an opening of your hips and a stretch of your obliques, thighs, quads, and calves.

HOW TO DO IT

• Sit upright with your knees bent.

• Keeping your right knee bent, open it up so that it touches the floor. Draw your right foot in toward your core.

• Extend your left leg straight out to the side of your body.

• Plant your arms on the floor behind you to support your lower back as you stretch.

• Hold for the recommended breaths, release the stretch, and then repeat on the opposite side.

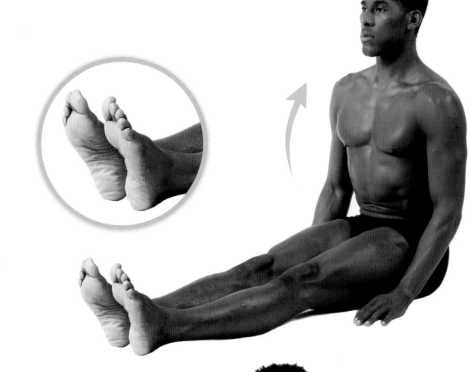

DO IT RIGHT

• Lean against a sofa, if necessary, to stabilize yourself and correctly align your hip bones on the floor.
• Avoid raising your grounded thigh from the floor.

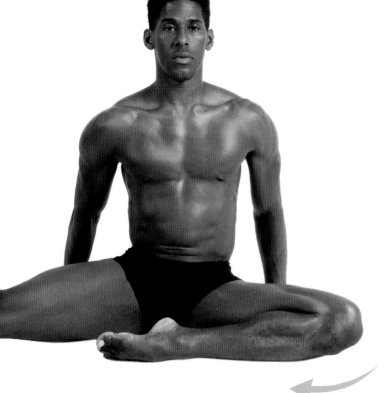

SANSKRIT
- Samakonasana

TARGETS
- Hamstrings
- Quadriceps
- Inner thighs
- Calves
- Obliques

BENEFITS
- Stretches obliques, quads, and hamstrings
- Improves lower-body flexibility

CAUTIONS
- Groin injury
- Lower-back issues

Annotation Key

Bold text indicates target muscles
Light text indicates other working muscles
* indicates deep muscles

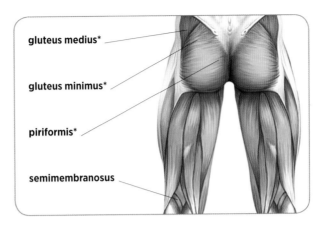

gluteus medius*

gluteus minimus*

piriformis*

semimembranosus

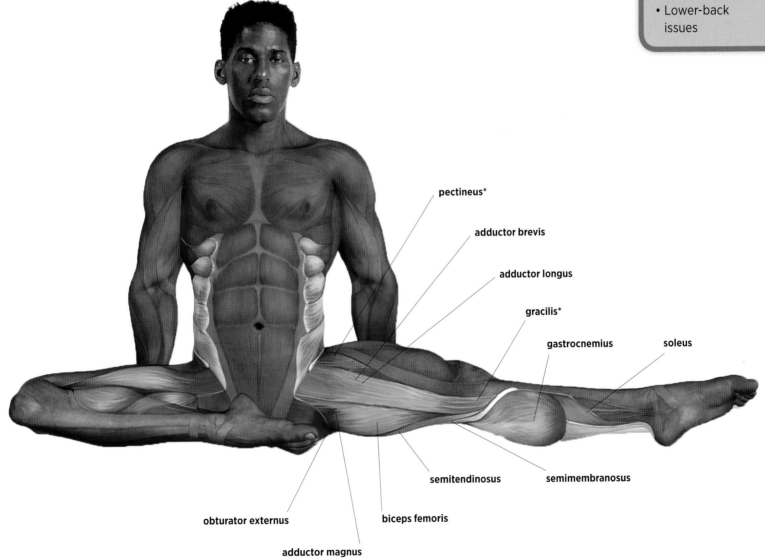

pectineus*

adductor brevis

adductor longus

gracilis*

gastrocnemius

soleus

semitendinosus

semimembranosus

obturator externus

biceps femoris

adductor magnus

Side-Leaning Half Straddle Pose

This pose increases the stretching benefits provided by the Half Straddle, deepening the effects on the obliques as you twist your torso to one side and then the other.

HOW TO DO IT

- Begin in the Half Straddle Pose (pages 152–53), seated upright, with your right leg bent on the floor and your left leg extended to the side. Bend your left elbow, and rest your left forearm on your left thigh.

- Raise your right arm over your head, palm inward.

- Slowly bend slightly forward at your hips, and lean toward your left side until you feel a comfortable stretch.

- Hold for the recommended breaths, release the stretch, and then repeat on the opposite side.

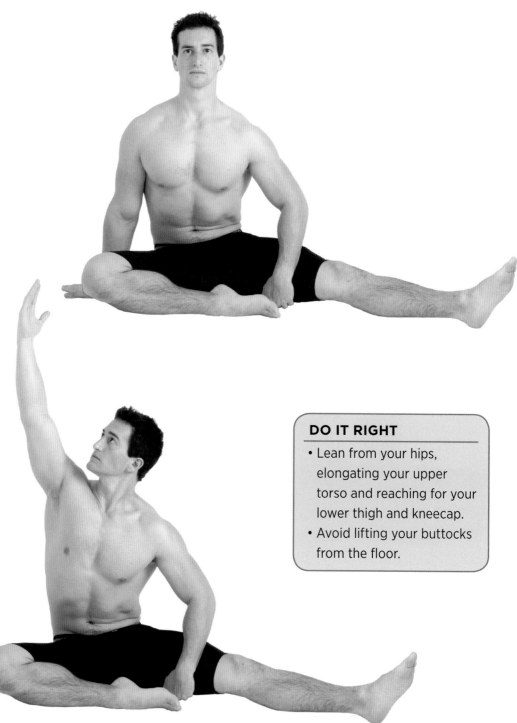

DO IT RIGHT

- Lean from your hips, elongating your upper torso and reaching for your lower thigh and kneecap.
- Avoid lifting your buttocks from the floor.

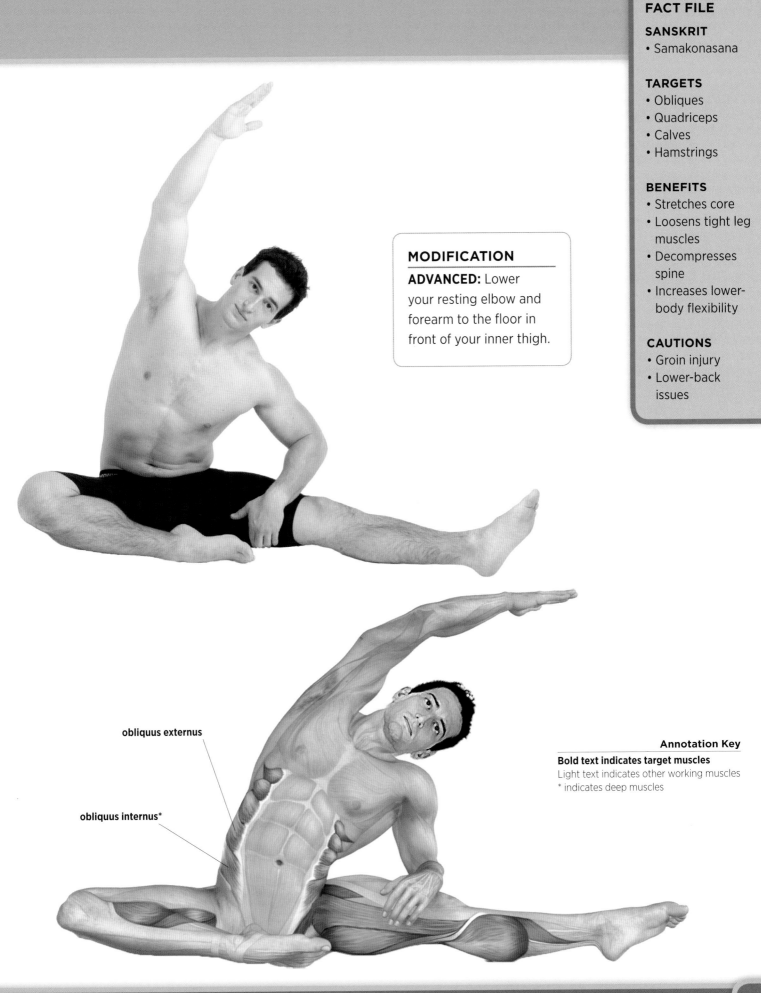

SANSKRIT
- Samakonasana

TARGETS
- Obliques
- Quadriceps
- Calves
- Hamstrings

BENEFITS
- Stretches core
- Loosens tight leg muscles
- Decompresses spine
- Increases lower-body flexibility

CAUTIONS
- Groin injury
- Lower-back issues

MODIFICATION

ADVANCED: Lower your resting elbow and forearm to the floor in front of your inner thigh.

obliquus externus

obliquus internus*

Annotation Key

Bold text indicates target muscles
Light text indicates other working muscles
* indicates deep muscles

Wide-Angle Seated Forward Bend

This pose is especially good for opening your hips and groin, strengthening your back, and stretching your upper legs and glutes.

HOW TO DO IT

- Sit in Staff Pose (pages 218–19), with your legs extended in front of you.

- Separate your legs as widely as is comfortable. Turn your thighs slightly outward so that your knees point up toward the ceiling. Flex your feet.

- Place your hands in front of your body, and walk them forward as you bring your upper body toward the floor.

- Hold for the recommended breaths, and then ease back into an upright position.

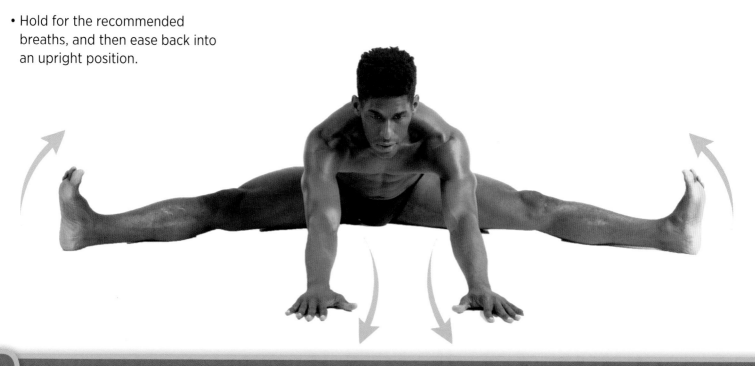

TARGETS
• Hamstrings
• Lower back
• Hip adductors
• Glutes

BENEFITS
• Stretches insides and backs of legs
• Strengthens spine
• Releases groin
• Stimulates internal organs
• Calms mind

CAUTIONS
• Groin injury
• Hip issues

Annotation Key

Bold text indicates target muscles
Light text indicates other working muscles
* indicates deep muscles

DO IT RIGHT

• Keep your torso long and flat, and your chest lifted.
• Lengthen your torso as you bend forward.
• Keep your legs turned out from your hips.
• Avoid overdoing this stretch—move carefully and slowly.

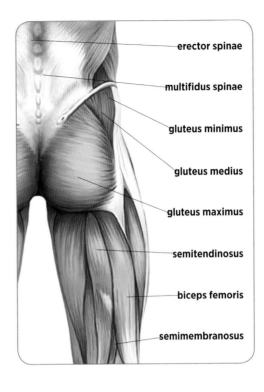

erector spinae

multifidus spinae

gluteus minimus

gluteus medius

gluteus maximus

semitendinosus

biceps femoris

semimembranosus

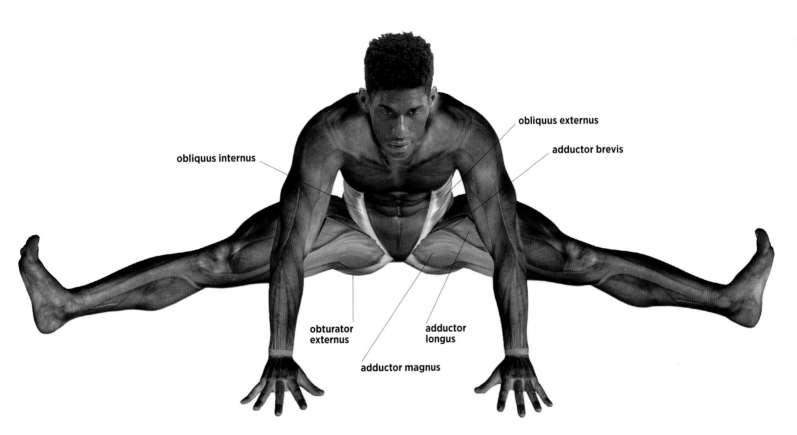

obliquus externus

adductor brevis

obliquus internus

obturator externus

adductor longus

adductor magnus

Chest-to-Thigh Straddle Split

This intermediate pose really opens up the pelvic area and provides a challenging stretch for your inner thighs and oblique muscles. It can also improve balance and mobility.

HOW TO DO IT

- Sit in Staff Pose (pages 218–19), with your legs extended in front of you.

- Open your legs wide. Turn your thighs slightly outward so that your knees point up toward the ceiling. Flex your feet. Place your right hand in front, and your left hand behind your torso, palms flat on the floor.

- Twist and lean your torso over your right thigh.

- With your hands on the floor on either side of your right calf, lower your chest toward your thigh.

- Hold for the recommended breaths, return to the center, and then repeat on the opposite side.

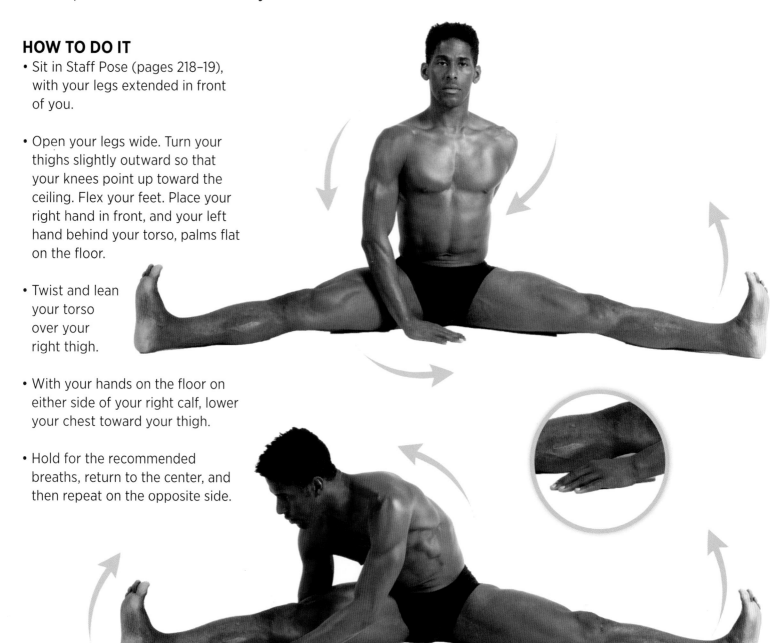

FACT FILE

SANSKRIT
- Konasana

TARGETS
- Inner thighs
- Hamstrings
- Glutes
- Rib cage
- Hip adductors

BENEFITS
- Increases hip and hamstring flexibility
- Strengthens glutes and inner thighs
- Improves movement and balance

CAUTIONS
- Hip issues
- Groin injury

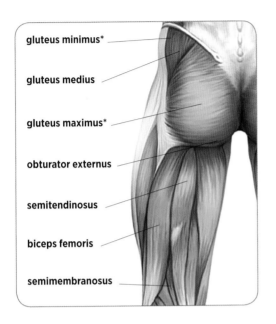

gluteus minimus*
gluteus medius
gluteus maximus*
obturator externus
semitendinosus
biceps femoris
semimembranosus

DO IT RIGHT
- Keep the external rotation in your legs, and aim your toes straight up.
- Avoid lifting your hip bones off the floor.
- Avoid allowing your legs to shift inward.

Annotation Key

Bold text indicates target muscles
Light text indicates other working muscles
* indicates deep muscles

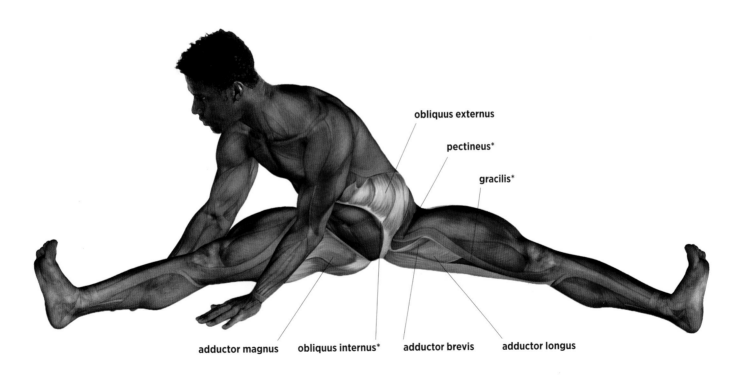

obliquus externus
pectineus*
gracilis*
adductor magnus
obliquus internus*
adductor brevis
adductor longus

Seated Straddle Split

This pose helps you overcome tight hip flexors that are often the result of spending hours in an office chair or in front of a computer. It also stretches your inner thighs and calves. The more you practice this pose, the wider you will be able to position your legs.

HOW TO DO IT

- Sit in Staff Pose (pages 218–19), with your legs extended in front of you.

- Turn your thighs slightly outward as you spread your legs wide so that your knees point up toward the ceiling. Flex your feet. Place your hands on the floor behind your buttocks to push them forward, separating your legs even farther.

- Place one hand on the floor directly in front of you and the other directly behind you. Align your hip bones on the floor.

- Hold for the recommended breaths, and then repeat on the opposite side.

MODIFICATION

EASIER: To take pressure off the lumbar region of your spine, sit up against a sofa or wall.

DO IT RIGHT

- Sit up as tall as possible, keeping your torso elongated.
- Avoid leaning back and rounding your lower back.
- Avoid bouncing your legs open—you want to feel the stretch but not pain.

MODIFICATION

ADVANCED: Press your hands down into the floor, lifting your body slightly upward. Carefully shift your pelvis forward, increasing the stretch, and then lower yourself back to the floor and point your toes. Repeat three times, holding each stretch for 20 to 30 seconds.

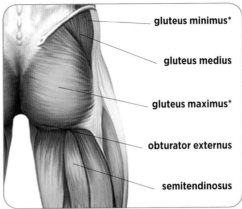

gluteus minimus*

gluteus medius

gluteus maximus*

obturator externus

semitendinosus

Annotation Key
Bold text indicates target muscles
Light text indicates other working muscles
* indicates deep muscles

FACT FILE

SANSKRIT
• Konasana

TARGETS
• Hip adductors
• Hamstrings

BENEFITS
• Opens hip and groin
• Stretches spine, inner thighs, and calf muscles
• Improves pelvic circulation

CAUTIONS
• Groin injury
• Hip issues

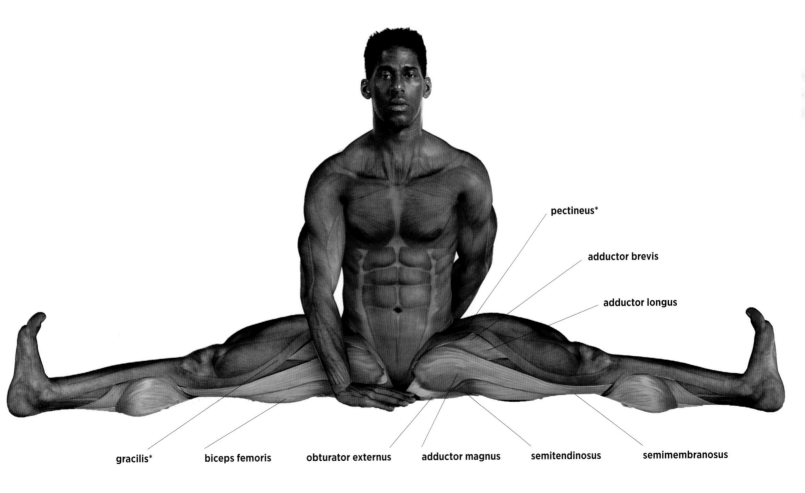

pectineus*

adductor brevis

adductor longus

gracilis*   biceps femoris   obturator externus   adductor magnus   semitendinosus   semimembranosus

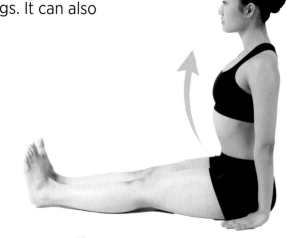

Chest-to-Floor Straddle Split Pose

This versatile straddle split increases the stretching benefits to your spine and hips as well as the backs and insides of your legs. It can also calm an overstressed mind.

HOW TO DO IT

- Sit in Staff Pose (pages 218–19), with your legs extended in front of you.

- Turn your thighs slightly outward so that your knees point up toward the ceiling. Flex your feet. Place your hands on the floor behind your buttocks to push them forward, separating your legs even farther.

- Inhale and raise your torso, placing your hands on the floor in front of you. Contract your leg muscles as you press the backs of your thighs and both sit bones into the floor.

- Exhale and bend forward from your waist, keeping your back flat. Walk your hands in front of you as you lower your torso slowly toward the floor. Keep your gaze forward. Stretch as far as possible without rounding your back.

- Hold for the recommended breaths.

DO IT RIGHT

- If you have trouble bending forward from your hips or sitting with your legs far apart, place a folded blanket beneath your buttocks.
- Keep your knees pointed up toward the ceiling.
- Avoid bending forward from your waist.

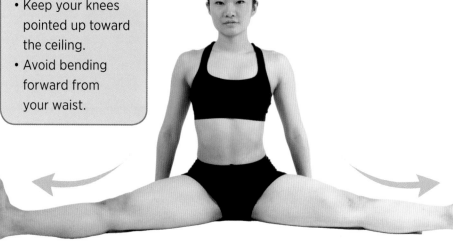

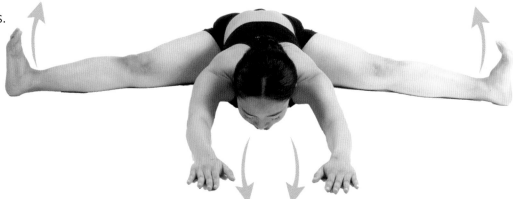

SANSKRIT
- Upavistha Konasana

TARGETS
- Back
- Hips
- Glutes
- Thighs

BENEFITS
- Stretches groin and hamstrings
- Strengthens spine

CAUTIONS
- Lower-back injury

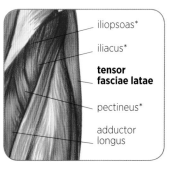

gluteus medius*
piriformis*
gluteus maximus
quadratus femoris*
obturator internus*
obturator externus*
adductor magnus
semitendinosus
biceps femoris
vastus lateralis
gracilis*
semimembranosus
plantaris
gastrocnemius

iliopsoas*
iliacus*
tensor fasciae latae
pectineus*
adductor longus

Annotation Key

Bold text indicates target muscles
Light text indicates other working muscles
* indicates deep muscles

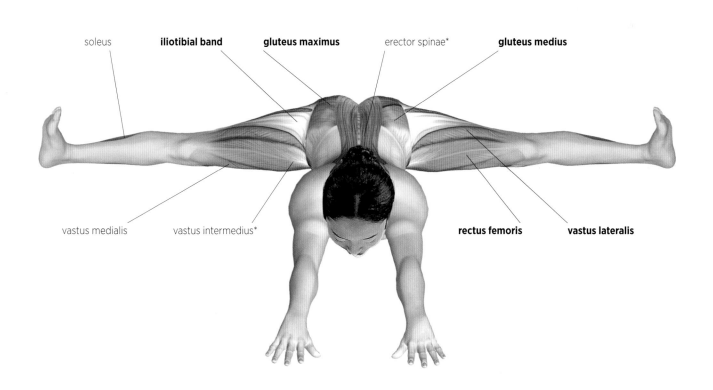

soleus
iliotibial band
gluteus maximus
erector spinae*
gluteus medius
vastus medialis
vastus intermedius*
rectus femoris
vastus lateralis

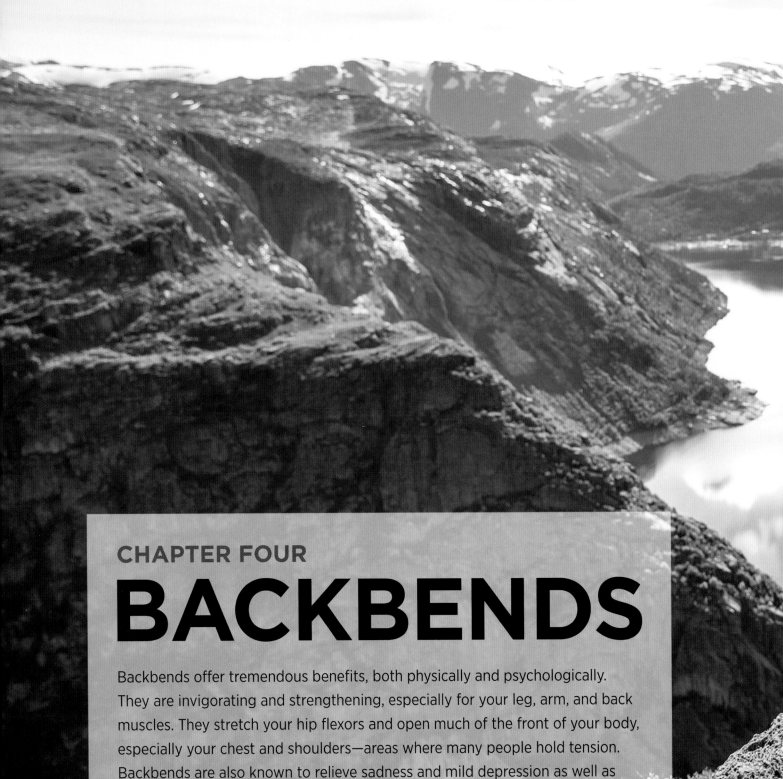

CHAPTER FOUR
BACKBENDS

Backbends offer tremendous benefits, both physically and psychologically. They are invigorating and strengthening, especially for your leg, arm, and back muscles. They stretch your hip flexors and open much of the front of your body, especially your chest and shoulders—areas where many people hold tension. Backbends are also known to relieve sadness and mild depression as well as boost energy levels and improve posture.

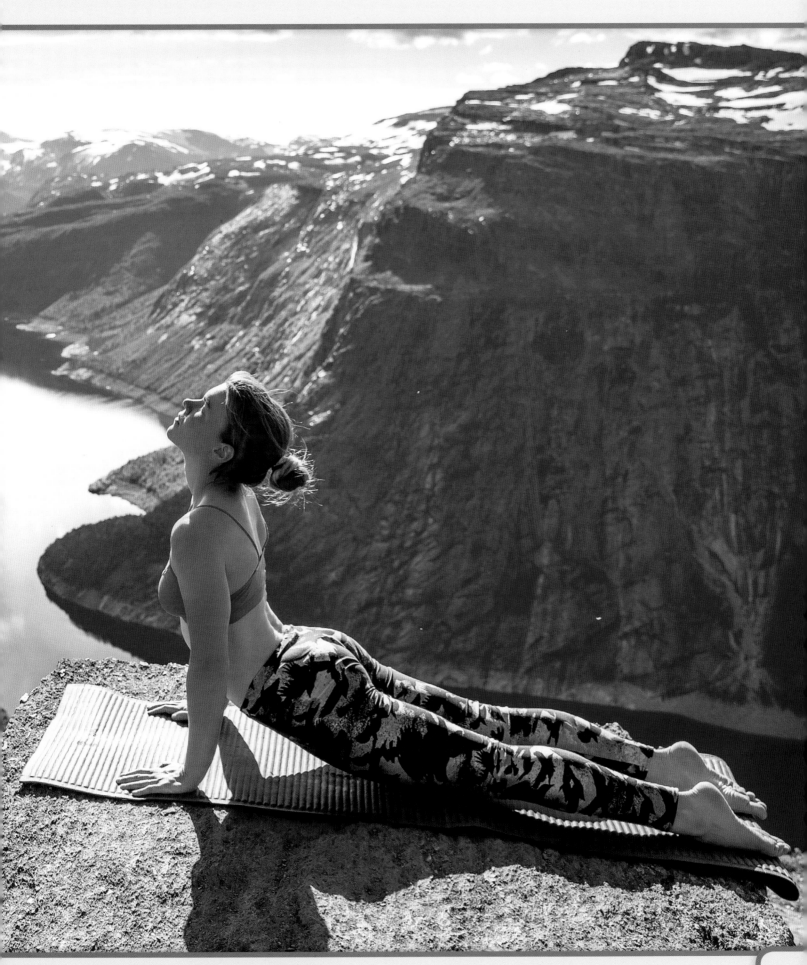

Cow Pose

Also known as Dog Tilt Pose, Cow Pose stretches your middle to lower back and hips and lengthens your spine. Pair it with Cat Pose (pages 102–03) to warm up your spine and increase your energy levels.

HOW TO DO IT

• Begin on all fours, with your hands planted directly below your shoulders and your knees aligned beneath your hips. Your hips should be in a neutral position and your feet up on your toes.

• Spread your fingers wide, pressing down through your knuckles.

• Inhale, lift your sternum, and arch your upper back, raising your sit bones toward the ceiling. Hold for the recommended breaths, and then exhale to release the stretch.

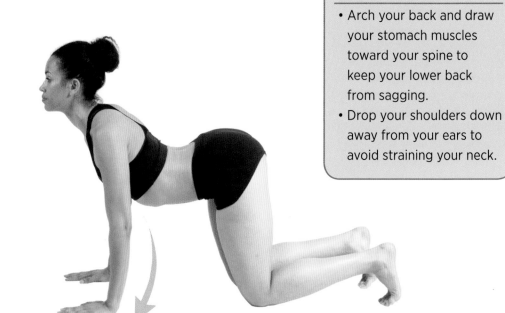

DO IT RIGHT

• Arch your back and draw your stomach muscles toward your spine to keep your lower back from sagging.
• Drop your shoulders down away from your ears to avoid straining your neck.

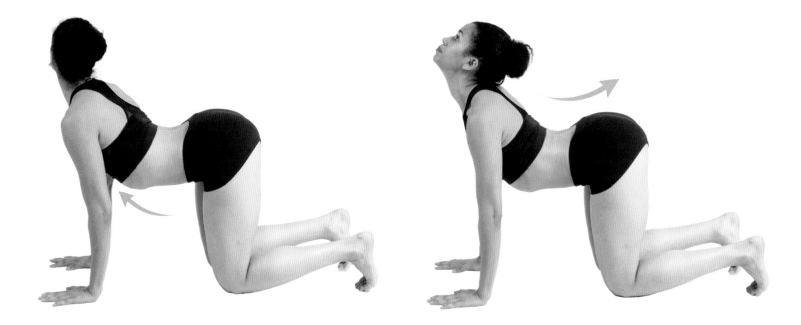

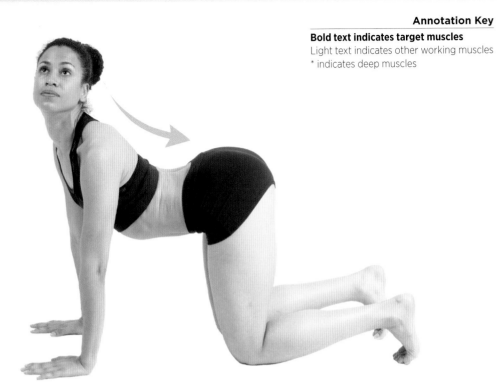

FACT FILE

SANSKRIT
• Bitilasana

TARGETS
• Spine
• Chest
• Neck

BENEFITS
• Stretches upper body and back
• Strengthens the muscles in the hands and wrists
• Massages spine
• Increases mobility

CAUTIONS
• Neck issues
• Wrist issues

Annotation Key

Bold text indicates target muscles
Light text indicates other working muscles
* indicates deep muscles

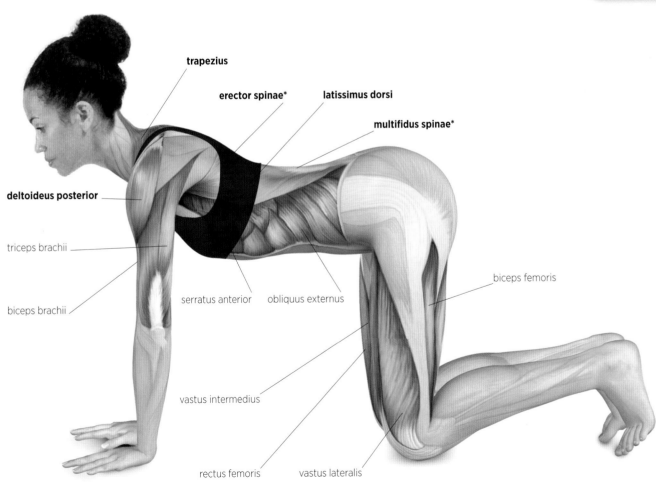

trapezius

erector spinae*

latissimus dorsi

multifidus spinae*

deltoideus posterior

triceps brachii

biceps brachii

serratus anterior

obliquus externus

biceps femoris

vastus intermedius

rectus femoris

vastus lateralis

Bridge Pose

An effective preparation for the full spinal lift of Wheel Pose (pages 194–95), Bridge Pose is a restorative asana with much to offer on its own. While preparing you for more challenging backbends, this exercise relies on the strength of your quads, glutes, and abdomen while opening your chest and stretching your spine.

HOW TO DO IT

• Lie faceup on the floor. Bend your knee, and draw you heels close to your buttocks. Place your arms flat on the floor at your sides.

• Exhale and press down through your feet to lift your buttocks off the floor. With your feet and thighs parallel, push your arms into the floor while extending through your fingertips.

• Lengthen your neck away from your shoulders. Lift your hips higher so that your torso rises from the floor.

• Hold for the recommended breaths, exhale, and release your spine onto the floor, one vertebra at a time.

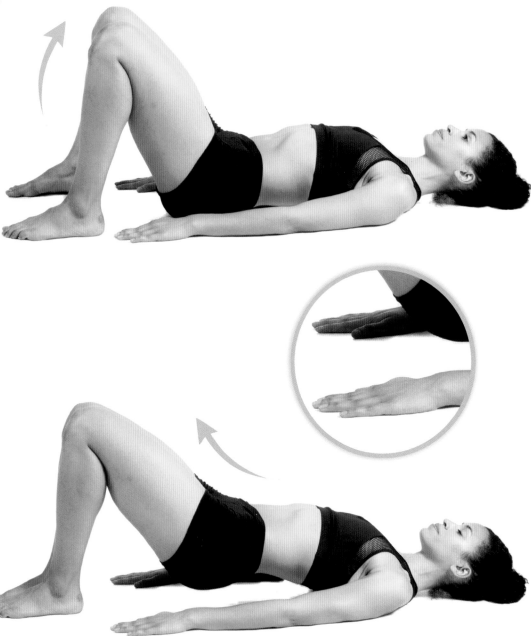

SANSKRIT
- Setu Bandha Sarvangasana

TARGETS
- Spine
- Chest
- Thighs
- Glutes

BENEFITS
- Stretches chest and spine
- Strengthens thighs and buttocks
- Stimulates digestion
- Stimulates thyroid
- Reduces stress

CAUTIONS
- Shoulder issues
- Back issues
- Neck issues

DO IT RIGHT

- Keep your knees over your heels.
- Focus on bending your upper back and chest.
- Place a block beneath your sacrum if you need support under your back.
- Contract your hamstrings to keep your legs active.
- Avoid sticking out your stomach or ribs.
- Avoid bending from your lower back.
- Avoid clenching your buttocks.

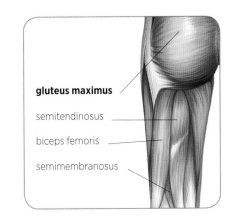

gluteus maximus

semitendinosus

biceps femoris

semimembranosus

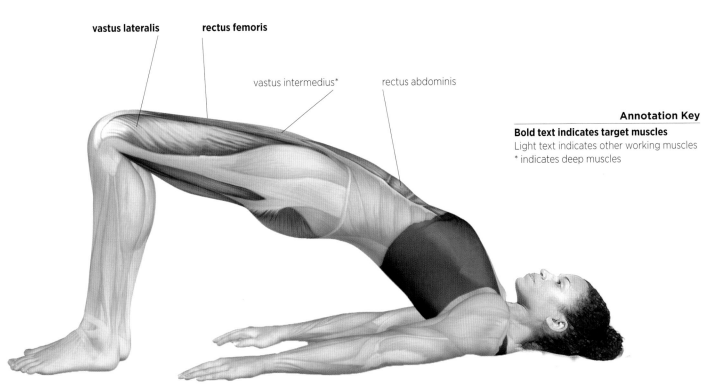

vastus lateralis

rectus femoris

vastus intermedius*

rectus abdominis

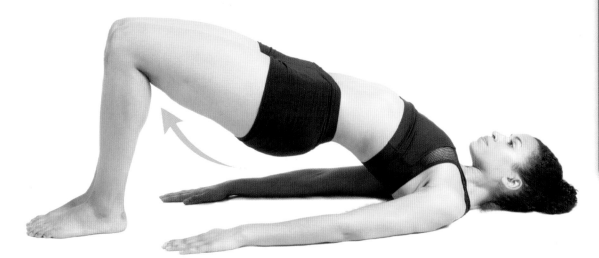

Annotation Key

Bold text indicates target muscles
Light text indicates other working muscles
* indicates deep muscles

Upward-Facing Dog

This moderate backbend is perfect for relieving stiff or aching muscles after hours spent hunched over a computer or desk. It is also an important pose in Sun Salutations.

HOW TO DO IT

• Lie facedown, and then bend your elbows as you place your hands flat on the mat on either side of your chest, fingers pointing forward. Keep your elbows pulled in toward your body. Spread your legs hip-width apart, extending them through your toes. Your toes should be touching the floor.

• Inhale as you press downward with your palms and the tops of your feet, lifting your torso and hips off the floor. Contract your thighs, and then tuck your tailbone toward your pubis.

• Lift up through the top of your chest by extending your arms and arching your back. Push your shoulders down and back, and then elongate your neck as you gaze slightly upward.

• Hold for the recommended breaths, and then exhale as you lower yourself to the floor.

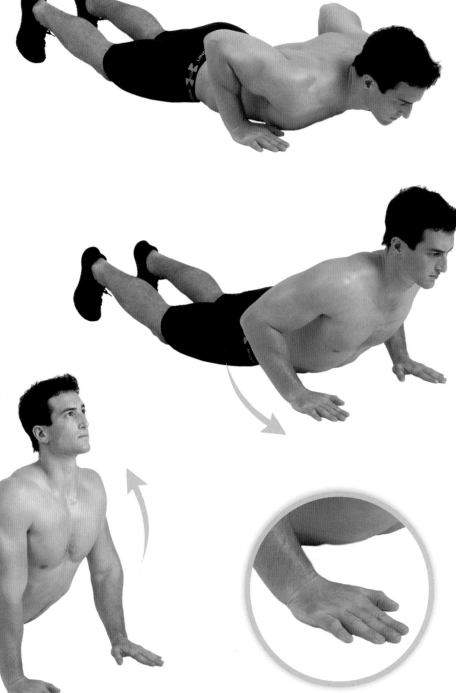

DO IT RIGHT

- Elongate your legs and arms to create full extension.
- Position your wrists directly below your shoulders, not in front of them, to avoid placing too much pressure on your lower back.
- Avoid shrugging your shoulders up toward your ears, hyperextending your elbows, poking your rib cage out of your chest, or dropping your thighs to the floor.
- Keep your chin tucked down slightly to keep your neck elongated.

Annotation Key

Bold text indicates target muscles
Light text indicates other working muscles
* indicates deep muscles

FACT FILE

SANSKRIT
- Urdhva Mukha Svanasana

TARGETS
- Spine
- Arms and wrists
- Chest
- Abdominals

BENEFITS
- Strengthens upper body and back
- Improves posture

CAUTIONS
- Back issues
- Wrist issues
- Carpal tunnel syndrome

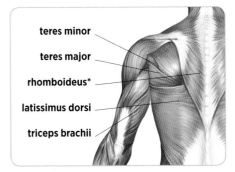

teres minor
teres major
rhomboideus*
latissimus dorsi
triceps brachii

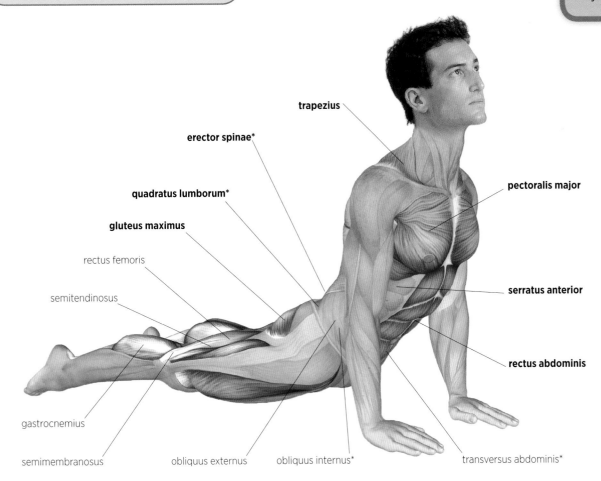

trapezius
erector spinae*
quadratus lumborum*
gluteus maximus
rectus femoris
semitendinosus
gastrocnemius
semimembranosus
obliquus externus
obliquus internus*
transversus abdominis*
pectoralis major
serratus anterior
rectus abdominis

Cobra Pose

Cobra Pose is quite effective for stretching and strengthening your spine. Try not to force your chest and shoulders too high at first. Go gradually—and focus on each incremental advance.

HOW TO DO IT

- Lie facedown on your stomach. Bend your arms and place your wrists underneath your elbows, with your fingers facing toward the front of your mat. Draw your elbows in close to your body.

- On an inhalation, press your hands into the mat and lift your chest and shoulders upward, propelling your sternum forward and drawing your shoulder blades together.

- Press into the floor with your toenails, especially those of your pinky toes, to help you find internal rotation in your thighs.

- Firm your buttocks as you straighten your legs and roll your inner thighs toward the ceiling. Feel your pubic bone pressing down to the floor as you draw your tailbone down toward your feet. Hold for the recommended breaths.

- On an exhalation, lead with your forehead as you lower yourself back to the mat.

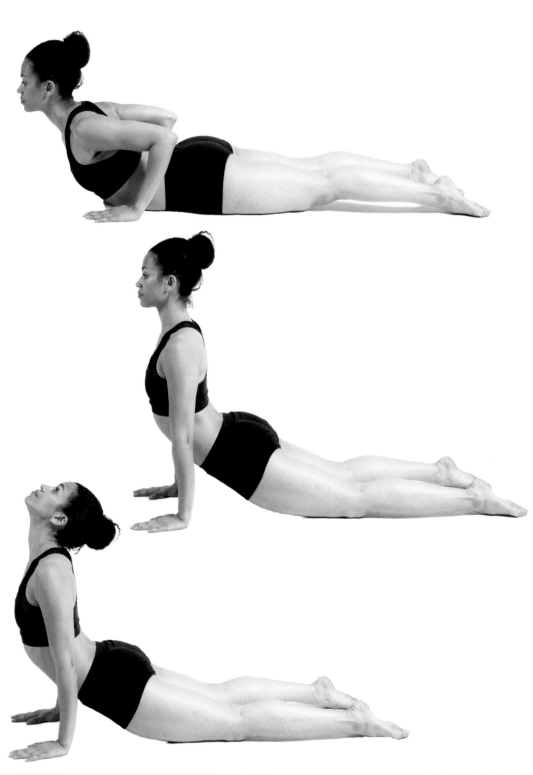

FACT FILE

SANSKRIT
• Bhujangasana

TARGETS
• Spine

BENEFITS
• Stretches and strengthens spine and upper arms
• Stretches front of body
• Improves posture

CAUTIONS
• Lower-back issues
• Pregnancy

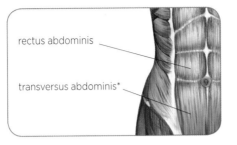

rectus abdominis

transversus abdominis*

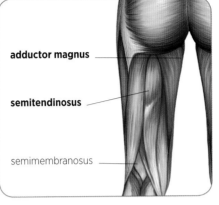

adductor magnus

semitendinosus

semimembranosus

Annotation Key

Bold text indicates target muscles
Light text indicates other working muscles
* indicates deep muscles

infraspinatus*

supraspinatus*

subscapularis*

teres minor

teres major

latissimus dorsi

erector spinae*

quadratus lumborum

gluteus medius*

DO IT RIGHT

• Keep the back of your neck long.
• Draw your belly button in toward your spine even though your stomach is resting on the floor.
• Avoid turning your legs outward.
• Avoid lifting your feet off the floor as your raise your chest.
• Don't squeeze your buttocks so hard that your lower back feels tense or crunched.

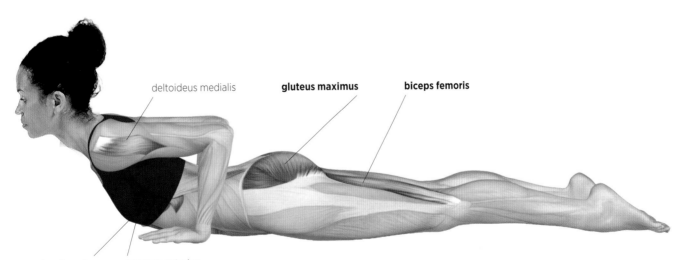

deltoideus medialis

gluteus maximus

biceps femoris

pectoralis major

serratus anterior

Locust Pose

Also known as Grasshopper Pose, Locust Pose is a mild backbend that strengthens your upper and lower back as well as your arms and legs. It also stretches your chest, shoulders, and abdominals. Practicing this pose will prepare your body for deeper backbends.

HOW TO DO IT

- Lie facedown on the floor with your arms resting at your sides and the palms of your hands facing downward. Turn your legs in toward each other so that your knees point directly into the floor.

- Squeezing your buttocks, inhale and simultaneously lift your head, chest, arms, and legs. Extend your arms and legs behind you, with your arms parallel to the floor. Lift up as high as possible, with your pelvis and lower abdominals stabilizing your body on the floor. Keep your head in a neutral position.

- Hold for the recommended breaths, and then release the stretch.

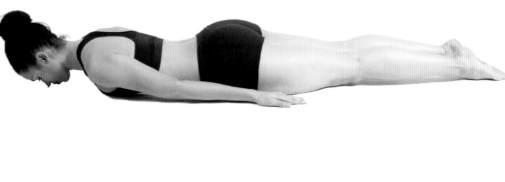

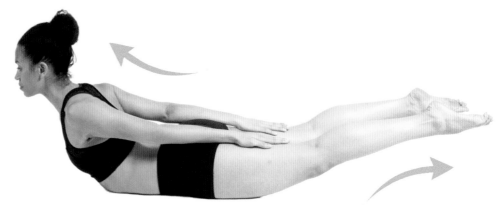

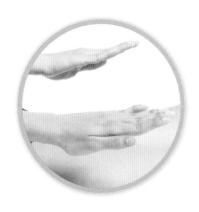

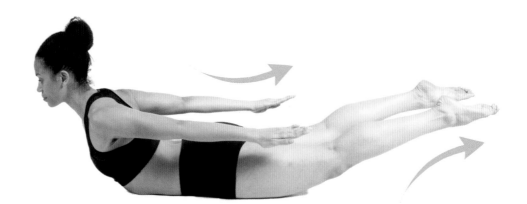

SANSKRIT
- Salabhasana

TARGETS
- Chest
- Shoulders
- Abdominals
- Hips
- Spine

BENEFITS
- Stretches hip flexors, chest, and abdomen
- Strengthens spine, buttocks, arms, and legs
- Stimulates digestion

CAUTIONS
- Back issues

DO IT RIGHT
- Elongate the back of your neck.
- Open your chest to extend the arch through your entire spine.
- Avoid bending your knees.
- Keep your breath even and steady.

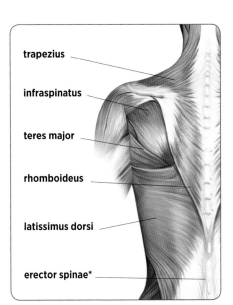

trapezius

infraspinatus

teres major

rhomboideus

latissimus dorsi

erector spinae*

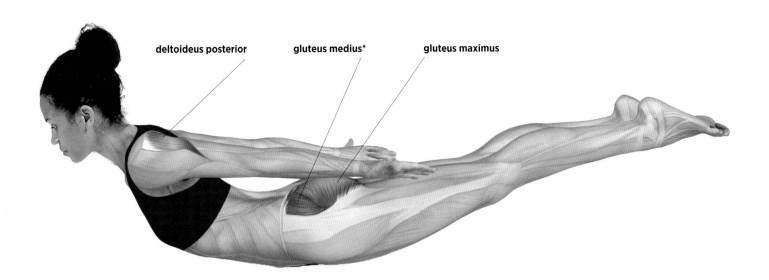

deltoideus posterior

gluteus medius*

gluteus maximus

Annotation Key

Bold text indicates target muscles

Light text indicates other working muscles

* indicates deep muscles

Swimming Locust Pose

The Swimming Locust Pose engages a wide variety of muscles in your body, but it especially targets your hip extensors, both stretching and strengthening them. It is also an effective exercise for the muscles that support your spine.

HOW TO DO IT

• Lie facedown with your legs hip-width apart. Stretch your arms beside your ears on the floor. Engage your pelvic floor, and draw your navel into your spine.

• Extend through your upper back as you simultaneously lift your left arm and right leg. Lift your head and shoulders off the floor.

• Lower your arm and leg to the starting position, maintaining a stretch in your limbs throughout.

• Extend your opposite arm and leg off the floor, lengthening and lifting your head and shoulders.

• Elongate your limbs as you return to the starting position, and perform the recommended repetitions.

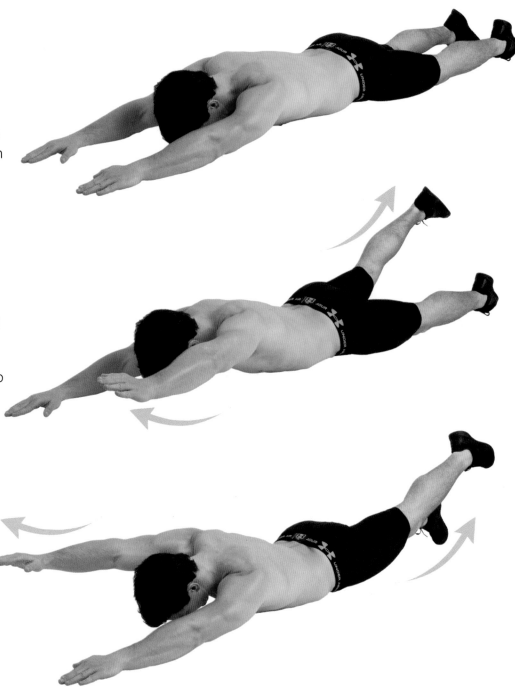

FACT FILE

SANSKRIT
• None

TARGETS
• Hips
• Spine

BENEFITS
• Strengthens hip and spine extensors
• Challenges stabilization of the spine against rotation

CAUTIONS
• Lower-back pain
• Extreme curvature of upper spine
• Curvature of lower spine

DO IT RIGHT

• Extend your limbs as long as possible in opposite directions.
• Make sure your glutes remain tightly squeezed and draw in your navel.
• Keep your neck long and relaxed.
• Avoid lifting your shoulders toward your ears.

Annotation Key

Bold text indicates target muscles
Light text indicates other working muscles
* indicates deep muscles

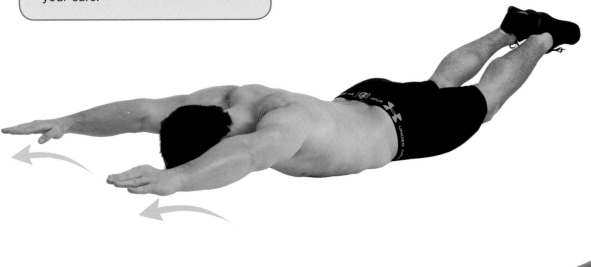

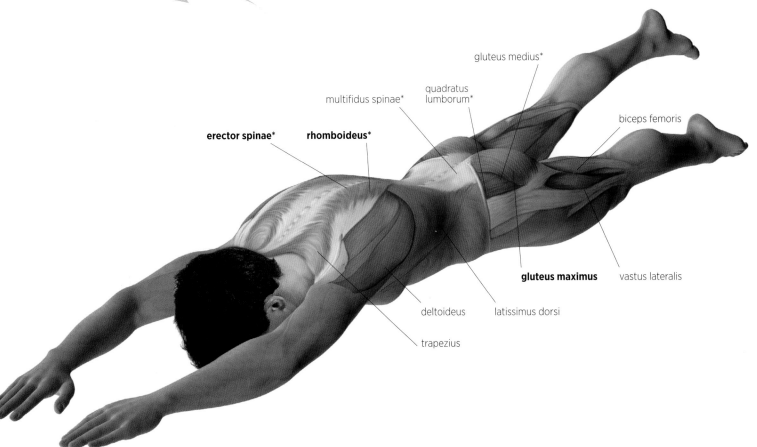

gluteus medius*

quadratus lumborum*

multifidus spinae*

biceps femoris

erector spinae*   **rhomboideus***

gluteus maximus

vastus lateralis

deltoideus   latissimus dorsi

trapezius

Half Frog Prep

This pose readies you for the slightly more challenging Half Frog Pose. It opens your shoulders and chest, and stretches your hips, quads, and abdominals. Half Frog Prep also helps improve your posture.

HOW TO DO IT

• Lie facedown on a mat with your forearms and legs flat on the mat.

• Prop yourself up onto your forearms with your elbows positioned directly beneath your shoulders.

• Bend your left knee, bringing your heel toward your left buttock. Reach your left arm behind you, and grasp the outside of your foot as you continue to press your foot toward your left hip.

• Press your right forearm and elbow down into the floor to avoid collapsing into your left shoulder. Square your shoulders toward the front of the mat.

• Hold for the recommended breaths, and then repeat on the opposite side.

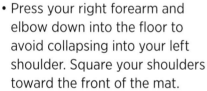

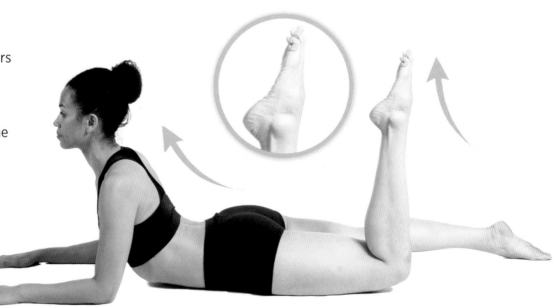

FACT FILE

SANSKRIT
- Ardha Bhekasana

TARGETS
- Hips
- Chest
- Shoulders
- Abdominals
- Thighs
- Ankles

BENEFITS
- Stretches upper body, hips, and thighs
- Strengthens back muscles
- Improves posture

CAUTIONS
- Lower-back issues
- Shoulder issues
- High or low blood pressure

Annotation Key

Bold text indicates target muscles
Light text indicates other working muscles
* indicates deep muscles

DO IT RIGHT
- Engage your stomach muscles.
- Avoid sinking into your supporting shoulder.
- Avoid twisting your neck.

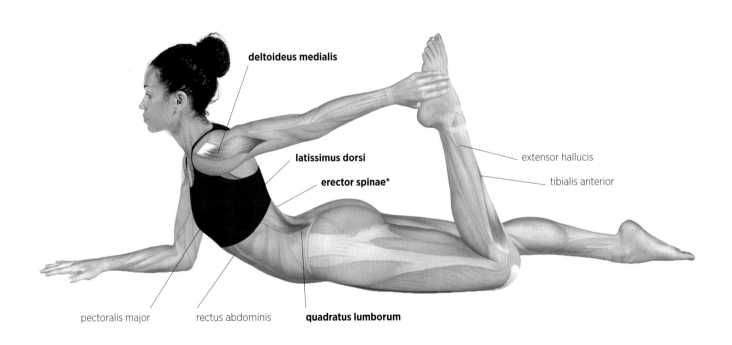

deltoideus medialis

latissimus dorsi

erector spinae*

extensor hallucis

tibialis anterior

pectoralis major

rectus abdominis

quadratus lumborum

Half Frog Pose

Half Frog Pose is an excellent preparation for Bow Pose (pages 192–93). It helps stretch and strengthen the muscles that will be used in the full expression of the pose.

HOW TO DO IT

- Lie facedown on a mat with your forearms and legs flat on the floor.

- Prop yourself up onto your forearms with your elbows directly beneath your shoulders.

- Bend your left knee, bringing your heel toward your left buttock. Shift your weight onto your right hand, and reach behind you with your left hand to grasp the inside of your left foot. Continue to lift your chest and push down with your right shoulder.

- Bend your left elbow up toward the ceiling, and rotate your hand so that it rests on top of your foot, with your fingers facing forward. Exhale and press down on your foot to stretch it toward your left buttock.

- Without separating your legs more than hip-width apart, deepen the stretch by moving your left foot slightly to the outside of your left thigh, aiming the sole of your foot toward the floor.

- Hold for the recommended breaths, and then repeat on the opposite side.

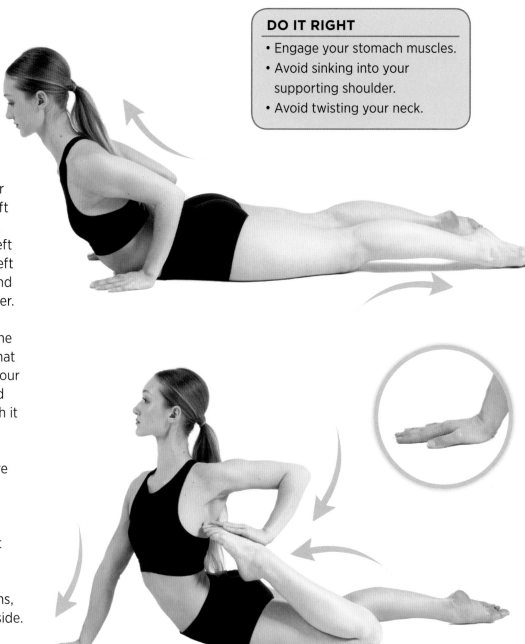

DO IT RIGHT

- Engage your stomach muscles.
- Avoid sinking into your supporting shoulder.
- Avoid twisting your neck.

TARGETS
• Hips
• Chest
• Shoulders
• Abdominals
• Thighs
• Ankles

BENEFITS
• Stretches shoulders, torso, neck, abdomen, thighs, hips, and ankles
• Strengthens back muscles
• Improves posture

CAUTIONS
• Lower-back issues
• Shoulder issues
• High or low blood pressure

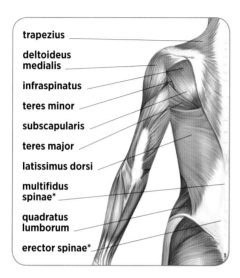

trapezius
deltoideus medialis
infraspinatus
teres minor
subscapularis
teres major
latissimus dorsi
multifidus spinae*
quadratus lumborum
erector spinae*

MODIFICATION
HARDER: Straighten your supporting arm, pressing away from the floor with your palm as you lift your chest upward.

Annotation Key
Bold text indicates target muscles
Light text indicates other working muscles
* indicates deep muscles

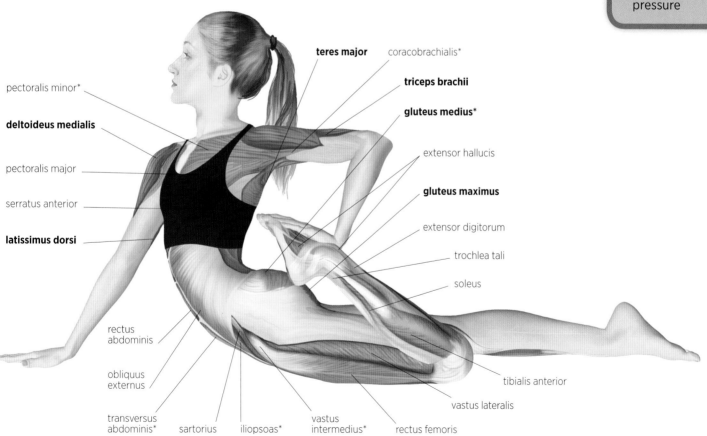

pectoralis minor*
deltoideus medialis
pectoralis major
serratus anterior
latissimus dorsi
rectus abdominis
obliquus externus
transversus abdominis*
sartorius
iliopsoas*
vastus intermedius*
rectus femoris
vastus lateralis
tibialis anterior
soleus
trochlea tali
extensor digitorum
gluteus maximus
extensor hallucis
gluteus medius*
triceps brachii
coracobrachialis*
teres major

Camel Pose

Camel Pose is a heart-opening backbend that stretches your shoulders and lower back. It also strengthens your thighs and expands your abdominal region, helping to improve digestion.

HOW TO DO IT

- Begin by kneeling with your body upright. Position your knees hip-width apart with your shins and feet aligned behind them. The tops of your feet should be on the floor, your toes pointing straight back.

- Bend your elbows, and bring your hands to your lower back, with your fingers pointing upward. Draw your elbows together, opening your chest. Internally rotate your thighs, and use the heels of your palms to draw your buttocks toward the floor as you lift out of your lower back.

- Bend from your upper back, and straighten your arms as you reach behind you to grasp your heels. Keep your hips directly above your knees; if your hips shift backward as you reach for your toes, keep your hands on your lower back. With practice, you will eventually be able to bend back to reach your heels.

- Broaden across your collarbones and press your shoulder blades in and up to open your chest and shoulders. Allow your head to drop back. Hold for the recommended breaths.

- To come out of the pose, exhale to lift your head and torso, and ease into Child's Pose (pages 132–33).

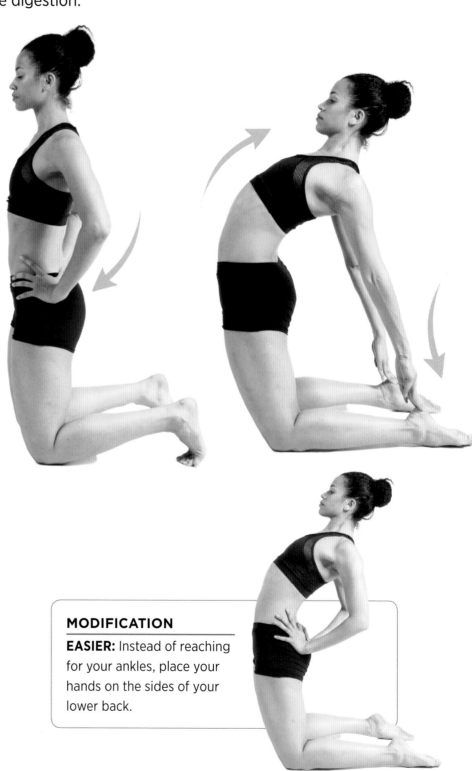

MODIFICATION

EASIER: Instead of reaching for your ankles, place your hands on the sides of your lower back.

SANSKRIT
- Ustrasana

TARGETS
- Hips
- Chest
- Shoulders
- Abdominals
- Thighs

BENEFITS
- Stretches hip flexors, thighs, and abdomen
- Opens shoulders and chest
- Improves posture

CAUTIONS
- Knee issues
- Lower-back issues
- Neck issues

DO IT RIGHT
- While bending backward, keep your thighs perpendicular to the floor.
- If your neck feels stressed when you drop your head back, just keep your head lifted and gaze forward.
- Avoid bending from your hips or arching your lower back.

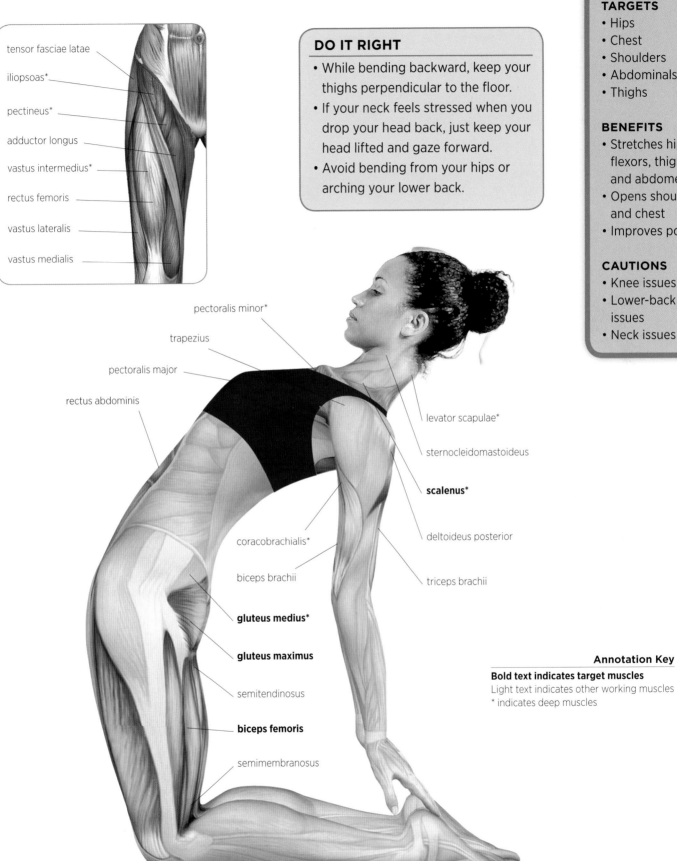

tensor fasciae latae

iliopsoas*

pectineus*

adductor longus

vastus intermedius*

rectus femoris

vastus lateralis

vastus medialis

pectoralis minor*

trapezius

pectoralis major

rectus abdominis

levator scapulae*

sternocleidomastoideus

scalenus*

deltoideus posterior

coracobrachialis*

biceps brachii

triceps brachii

gluteus medius*

gluteus maximus

semitendinosus

biceps femoris

semimembranosus

Annotation Key

Bold text indicates target muscles
Light text indicates other working muscles
* indicates deep muscles

Half Camel Pose

Practice this backbend to create flexibility along the front of your body and to increase your energy and vibrancy.

FACT FILE

SANSKRIT
• Ardha Ustrasana

TARGETS
• Hips
• Chest
• Shoulders
• Abdominals
• Thighs

BENEFITS
• Stretches hip flexors, thighs, and abdomen
• Opens shoulders and chest
• Improves posture

CAUTIONS
• Knee issues
• Lower-back issues
• Neck issues

HOW TO DO IT

• Begin in Camel Pose (pages 182–83), with your legs hip-width apart.

• Reach back with your left arm and place your left palm on the heel of your left foot, holding your foot lightly.

• Reach straight back with your right arm, and bring your thumb and index finger together, forming a circle. This hand position is called the Gyan Mudra, perhaps the most popular hand gesture in yoga. It symbolizes fire and air.

• Hold for the recommended breaths, and then repeat on the opposite side.

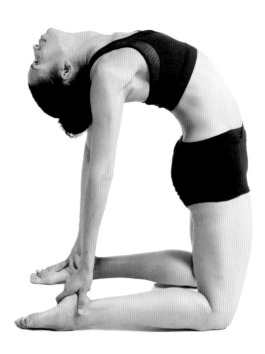

DO IT RIGHT

• Keep your outstretched arm parallel to the floor.

• Avoid widening your knees too much; they should be hip-width apart.

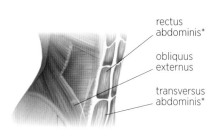

rectus abdominis*

obliquus externus

transversus abdominis*

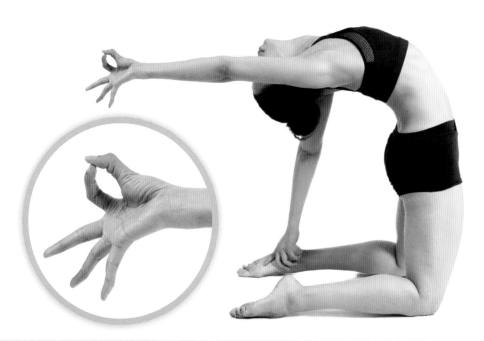

Extended Hand-to-Toe in Camel Pose

This variation of Camel Pose, which strengthens your back and hamstrings, requires good balance and excellent flexibility. Make sure you have warmed up with some basic arm and leg stretches before attempting this pose.

HOW TO DO IT

- Begin in Camel Pose (pages 182–83), with your legs hip-width apart.

- Swing your right leg out in front of you, and grab your big toe with your fingers. Begin to raise your leg with your knee locked.

- Balancing on your left hand, swing your leg around and up as straight and high as you can comfortably manage.

- Hold for the recommended breaths, and then repeat on the opposite side.

TARGETS
- Hips
- Chest
- Shoulders
- Abdominals
- Thighs

BENEFITS
- Stretches hip flexors, hamstrings, and abdomen
- Opens shoulders and chest
- Improves posture

CAUTIONS
- Knee issues
- Lower-back issues
- Neck issues

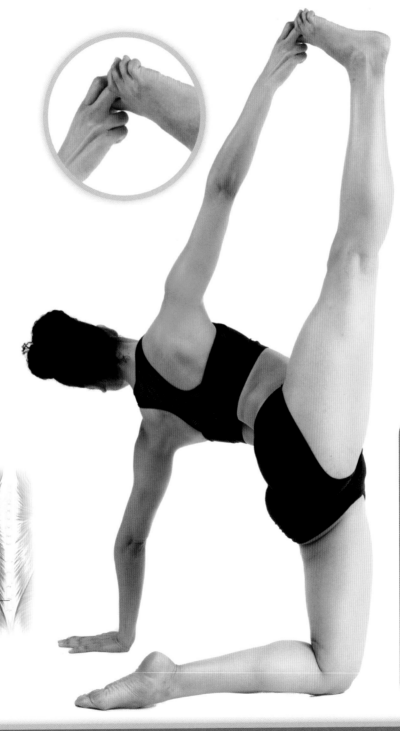

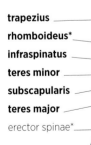

trapezius
rhomboideus*
infraspinatus
teres minor
subscapularis
teres major
erector spinae*

DO IT RIGHT

- Ease into this pose. Never force yourself into a position—that's a sure way to invite injury. Instead, concentrate on increasing flexibility and relaxing tense muscles.
- Avoid bending your raised leg or your raised arm.

Bridge Pose
Eye of the Needle

This variation of Bridge Pose targets the piriformis, one of the gluteal muscles. It requires deep muscle work to rotate your hip, turning your leg and foot outward as you raise your torso.

HOW TO DO IT

- Lie on your back with your arms extended at your sides. Bend your knees and place your feet flat on the mat. Raise your left leg and place your calf across your right knee.

- Press your palms into the floor and engage your abdominals as you lift your torso. Align your shoulders with your knees; your body should form a diagonal line.

- Hold for the recommended breaths, then slowly and with control, return to the starting position. Repeat on the opposite side.

DO IT RIGHT

- Squeeze your buttocks as you lift and lower.
- Draw your navel toward your spine.
- Press your shoulders down toward your back.
- Anchor your arms to the floor.
- Avoid tensing your neck; keep it relaxed.
- Avoid lifting your shoulders toward your ears.

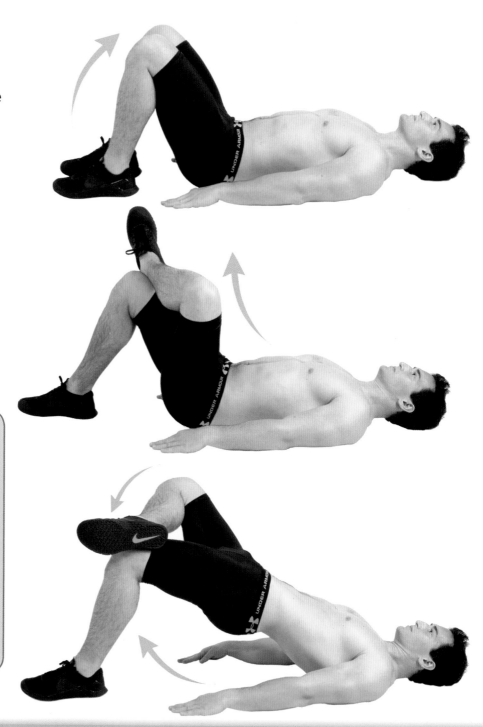

TARGETS
• Piriformis
• Spine
• Chest
• Thighs

BENEFITS
• Stretches piriformis
• Stretches chest and spine
• Strengthens thighs and buttocks
• Stimulates digestion
• Stimulates thyroid
• Reduces stress
• Stabilizes core

CAUTIONS
• Shoulder issues
• Back issues
• Neck issues

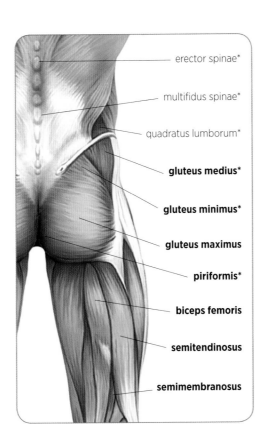

erector spinae*

multifidus spinae*

quadratus lumborum*

gluteus medius*

gluteus minimus*

gluteus maximus

piriformis*

biceps femoris

semitendinosus

semimembranosus

Annotation Key
Bold text indicates target muscles
Light text indicates other working muscles
* indicates deep muscles

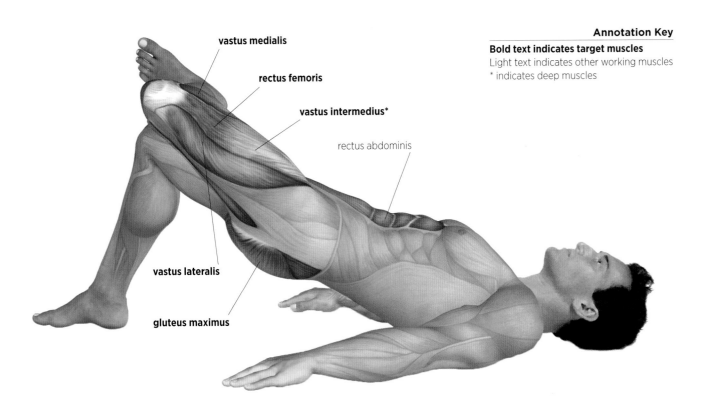

vastus medialis

rectus femoris

vastus intermedius*

rectus abdominis

vastus lateralis

gluteus maximus

One-Legged Bridge I

This Bridge Pose stretches your chest, spine, and thighs while strengthening your core and buttocks. It also eases stress by relieving tension in your back and shoulders.

HOW TO DO IT

- Lie on your back with your arms out to your sides. Bend your knees and align your feet directly under your knees.

- Exhale and press down through your feet to lift your buttocks off the floor. With your feet and thighs parallel, push your arms into the floor while extending through your fingertips.

- Lengthen your neck away from your shoulders. Lift your hips higher so that your torso rises from the floor.

- Straighten your right leg so that it is fully extended, forming a straight line from hip to toe.

- Hold for the recommended breaths, return to the starting position, and then repeat on the opposite side.

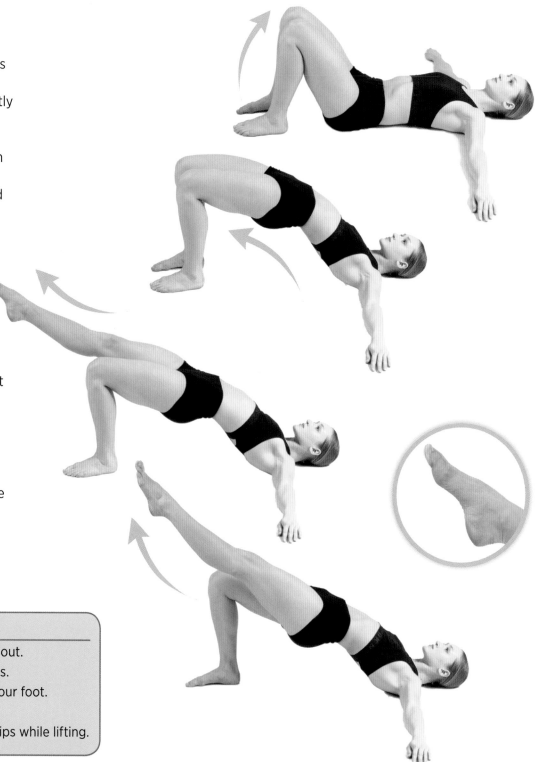

DO IT RIGHT
- Engage your buttocks throughout.
- Keep your hips level at all times.
- Extend your leg out through your foot.
- Avoid arching your back.
- Avoid twisting or tilting your hips while lifting.

SANSKRIT
• Setu Bandha
  Sarvangasana

TARGETS
• Spine
• Adominals
• Thighs
• Glutes

BENEFITS
• Stretches chest
  and spine
• Strengthens
  thighs and
  buttocks
• Stimulates
  digestion
• Stimulates thyroid
• Reduces stress

CAUTIONS
• Shoulder issues
• Back issues
• Neck issues
• Lower-back
  issues

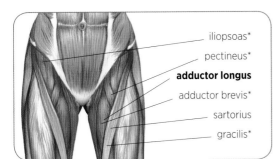

iliopsoas*
pectineus*
adductor longus
adductor brevis*
sartorius
gracilis*

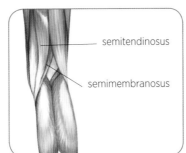

semitendinosus
semimembranosus

MODIFICATION

HARDER: Follow the first four steps and then draw your hands together above your chest, keeping your elbows straight. Hold for the recommended breaths, and then repeat on the opposite side.

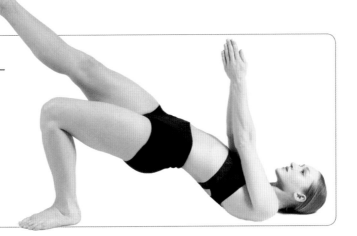

Annotation Key
Bold text indicates target muscles
Light text indicates other working muscles
* indicates deep muscles

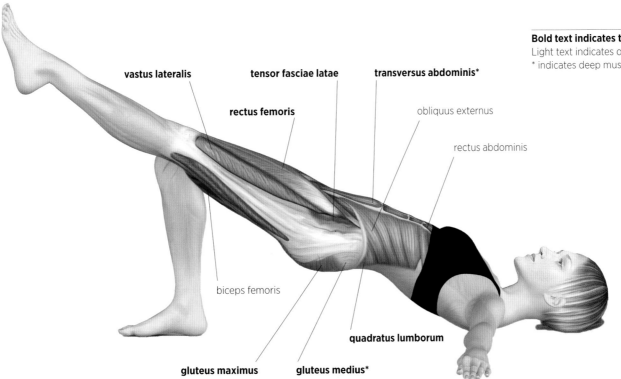

vastus lateralis
tensor fasciae latae
transversus abdominis*

rectus femoris

obliquus externus

rectus abdominis

biceps femoris

quadratus lumborum

gluteus maximus
gluteus medius*

One-Legged Bridge II

Yoga is known for developing sleek and strong torsos, and this variation of the Bridge Pose can help you develop strong abdominals and tight buttocks. When lifting, raise your body only as high as you can go while maintaining correct alignment. If you feel any straining in your lower back, you're going too far.

HOW TO DO IT

- Lie on your back with your arms at your sides. Bend your knees and align your feet directly under your knees. Extend one leg upward, pointing through your toes.

- Engage your abdominals to raise your torso from shoulders to hips into a stable one-legged bridge.

- Maintain this position, focusing on keeping your hips level, your navel pressing into your spine, and your free leg extending from your hip joint.

- Hold for the recommended breaths before lowering back to the mat, keeping your leg extended.

- Return to the starting position, and then repeat on the opposite side.

DO IT RIGHT
- Engage your buttocks throughout.
- Keep your hips level at all times.
- Extend your leg through your foot.
- Avoid arching your back.
- Avoid twisting or tilting your hips while lifting.

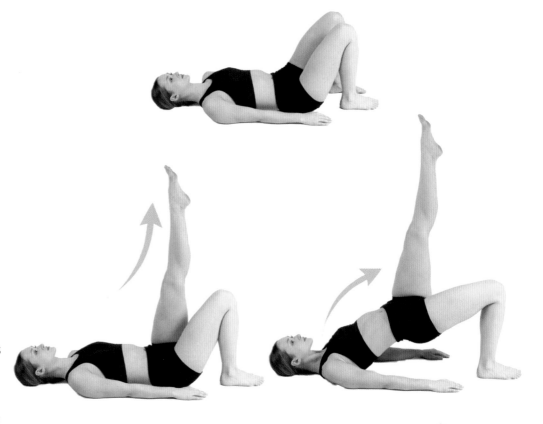

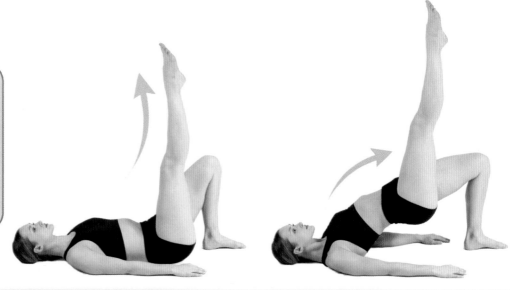

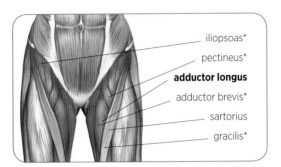

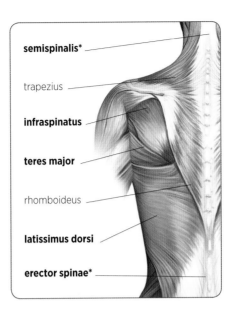

TARGETS
• Spine
• Adominals
• Thighs
• Glutes
• Lower back

BENEFITS
• Stretches chest and spine
• Strengthens thighs and buttocks
• Stimulates digestion
• Stimulates thyroid
• Reduces stress

CAUTIONS
• Shoulder issues
• Back issues
• Neck issues
• Lower-back issues

semispinalis*
trapezius
infraspinatus
teres major
rhomboideus
latissimus dorsi
erector spinae*

iliopsoas*
pectineus*
adductor longus
adductor brevis*
sartorius
gracilis*

Annotation Key

Bold text indicates target muscles
Light text indicates other working muscles
* indicates deep muscles

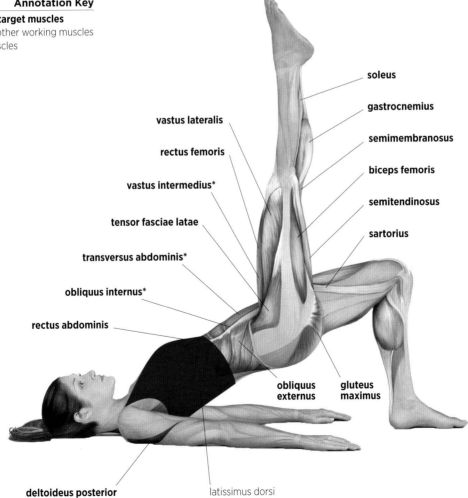

soleus
gastrocnemius
semimembranosus
biceps femoris
semitendinosus
sartorius

vastus lateralis
rectus femoris
vastus intermedius*
tensor fasciae latae
transversus abdominis*
obliquus internus*
rectus abdominis

obliquus externus
gluteus maximus

deltoideus posterior
latissimus dorsi

Bow Pose

Bow Pose works to strengthen your whole body, engaging your back, arms, abdominals, and legs, while stretching your neck, chest, hips, groin, thighs, and ankles. It also increases your circulation. In the Sanskrit name, Dhanurasana, "Dhanur" means "bow-shaped." This pose resembles the image of a bow ready to shoot an arrow.

HOW TO DO IT

• Begin by lying on your stomach, with your forehead resting on a mat and your arms and legs extended straight behind you. Ground your pelvis and lower abdomen into the mat to create a foundation for the pose.

• Keep your legs hip-width apart and bend both knees at the same time until your ankles and shins are in line over your knees.

• On an inhale, reach your arms back and wrap your hands around the outsides of your ankles.

• As you exhale, lift your chest and thighs away from the mat, keeping your arms straight. Ease your feet away from your head to help lift your chest higher.

• Create internal rotation in both thighs, allowing your inner thighs to move up toward the ceiling. Draw your tailbone slightly downward to alleviate any crunching in your lower back. Balance on your navel as you find equal extension between the lift of your chest and that of your legs. Hold for the recommended breaths.

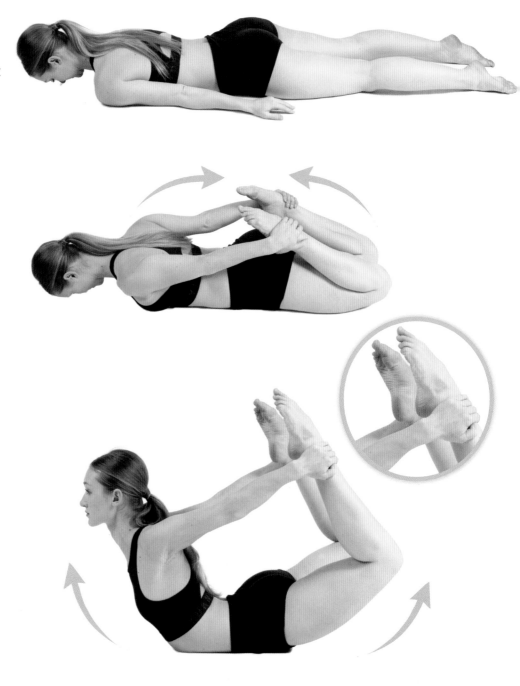

TARGETS
• Back
• Spine
• Chest
• Shoulders

BENEFITS
• Stretches shoulders, chest, abdomen, and thighs
• Strengthens spine
• Aids digestion and circulation
• Massages the abdominal organs

CAUTIONS
• Lower-back issues
• Knee pain
• Shoulder issues
• Pregnancy

DO IT RIGHT

• Lengthen your tailbone to create space for your lower back.
• Squeeze your shoulder blades toward each other to help lift your chest.
• Lift your chest and thighs simultaneously.
• Avoid externally rotating your thighs.

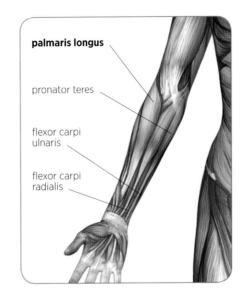

palmaris longus

pronator teres

flexor carpi ulnaris

flexor carpi radialis

Annotation Key

Bold text indicates target muscles
Light text indicates other working muscles
* indicates deep muscles

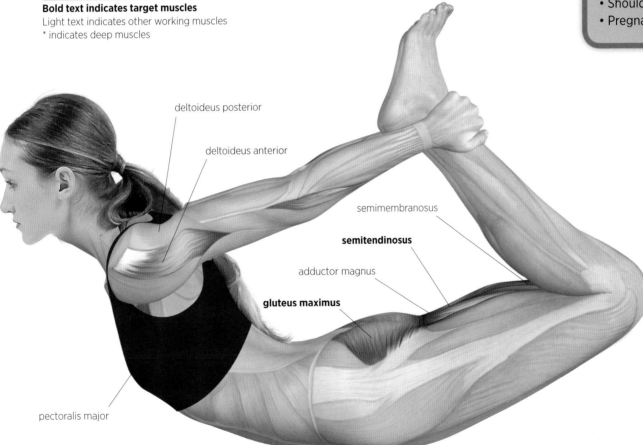

deltoideus posterior

deltoideus anterior

semimembranosus

semitendinosus

adductor magnus

gluteus maximus

pectoralis major

Wheel Pose

The invigorating and energizing Wheel Pose is a deep, challenging backbend that strengthens the entire body, and stretches the chest and rib cage. It is excellent for the heart, liver, and kidneys, and can be beneficial to those who suffer from asthma and osteoporosis.

HOW TO DO IT

- Begin by lying on your back, with your knees bent and your feet hip-width apart. Inhale and stretch your arms straight up to the ceiling, with your palms facing away from you. Then, bend your arms and place your hands on the floor next to your ears, shoulder-width apart, with your fingers facing the same direction as your toes.

- Press your hands and feet into the floor as you lift your hips up, as if you were coming into Bridge Pose (pages 168–69).

- Lift yourself onto the crown of your head. Pause and press your palms into the floor, spreading your fingers wide and grounding down through every knuckle and through the base of your thumb and index finger.

- Straighten your arms, and move your outer upper arms inward to find external rotation. Press down through all four corners of your feet, shifting your weight onto your heels. Roll your inner thighs toward the floor as you firm your outer hips inward. Let your head fall between your shoulders in a comfortable position. Hold for the recommended breaths.

- To come out of the pose, bend your arms and shift your body weight toward your shoulders as you slowly descend, landing on the back of your head and your shoulder blades.

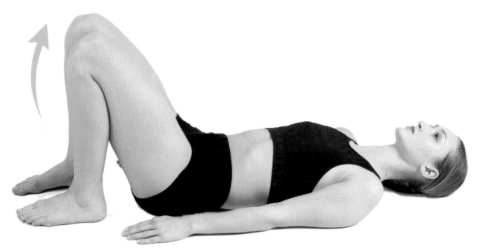

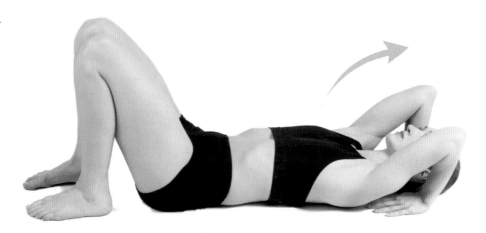

DO IT RIGHT

- Keep your feet parallel, even as you transition into and out of the pose.
- After lifting yourself onto the crown of your head, squeeze your elbows toward each other to keep them positioned over your wrists.
- While holding the pose, draw your tailbone down toward your knees and lift your frontal hip bones up toward your ribs.
- Avoid letting your thighs externally rotate, which can cause compression in your lower back.

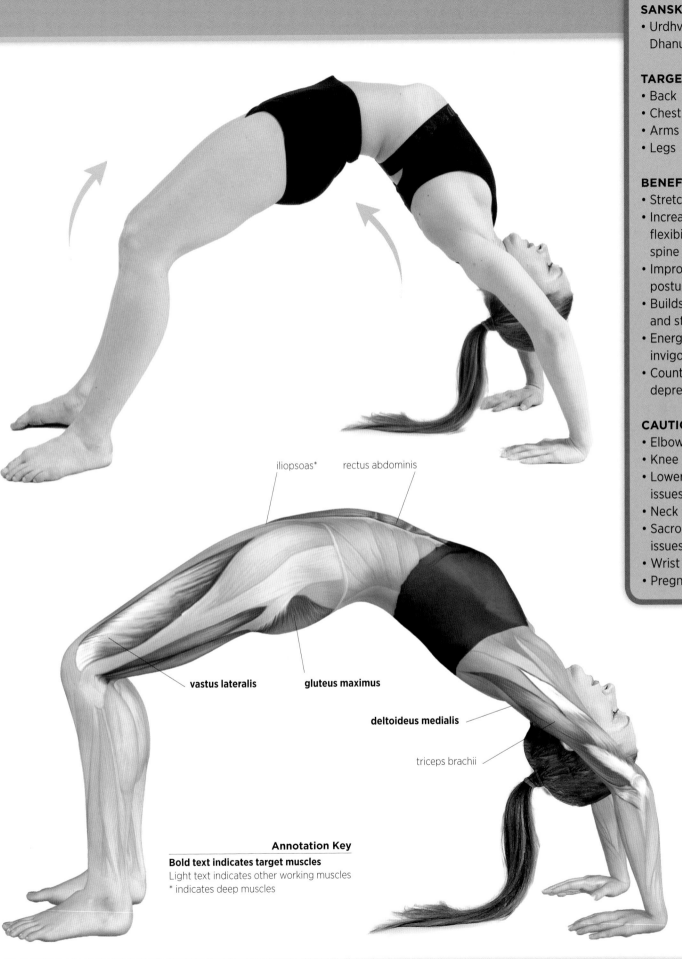

FACT FILE

SANSKRIT
• Urdhva Dhanurasana

TARGETS
• Back
• Chest
• Arms
• Legs

BENEFITS
• Stretches chest
• Increases flexibility in spine
• Improves posture
• Builds stamina and strength
• Energizes and invigorates
• Counteracts depression

CAUTIONS
• Elbow issues
• Knee issues
• Lower-back issues
• Neck issues
• Sacroiliac joint issues
• Wrist issues
• Pregnancy

iliopsoas*

rectus abdominis

vastus lateralis

gluteus maximus

deltoideus medialis

triceps brachii

Annotation Key

Bold text indicates target muscles
Light text indicates other working muscles
* indicates deep muscles

Fish Pose

Fish Pose, often used as a counterpose to Shoulderstand, stretches the front of your body, including your neck, chest, abdominals, and hip flexors as well as your intercostal muscles between your ribs. It also strengthens your upper back and the muscles at the back of your neck, improving mobility and posture.

HOW TO DO IT

- Begin by lying on your back with your knees bent and your feet on your mat. Place your hands slightly underneath your buttocks and ease your hips off the mat.

- Press your palms, elbows, and forearms into the mat and draw your shoulder blades together as you lift your head and chest off the mat.

- With the top of your head resting on the mat, extend your legs straight. Internally rotate your thighs and press them downward. Reach out through the balls of your feet as you hold for the recommended breaths.

DO IT RIGHT

- While holding the pose, engage your stomach muscles to support your lower back.
- Avoid letting your torso sink into your lower back.

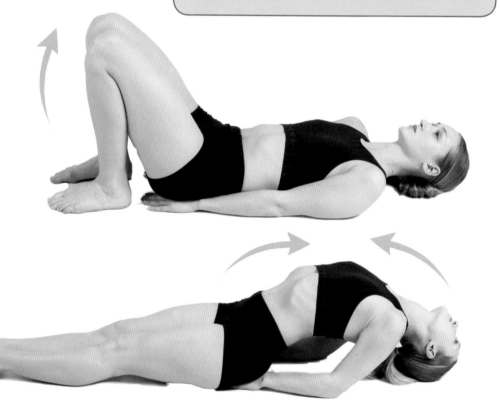

MODIFICATION

EASIER: Try placing a block underneath your thoracic spine and another beneath your head, to turn Fish Pose into a restorative backbend.

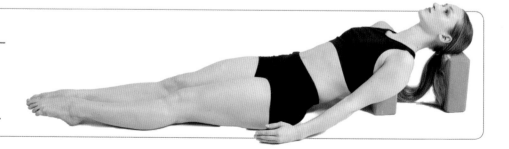

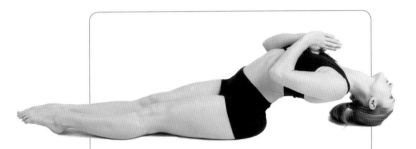

MODIFICATION

HARDER: Instead of resting your forearms and hands on the mat, bring your hands to your chest with your palms together in prayer position.

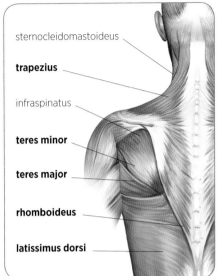

sternocleidomastoideus

trapezius

infraspinatus

teres minor

teres major

rhomboideus

latissimus dorsi

FACT FILE

SANSKRIT
• Matsyasana

TARGETS
• Anterior torso
• Upper back
• Back of neck

BENEFITS
• Opens chest
• Relieves tightness in upper back and neck
• Stretches hip flexors and muscles between ribs
• Improves posture

CAUTIONS
• Lower-back issues
• Neck issues

Annotation Key

Bold text indicates target muscles
Light text indicates other working muscles
* indicates deep muscles

serratus anterior   pectoralis major

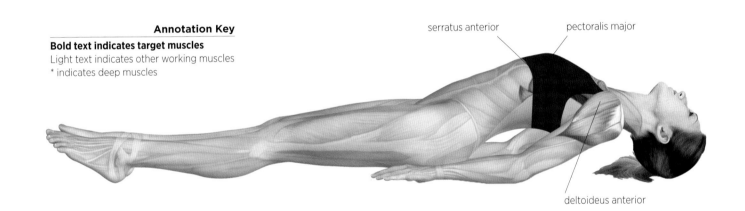

deltoideus anterior

MODIFICATION

HARDER: To make the pose even more challenging, keep your legs together and extended as you lift them off the mat—making sure that you maintain your form.

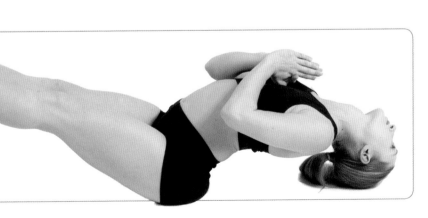

One-Legged King Pigeon Pose Prep

This pose allows the student to prepare for the more challenging series of advanced One-Legged Pigeon Poses. It opens up your chest and shoulders, stretches your thighs, groin, and abdominals, and can be used to relieve stress, anxiety, and fatigue.

HOW TO DO IT

- Begin by kneeling with your buttocks resting lightly on your heels and your arms at your sides, supporting some of your weight.

- Extend your left leg behind you, keeping your leg aligned with your body, including your right knee, which should be facing straight forward.

- Move your arms forward to rest slightly in front of your right knee. Your hands should be shoulder-width apart, and your palms flat on the mat.

- Move your right foot under your left hip.

- Hold for the recommended breaths, and then repeat on the opposite side.

DO IT RIGHT

- Be sure to maintain a slight bend in your elbows.
- Lean primarily on your bent leg.
- Avoid hyperextending your elbows.

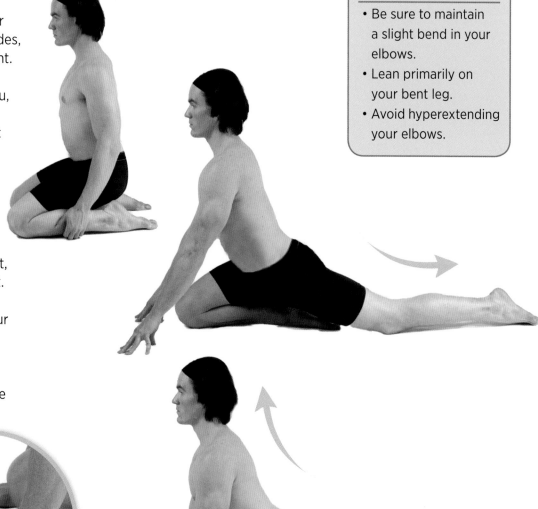

SANKRIT
• None

TARGETS
• Gluteal area
• Groin muscles
• Hamstrings
• Quadriceps

BENEFITS
• Stretches lower
  body and
  upper legs
• Opens chest
  and shoulders

CAUTIONS
• Groin injury
• Hamstring
  issues

MODIFICATION

HARDER: For an even
more advanced stretch,
lean your torso forward
until your head is resting
on your crossed forearms.

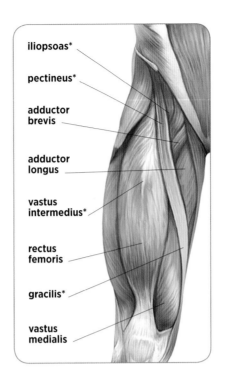

iliopsoas*
pectineus*
adductor brevis
adductor longus
vastus intermedius*
rectus femoris
gracilis*
vastus medialis

Annotation Key

Bold text indicates target muscles
Light text indicates other working muscles
* indicates deep muscles

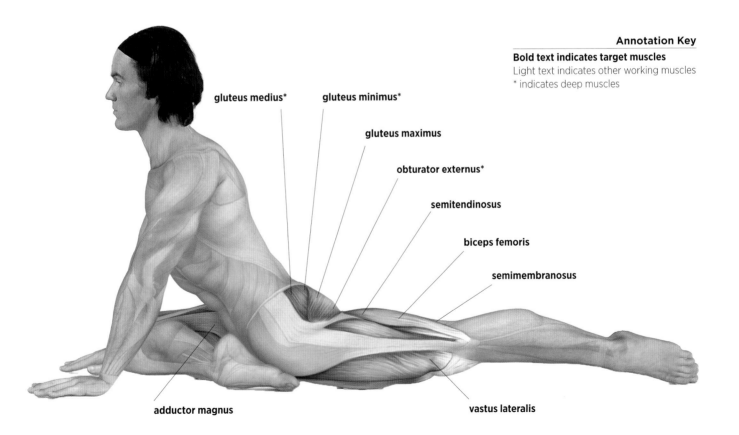

gluteus medius*
gluteus minimus*
gluteus maximus
obturator externus*
semitendinosus
biceps femoris
semimembranosus
adductor magnus
vastus lateralis

One-Legged King Pigeon Pose I

This advanced pose requires a great deal of flexibility; it stretches the thighs, groin, and abdominals while relieving tension in the chest and shoulders. By stimulating the abdominal organs, it also aids digestion.

HOW TO DO IT

• Begin in Downward-Facing Dog (pages 268–69). Bend your left knee, and bring it forward, in between your hands. Place your left leg on the mat with your knee still bent, lowering your shin and thigh to the floor. Your left heel should point toward your pubis.

• Extend your right leg behind you. Your hips should be squared forward, and your right knee should point down toward the mat.

• Lift your chest, using your fingertips to bring your torso to an upright position. Press down into the mat with your hips and pubis, and lift up with your chest.

• Bend your right knee and flex your foot, drawing your right heel toward your buttock. Reach back with your right hand, your palm facing up, and grasp your toes from the outside of your foot. You may keep your left fingertips on the mat in front of you for balance.

• Point your right elbow up toward the ceiling, pull your sternum upward, and point your toes. Drop your head back, and reach your left arm over your head to grasp your toes with your left hand. Pull your foot toward your head.

• Hold for the recommended breaths. Return to Downward-Facing Dog, and repeat on the opposite side.

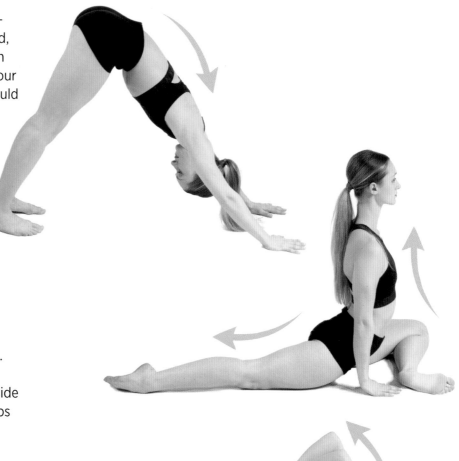

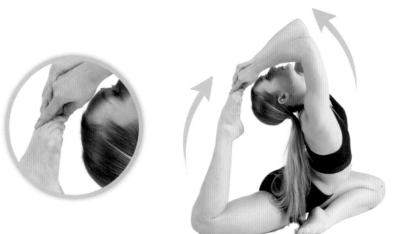

TARGETS
• Chest
• Shoulders
• Hips
• Groin

BENEFITS
• Stretches upper body
• Strengthens spine
• Opens hips and groin
• Eases digestion

CAUTIONS
• Hip injury
• Back issues
• Knee injury

DO IT RIGHT

• Keep your hips squared forward throughout the pose.
• Sit as deeply as possible into the leg position, drawing your groin toward the floor.
• Avoid compensating for tight shoulders and chest by compressing your lower back.
• Avoid rolling your rear knee to either side.

Annotation Key

Bold text indicates target muscles
Light text indicates other working muscles
* indicates deep muscles

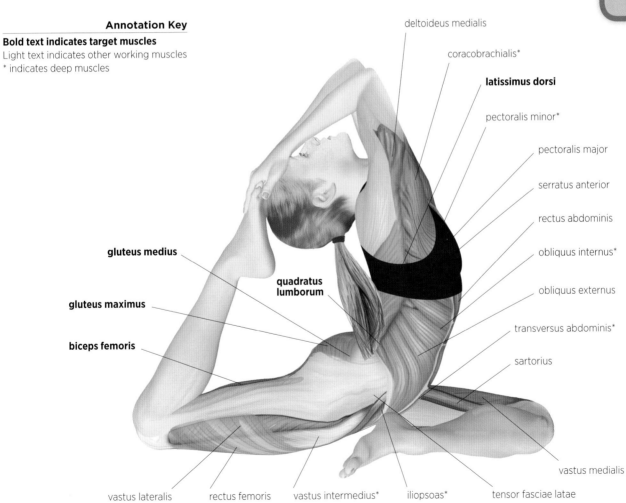

deltoideus medialis

coracobrachialis*

latissimus dorsi

pectoralis minor*

pectoralis major

serratus anterior

rectus abdominis

obliquus internus*

obliquus externus

transversus abdominis*

sartorius

vastus medialis

tensor fasciae latae

iliopsoas*

vastus intermedius*

rectus femoris

vastus lateralis

biceps femoris

gluteus maximus

gluteus medius

quadratus lumborum

One-Legged King Pigeon Pose II

This is another challenging pose that requires flexibility in your hips, thighs, spine, and shoulders. Make sure that you have prepared for this pose by practicing the Prep and by warming up with other poses that focus on flexibility.

HOW TO DO IT

- From Downward-Facing Dog (pages 268–69), inhale and raise your right leg up behind you.

- On an exhale, bend your right knee into your chest and then lower your body so that your right knee is on the mat in front of you. Your right foot should be facing left, and your right shin and foot should be on the floor. Draw your right shin slightly forward, and flex your right ankle to keep your knee in alignment.

- Extend your left leg behind you, with the top of your foot on the floor and your toes pointing straight back.

- Slowly lift your torso upright, bend your left knee, and hold your foot with your left hand. Lift up out of your lower back by drawing your tailbone down as you tilt your pubic bone toward your frontal hip bones.

- Bring your foot into the crook of your left elbow. Reach your right arm up, bending your elbow toward the ceiling, and clasp your hands together as you continue to square your hips and shoulders. Hold for the recommended breaths, and then repeat on the opposite side.

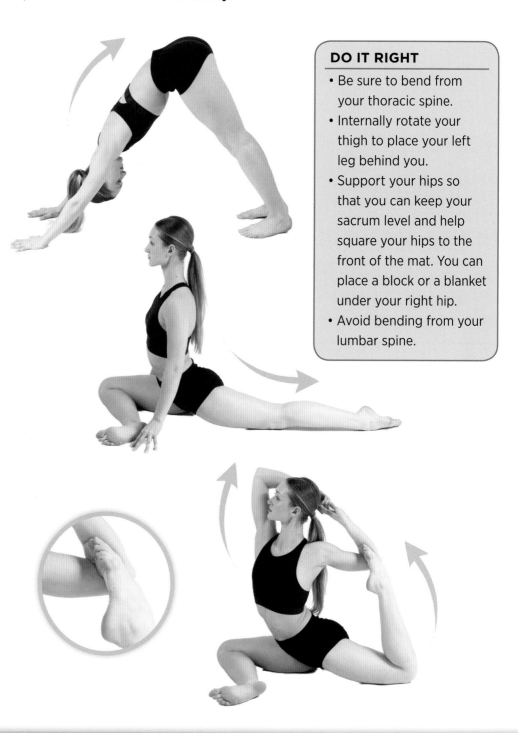

DO IT RIGHT

- Be sure to bend from your thoracic spine.
- Internally rotate your thigh to place your left leg behind you.
- Support your hips so that you can keep your sacrum level and help square your hips to the front of the mat. You can place a block or a blanket under your right hip.
- Avoid bending from your lumbar spine.

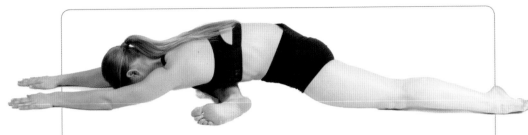

MODIFICATION

EASIER: Try making the pose more restorative by "walking" your hands in front of you and releasing your torso into a forward bend. Place your forehead on the floor and hold for the recommended breaths.

FACT FILE

SANSKRIT
• Eka Pada Rajakapotasana

TARGETS
• Chest
• Shoulders
• Hips
• Spine

BENEFITS
• Stretches thighs, hips, groin, abdomen, chest, shoulders, and spine
• Opens chest and shoulders
• Improves posture

CAUTIONS
• Ankle issues
• Hip or quadricep stiffness
• Knee issues
• Lower-back issues

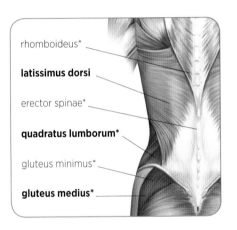

rhomboideus*
latissimus dorsi
erector spinae*
quadratus lumborum*
gluteus minimus*
gluteus medius*

Annotation Key

Bold text indicates target muscles
Light text indicates other working muscles
* indicates deep muscles

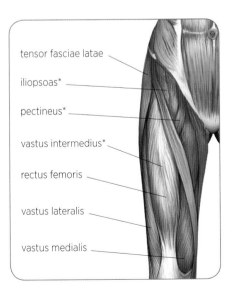

tensor fasciae latae
iliopsoas*
pectineus*
vastus intermedius*
rectus femoris
vastus lateralis
vastus medialis

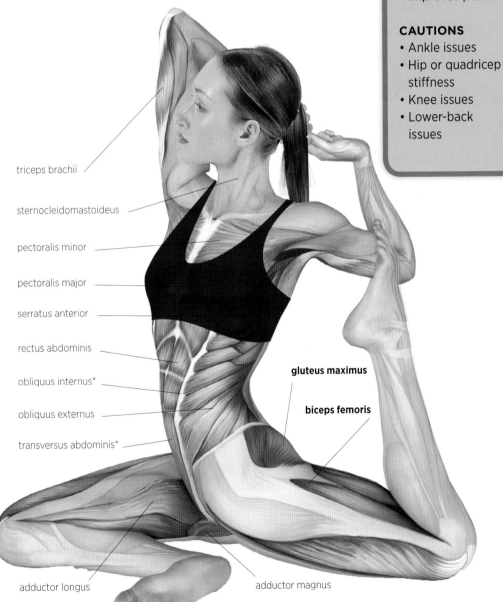

triceps brachii
sternocleidomastoideus
pectoralis minor
pectoralis major
serratus anterior
rectus abdominis
obliquus internus*
obliquus externus
transversus abdominis*

gluteus maximus

biceps femoris

adductor longus
adductor magnus

One-Legged King Pigeon Pose III

This advanced version of the One-Legged King Pigeon Pose deeply stretches your hips, legs, and groin, while opening your chest and shoulders.

HOW TO DO IT

- While in basic King Pigeon Pose I (pages 200–01), unbend your right leg and extend it forward, with your toes pointed. Release your right hand from your left foot, so that only your left hand is grasping your toes.

- Hold for the recommended breaths, and then repeat on the opposite side.

FACT FILE
SANSKRIT
- Eka Pada Rajakapotasana

TARGETS
- Arms
- Back
- Hips
- Core

BENEFITS
- Opens chest and shoulders
- Increases flexibility in spine and hips

CAUTIONS
- Neck injury
- Hip injury
- Back issues
- Groin issues

DO IT RIGHT
- Your chin should be pointed up as you hold the pose.
- Avoid rotating your extended leg inward.

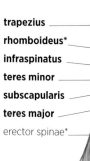

trapezius
rhomboideus*
infraspinatus
teres minor
subscapularis
teres major
erector spinae*

Annotation Key
Bold text indicates target muscles
Light text indicates other working muscles
* indicates deep muscles

One-Legged King Pigeon Pose IV

This pose stretches the thighs, abdominals, groin, shoulders, neck, and chest and is believed to stimulate the abdominal organs. Make sure to keep your glutes, hamstrings, and pelvic floor fully engaged.

HOW TO DO IT

- While in One-Legged King Pigeon Pose I (pages 200–01), holding the toes of your left foot with your hands, straighten your right leg and extend it forward.

- Decrease the amount of arch in your back and raise your head so that your neck is now in a neutral position.

- Hold for the recommended breaths, and then repeat on the opposite side.

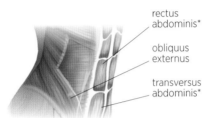

rectus abdominis*

obliquus externus

transversus abdominis*

Annotation Key

Bold text indicates target muscles
Light text indicates other working muscles
* indicates deep muscles

DO IT RIGHT

- Be sure to relax your head, but do not let it roll backward.
- Avoid letting the hip of your rear leg sink toward the mat.

FACT FILE

SANSKRIT
- Eka Pada Rajakapotasana

TARGETS
- Arms
- Spine
- Abdomen
- Hips
- Glutes

BENEFITS
- Opens chest and shoulders
- Stretches spine and hips

CAUTIONS
- Back injury
- Hip injury
- Groin issues

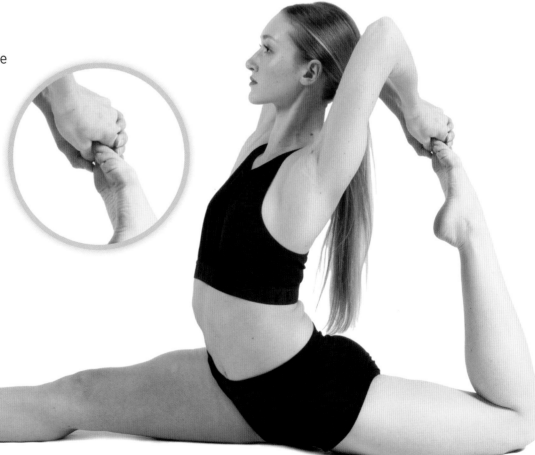

King Cobra Pose

This advanced pose provides a deep backbend and a powerful stretch across the front of your body. It is effective for increasing the flexibility of your spine and hips, while strengthening your abdomen and lengthening your hamstrings.

HOW TO DO IT

- Begin by lying facedown. Place your hands on the mat under your shoulders with your fingers spread and your arms snug against your body. Keep your legs straight, with your knees as wide as the mat. Concentrate on reaching your tailbone toward your knees and pressing your pubic bone into the mat. This supports your lower back.

- Roll your outer thighs toward the floor and your inner thighs toward the ceiling. Inhale and straighten your arms as you lift your upper torso from the mat. Draw your shoulder blades back and relax them away from your ears.

- Bend your knees and squeeze your heels toward your glutes. You should feel your back muscles lighting up.

- Tilt your head back, point your feet, and bring your head and toes toward each other. Do not collapse your neck into your shoulders; rather, lift up from your shoulders. Hold for the recommended breaths.

DO IT RIGHT

- During the pose, your chin should be pointed at the ceiling.
- Don't let your neck collapse down into your shoulders.

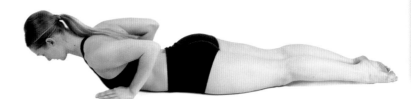

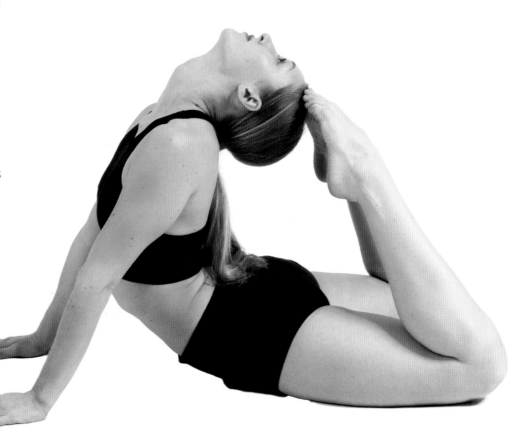

FACT FILE

SANSKRIT
- Raja Bhujangasana

TARGETS
- Upper body
- Spine
- Thighs

BENEFITS
- Stretches shoulders, chest, abdomen, and thighs
- Strengthens spine
- Aids digestion
- Massages the abdominal organs

CAUTIONS
- Lower-back issues
- Knee pain
- Shoulder issues
- Pregnancy

Big Toe Bow Pose

You will become truly extended in the Big Toe Bow Pose, so prepare before you attempt it by doing several basic stretching poses. Big Toe Bow Pose is very effective in opening your chest and broadening your shoulders. It also improves flexibility in your spine and hips.

HOW TO DO IT

- While in Bow Pose (pages 192–93)—with your legs raised, your back arched, and your hands on your ankles—slide your hands up to grasp your toes.

- Increase the arch of your back, extend your neck, and tilt your head back so that your gaze is on the ceiling.

- Draw your legs high above your back, as far as is comfortable. Hold for the recommended breaths.

FACT FILE

SANSKRIT
- Padangustha Dhanurasana

TARGETS
- Hips
- Back
- Legs
- Abdominals

BENEFITS
- Stretches hamstrings, spine, and glutes
- Strengthens abdomen
- Increases hip flexibility

CAUTIONS
- Neck issues
- Lower-back issues
- Groin injury

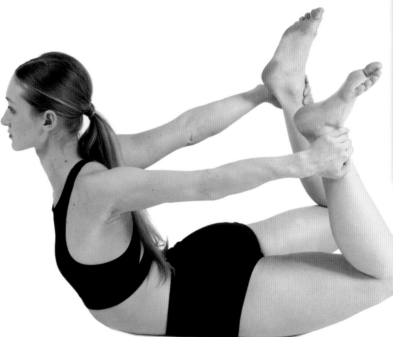

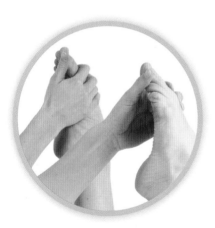

DO IT RIGHT

- Make sure you are comfortably flexed and not straining in the pose.
- Avoid rolling your head too far back.

Toes-to-Elbow Bow Pose

In this version of the Bow Pose, be sure that you keep your neck relaxed; do not tilt your head back. The arching should take place only with your back.

HOW TO DO IT

• Lie prone on a mat with your arms at your sides.

• Place your chin on the mat, and exhale as you bend your knees. Reach your arms behind you, and grasp the outside of your ankles.

• Inhale and lift your chest off the mat. Simultaneously lift your thighs by pulling your ankles up with your hands. Shift your weight onto your abdominals.

• Slide your hands along the tops of your shins until your toes reach under your inner elbows, positioning your calves and feet as close to your buttocks as is comfortable.

• Keep your head in a neutral position. Tuck your tailbone into your pubis.

• Hold for the recommended breaths. Exhale and release your legs, gently returning them to the mat.

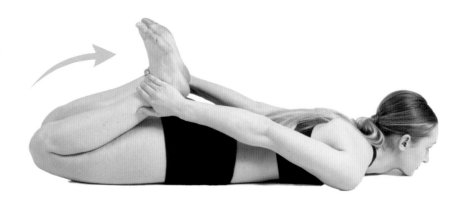

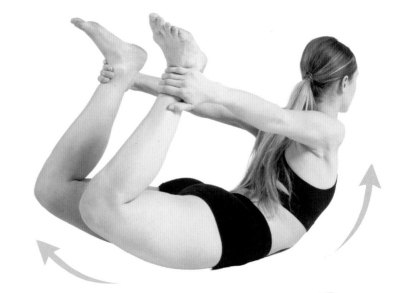

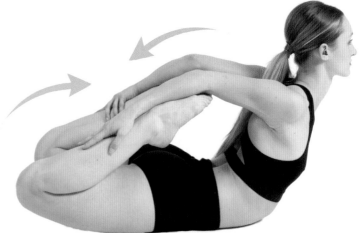

SANSKRIT
• Dhanurasana

TARGETS
• Upper body
• Back
• Thighs
• Hips

BENEFITS
• Strengthens spine
• Stretches chest, abdomen, hip flexors, and quadriceps
• Stimulates digestion

CAUTIONS
• Headache
• High or low blood pressure
• Back injury

DO IT RIGHT

• Keep your knees close together; they should not separate more than hip-width.
• Avoid holding your breath. Breathing in this pose can be difficult, so take short, controlled breaths.
• Avoid rolling back onto your pelvis to support your weight.

brachioradialis

rhomboideus*

anconeus

deltoideus posterior

palmaris longus

triceps brachii

pronator teres

pectoralis minor*

flexor carpi pollicis longus

deltoideus anterior

pectoralis major

multifidus spinae*

erector spinae*

extensor digitorum

brachialis

gluteus medius*

gluteus maximus

gemellus superior*

iliopsoas*

obturator externus*

rectus femoris

vastus medialis

biceps femoris

semitendinosus

Annotation Key

Bold text indicates target muscles
Light text indicates other working muscles
* indicates deep muscles

Lord of the Dance Pose

The Sanskrit name of this pose, Natarajasana, refers to the Hindu god Shiva, who is known as the Lord of the Dance. This pose requires a strong sense of balance and is very effective at opening your hips and shoulders.

HOW TO DO IT

• Begin standing in Mountain Pose (pages 32–33). Bend your right knee, and draw your right heel toward your buttocks. Contract the muscles of your left thigh. Keep both hips open.

• Turn your right palm outward, reach behind your back, and grasp the inside of your right foot. Lift through your spine, from your tailbone to the top of your neck.

• Raise your right foot toward the ceiling, and push back against your right hand. At the same time, lift your left arm up toward the ceiling, and bring your left thumb and index finger together in Gyan Mudra, a gesture of unity.

• Lift your chest and arm to help you stand upright and increase your flexibility, rather than tilting your torso forward as you raise your back leg.

• Hold for the recommended breaths. Release your foot, and repeat on the opposite side.

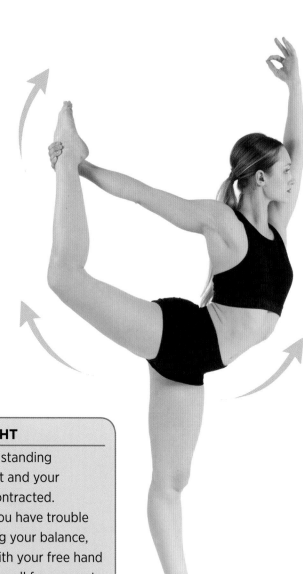

DO IT RIGHT

• Keep your standing leg straight and your muscles contracted.
• If at first you have trouble maintaining your balance, practice with your free hand touching a wall for support.
• Avoid looking down at the floor, which can cause you to lose your balance.
• Avoid compressing your lower back.

SANSKRIT
• Natarajasana

TARGETS
• Thighs
• Groin
• Chest
• Shoulders

BENEFITS
• Stretches thighs, groin, abdomen, shoulders, and chest
• Strengthens spine, thighs, hips, and ankles
• Improves balance

CAUTIONS
• Back injury
• Low blood pressure

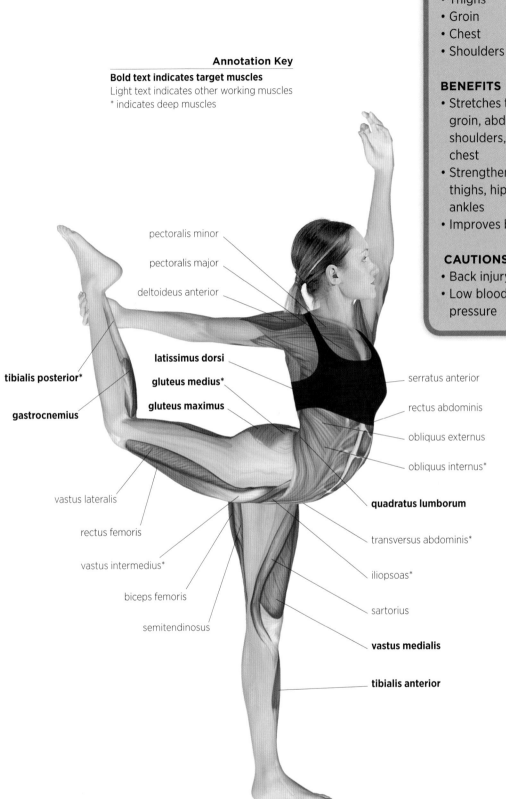

Annotation Key

Bold text indicates target muscles
Light text indicates other working muscles
* indicates deep muscles

pectoralis minor

pectoralis major

deltoideus anterior

latissimus dorsi

tibialis posterior*

gluteus medius*

gluteus maximus

gastrocnemius

serratus anterior

rectus abdominis

obliquus externus

obliquus internus*

quadratus lumborum

vastus lateralis

transversus abdominis*

rectus femoris

iliopsoas*

vastus intermedius*

sartorius

biceps femoris

vastus medialis

semitendinosus

tibialis anterior

MODIFICATION

HARDER: Follow the first step. Turn your right palm outward, but instead of grasping the inside of your right foot, reach for the outside of your foot. Rotate your shoulder so that your right elbow points up toward the ceiling. Lift your leg and open your chest. Reach over your head with your left arm, bending your elbow, and grasp the top of your raised foot. Slowly walk your fingers back until both hands are holding your toes.

Bound Lord of the Dance Pose

This more challenging variation of Lord of the Dance Pose stretches and strengthens your shoulders, chest, spine, legs, and ankles. It also opens your hips, and lengthens your hamstrings.

HOW TO DO IT

• Begin by standing in Mountain Pose (pages 32–33). Fix your gaze on something stationary nearby, such as a vase or lamp. Bend your right leg, and draw the heel toward your buttocks. Catch your right ankle with your right hand. It's okay to wobble until you find your balance.

• Bow by pressing your right foot into your right hand as you hinge forward at the waist.

• Continue to arch your spine as you reach your left arm around the front of your body to hold your right foot. Using your left hand, begin to work your right foot inside the crook of your right arm, all the while maintaining your balance.

• Once your right foot is firmly tucked in your right arm, press your right elbow behind you. Extend your left arm overhead to reach back to clasp the fingers of your right hand.

• Maintain an even breath as you continue to tuck your right foot into your arm, arching forward to deepen the backbend, and lifting your gaze.

• Hold for the recommended breaths, and then release your right hand, and lower your foot. Return to the starting position, and then repeat on the opposite side.

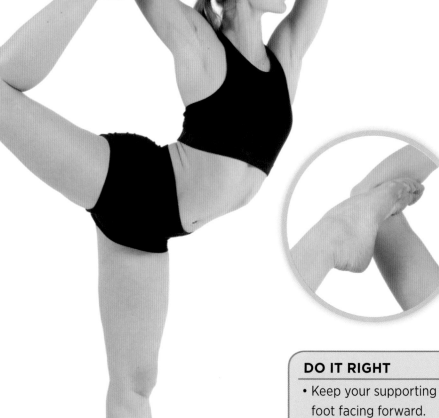

FACT FILE

SANSKRIT
• Natarajasana

TARGETS
• Shoulders
• Chest
• Back
• Legs

BENEFITS
• Opens hips and chest
• Stretches thighs
• Increases spinal flexibility

CAUTIONS
• Back issues
• Shoulder injury

DO IT RIGHT

• Keep your supporting foot facing forward.
• Engage the hamstrings of your extended leg to deepen the stretch.
• Avoid tipping your head too far back; your chin should be parallel to the floor.

Hand-to-Foot Lord of the Dance Pose

In this version of the pose, begin by consciously shifting the weight of your body to your stationary foot as you raise your other leg. It improves balance while stretching your shoulders, chest, thighs, and groin and strengthening your legs and ankles. Like all extended poses that involve opposite arm-leg connections, it works the muscles of your abdomen and sides.

HOW TO DO IT

- In Mountain Pose (pages 32–33), bend your right knee and raise your right heel toward your buttocks.

- Reach back with your right hand, palm outward, and grasp your toes.

- Rotate your shoulder so that your right elbow points to the ceiling.

- Rotate your left hand back to grasp your right wrist. Walk your left hand up until both hands are grasping your right toes.

- Hold for the recommended breaths, release your leg, and then repeat on the opposite side.

DO IT RIGHT
- Make sure you are flexing from your mid and lower back.
- If at first you have trouble grasping your raised foot in these poses, try using a foot strap until your flexibility improves.
- When in position, your thighs should almost form a straight vertical line.
- Avoid tipping your head back; your gaze should be facing straight ahead.

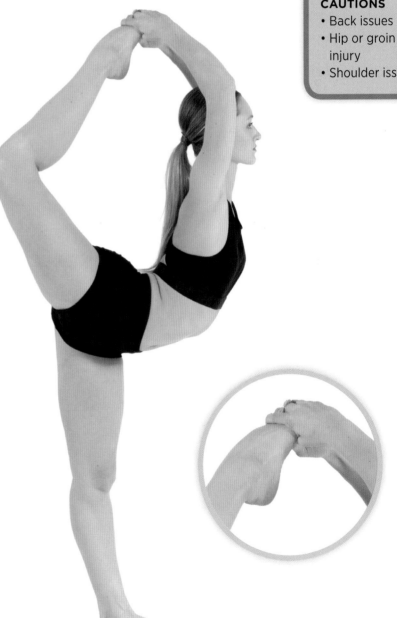

One-Legged Inverted Locust Pose

Extended lower-body leg lifts require intense focus, but they are a great way to work on your abdominals, obliques, and back muscles, while improving spinal flexibility.

HOW TO DO IT

- Start in a kneeling position. Bring your palms onto the mat with your fingers splayed on either side of your knees and facing the rear of the mat.

- Bend your arms and lean forward, putting the weight of your chest onto the backs of your upper arms and your chin, creating a tripod.

- Extend your left leg straight behind you, balancing on the top of your foot. Kick your right leg into a split above you.

- Hold for the recommended breaths, ease yourself back down to kneeling position, and repeat on the opposite side.

DO IT RIGHT

- Be sure to anchor yourself with downward pressure from your arms and hands.
- Don't overdo the width of the split until you have achieved the needed flexibility.
- Avoid swaying or wobbling.

FACT FILE

SANSKRIT
- Salabhasana

TARGETS
- Stomach
- Sides
- Back
- Thighs

BENEFITS
- Stretches abdominals, obliques, and spine
- Strengthens core and thighs
- Improves flexibility and balance

CAUTIONS
- Groin injury
- Neck injury
- Lower-back issues

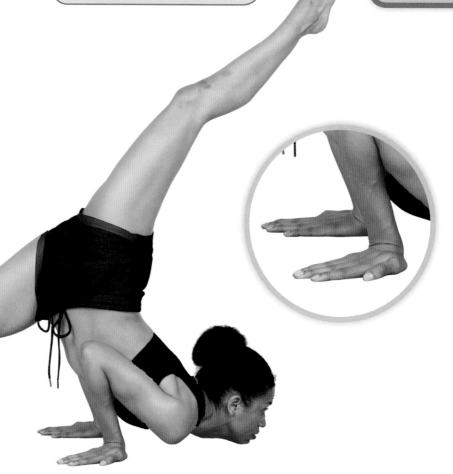

Raised Inverted Locust Pose

This challenging extended lower-body lift requires both upper-body and core strength, as well as flexibility in your back. Perform this pose at your own speed—raise your feet only as high as is comfortable. With time and practice, you will be able to increase the lift until your legs are fully extended.

HOW TO DO IT

• Start in a kneeling position.

• Bring your palms down to the floor with your fingers splayed on either side of your knees and facing the rear of the mat.

• Bend your arms and lean forward, putting the weight of your chest onto the backs of your upper arms and onto the side of your head, creating a tripod.

• Kick one leg at a time into Locust posture, keeping your toes pointed to the ceiling.

• Hold for the recommended breaths.

FACT FILE

SANSKRIT
• Salabhasana

TARGETS
• Shoulders
• Back
• Wrists
• Core

BENEFITS
• Strengthens upper body and core
• Increases spinal flexibility
• Improves balance

CAUTIONS
• Neck injury
• Wrist issues

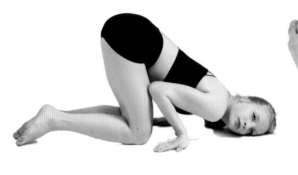

DO IT RIGHT

• Be sure to anchor yourself with pressure from your arms and hands.
• Avoid swaying or wobbling.

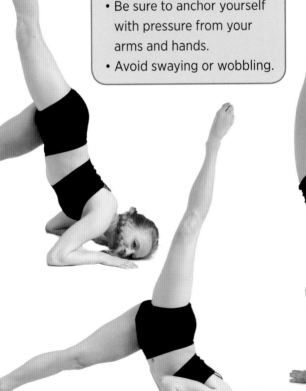

CHAPTER FIVE

SEATED POSES AND TWISTS

Seated poses are mainstays of yoga, typically the poses you assume when you practice meditation or work on breathing exercises. Many of these poses prepare you for more complicated postures. The seated twists are believed to detoxify the body: each time you twist your torso, you are "massaging" your internal organs, helping to improve your digestion.

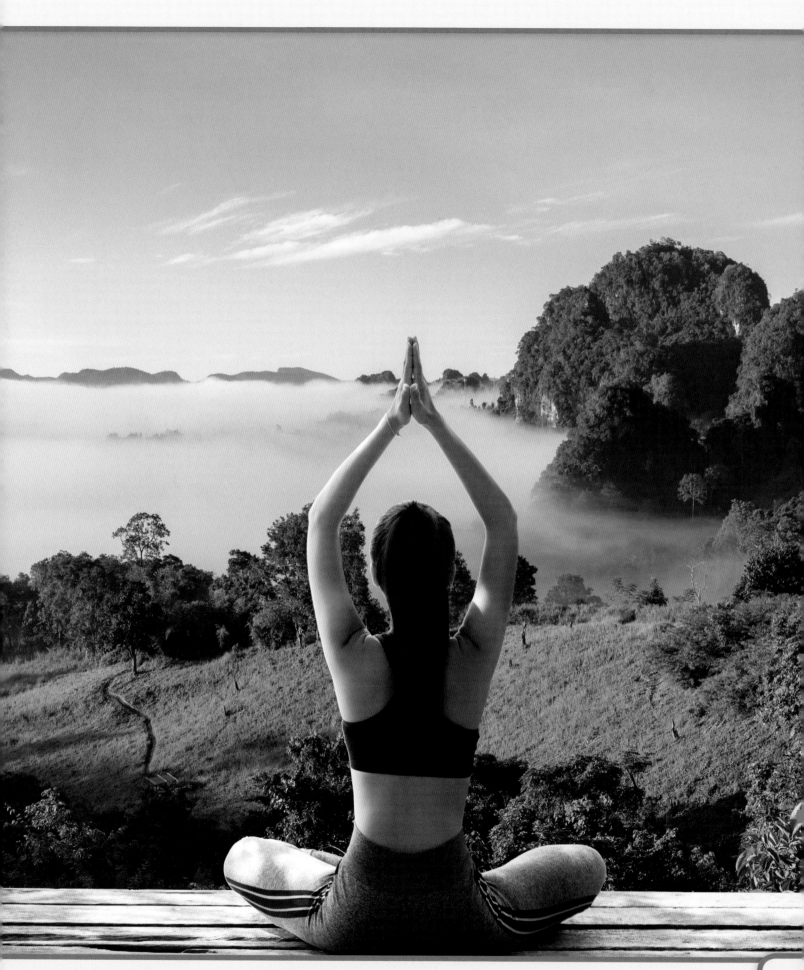

Staff Pose

Staff Pose is a foundational posture, forming the basis for many other seated poses. It is a deceptively easy pose, but keep in mind that you must perfect your form to receive its full benefits.

HOW TO DO IT

- Sit up tall, with your legs pressed together and extended in front of you. Firm your thighs into the floor, activating your legs. Flex your feet, drawing your toes back toward your torso as you press your heels forward.

- With your pelvis in a neutral position, sit toward the front of your sit bones as your tailbone roots into the floor. Position your arms by your sides, with your hands pressed into the floor.

- Engage your abdominals, lifting your energy upward—from the base of your tailbone to the crown of your head. Hold for the recommended breaths.

DO IT RIGHT

- Keep your legs firm and active.
- Draw your shoulder blades together.
- If you find that your lower back is rounding and your pelvis tucks under when your legs are straight, try sitting on a block or blanket.
- Avoid sticking out your ribs.

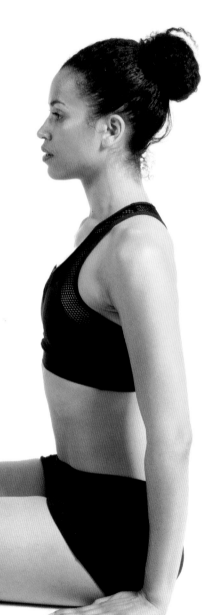

SANSKRIT
• Dandasana

TARGETS
• Spine
• Legs

BENEFITS
• Improves posture
• Stretches legs
• Strengthens spine

CAUTIONS
• Lower-back pain
• Tight hamstrings

Annotation Key

Bold text indicates target muscles
Light text indicates other working muscles
* indicates deep muscles

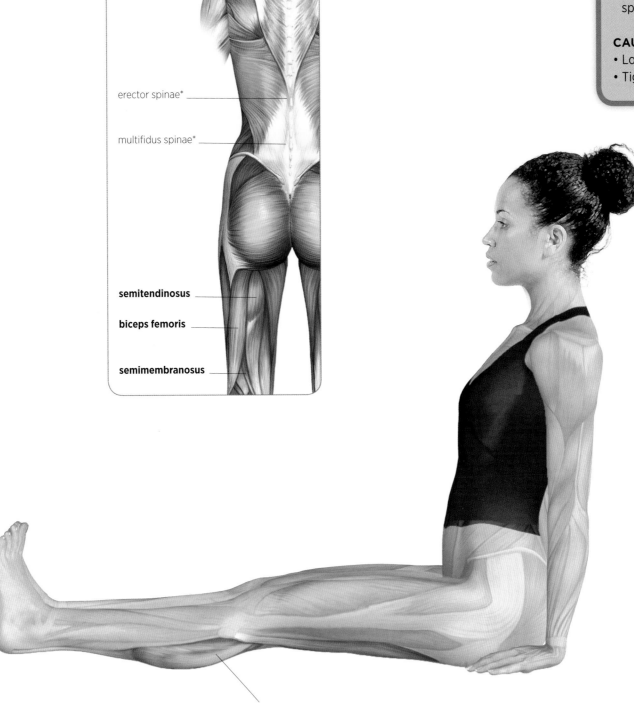

erector spinae*

multifidus spinae*

semitendinosus

biceps femoris

semimembranosus

gastrocnemius

Easy Pose

This beginner pose may look simple, but if your hamstrings, lower back, or hip flexors are tight, it might prove difficult. As you practice this pose, it will become increasingly more comfortable. Over time, you will be able to assume this pose and even sustain it during meditation.

HOW TO DO IT

• Sit on the floor, bend your knees, and cross your legs at the shins. Flex your feet to keep your knees in alignment. Press both sit bones firmly into the floor and find a neutral pelvis. Sit up straight to lengthen your spine and open your collarbones.

• Place your hands on your thighs with your palms facing either up or down.

• Close your eyes and draw your focus inward. Increase the length of your inhalations and exhalations, aiming for equal length. Hold the pose for the recommended breaths.

DO IT RIGHT

• If this is difficult at first, sit on a block or blanket to elevate your hips above your knees.
• Alternate your legs when crossing your shins. We all have a dominant side; allow your less dominant side to stretch, and find balance in your hips by alternating the top leg.
• Avoid letting your knees rise above your hips.
• Avoid rounding your shoulders.

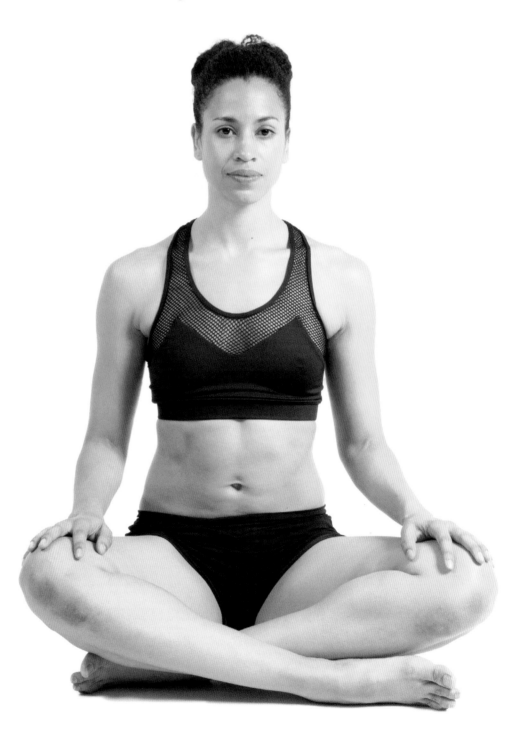

FACT FILE

SANSKRIT
- Sukhasana

TARGETS
- Hips
- Back
- Abdominals

BENEFITS
- Stretches hips
- Strengthens back
- Calms mind and body

CAUTIONS
- Knee issues

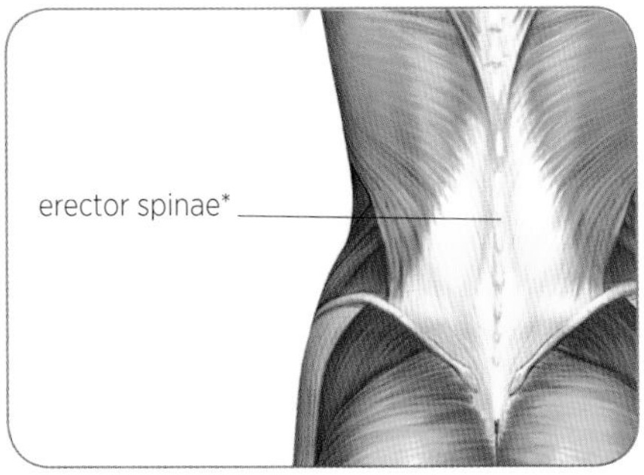

erector spinae*

Annotation Key

Bold text indicates target muscles
Light text indicates other working muscles
* indicates deep muscles

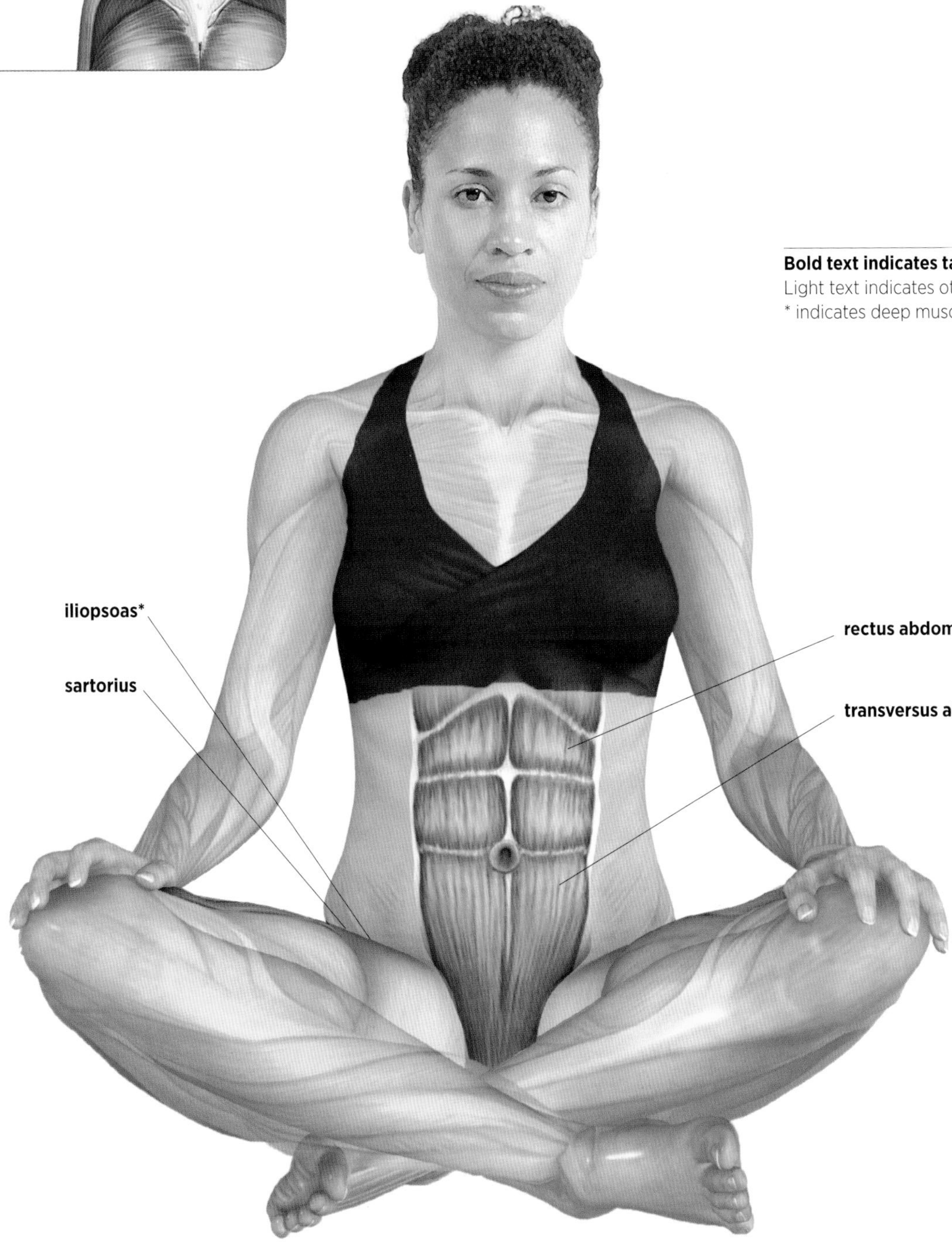

iliopsoas*
sartorius
rectus abdominis
transversus abdominis*

Bound Angle Pose

A beginner pose that benefits practitioners at all levels, Bound Angle Pose opens your hips. To execute this pose properly, try aiming your navel—not your head—toward your feet.

HOW TO DO IT

• Begin by sitting in Staff Pose (pages 218–19).

• Bend both knees, and bring the soles of your feet together as you draw your feet in toward your pelvis, keeping your knees apart.

• Hold your ankles, and press the pinkie-toe side of your feet together to open the insides of your feet, as if you were opening a book.

• Inhale as you lengthen your sternum and open your collarbones. Hold for the recommended breaths.

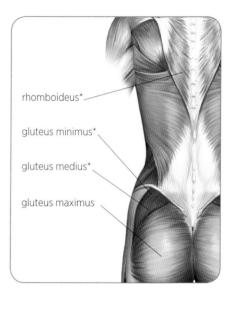

rhomboideus*

gluteus minimus*

gluteus medius*

gluteus maximus

DO IT RIGHT

• Create a straight line from your sit bones to your shoulders.
• Avoid rounding your upper back.
• Avoid forcing your knees down.

SANSKRIT
• Baddha Konasana

TARGETS
• Thighs
• Groin
• Spine

BENEFITS
• Stretches inner and outer thighs, groin, and spine
• Calms mind

CAUTIONS
• Groin issues

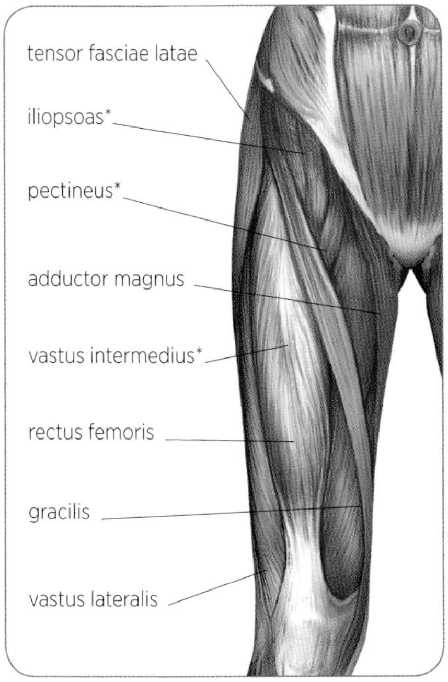

tensor fasciae latae

iliopsoas*

pectineus*

adductor magnus

vastus intermedius*

rectus femoris

gracilis

vastus lateralis

Annotation Key

Bold text indicates target muscles
Light text indicates other working muscles
* indicates deep muscles

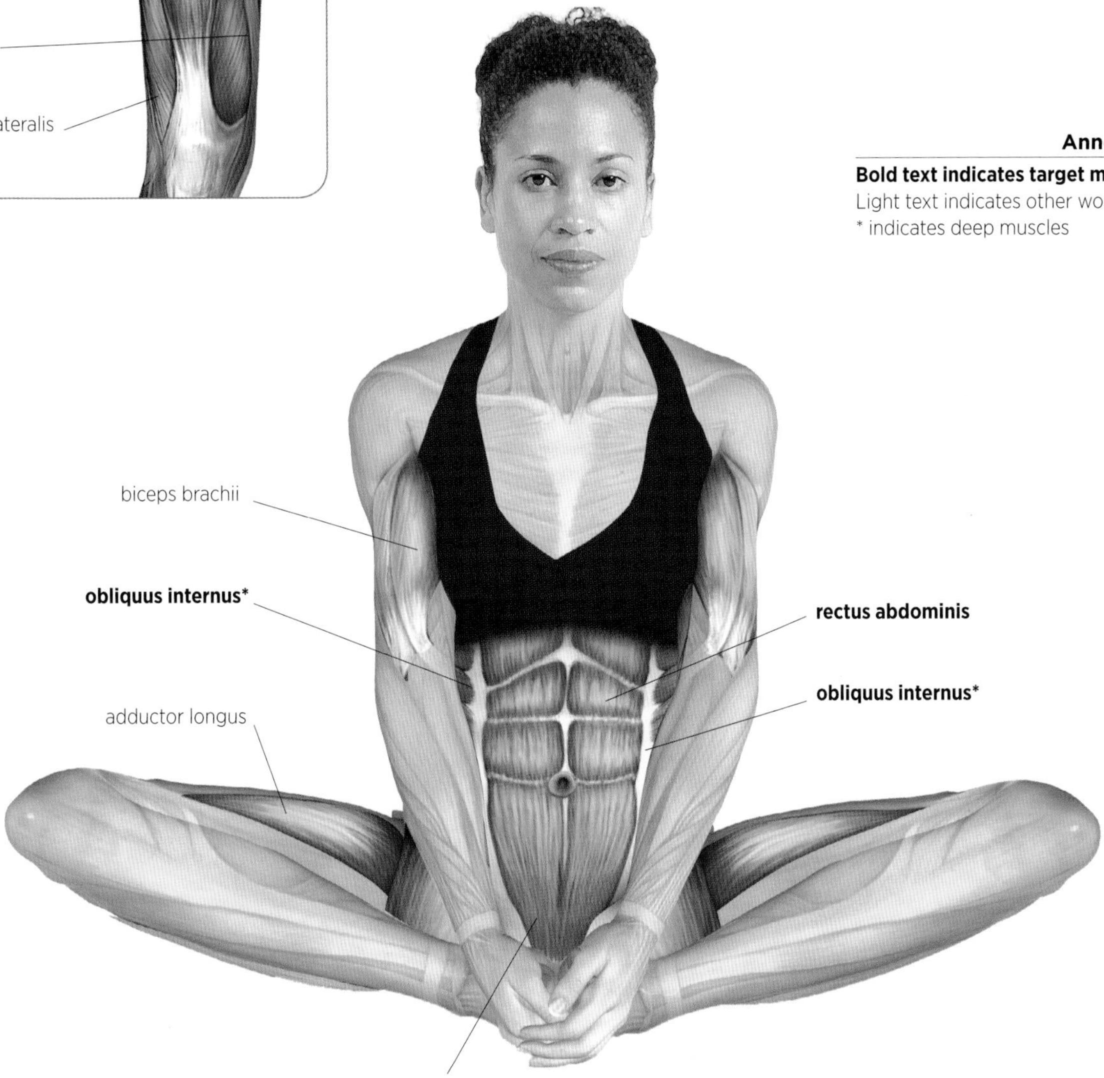

biceps brachii

obliquus internus*

rectus abdominis

obliquus internus*

adductor longus

transversus abdominis*

Hero Pose

This classical seated yoga posture stretches your thighs and ankles and also improves your posture. You can sit in Hero Pose to meditate as an alternative to Lotus Pose (pages 248–49) or Easy Pose (pages 220–21).

HOW TO DO IT

• Kneel on the floor, resting on your knees and shins, with the tops of your feet flat on the floor and toes pointing back.

• Bring your knees together while moving your feet to slightly wider than hip-width apart. You can use your fingers on the backs of your knees to roll the flesh of your calves down toward your heels.

• Sit your buttocks down between your heels, keeping your torso upright. Find internal rotation in your thighs, pressing them downward. Lengthen your tailbone down toward your heels as you lift your pubic bone up toward your navel.

• Rest your hands on your thighs, with your palms facing up in a gesture of receiving and energizing, or down for a more grounding and calming effect. Hold for the recommended breaths.

DO IT RIGHT

• Draw your shoulder blades together.
• Avoid sticking your ribs outward.

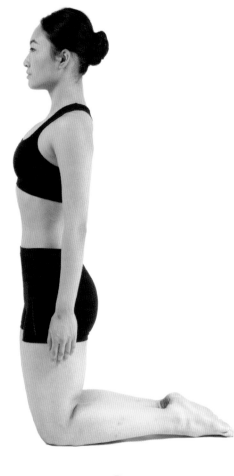

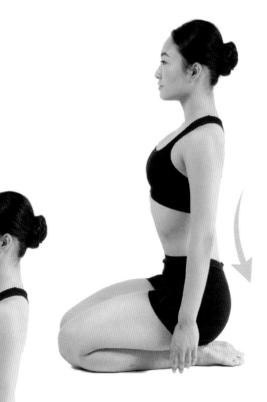

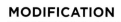

MODIFICATION

EASIER: If your thighs feel tight, try sitting on a block or two.

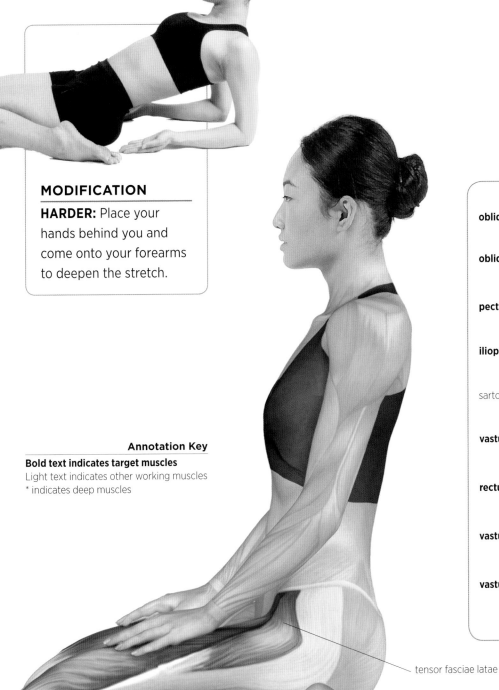

SANSKRIT
• Virasana

TARGETS
• Thighs
• Shins

BENEFITS
• Stretches
  thighs, knees,
  and ankles

CAUTIONS
• Ankle issues
• Knee issues

MODIFICATION

HARDER: Place your
hands behind you and
come onto your forearms
to deepen the stretch.

Annotation Key

Bold text indicates target muscles
Light text indicates other working muscles
* indicates deep muscles

obliquus internus*

obliquus externus

pectineus*

iliopsoas*

sartorius

vastus intermedius*

rectus femoris

vastus medialis

vastus lateralis

tensor fasciae latae

tibialis anterior

extensor hallucis

peroneus

Marichi's Pose

More formally known as Pose Dedicated to the Sage Marichi III, this asana takes its name from Marichi, a Hindu seer credited with intuiting the divine law of the universe. It is a beginner seated twist that conditions your hips and spine.

HOW TO DO IT

• Sit in Staff Pose (pages 218–19). Bend your right knee, pulling your heel toward your groin. Keep your left leg extended with your knee pointed up toward the ceiling, and focus on keeping your leg grounded. Place your hands on the floor by your sides.

• Pushing your right foot and left leg into the floor, inhale and lift up through your spine and chest. Keep both sit bones on the floor, and relax your shoulders.

• Exhale and begin twisting toward your right knee. Wrap your left hand around the outside of your right thigh, pulling your knee in toward your abdominals. Press the fingertips of your right hand into the floor behind your hips.

• Turn your head to the right, and place your left elbow on the outside of your right knee. Lean back slightly, leading with your upper torso to help twist your entire spine.

• Hold for the recommended breaths, and then gently untwist as you exhale, and repeat on the opposite side.

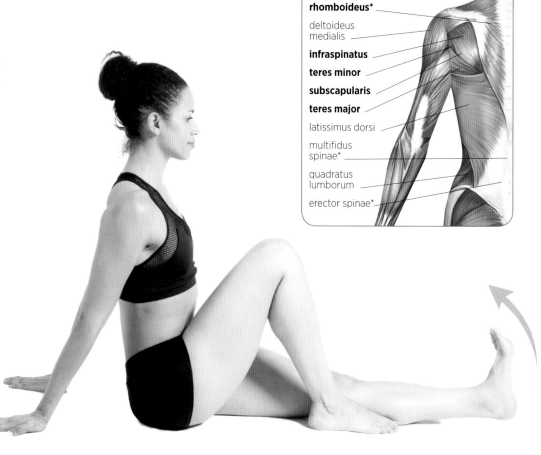

trapezius
rhomboideus*
deltoideus medialis
infraspinatus
teres minor
subscapularis
teres major
latissimus dorsi
multifidus spinae*
quadratus lumborum
erector spinae*

DO IT RIGHT

• Keep both sit bones on the floor.
• Twist from the bottom up—rotate from your lower spine, through your torso, and up through your chest.
• Avoid tensing your shoulders up toward your ears.
• Avoid rounding your spine.
• Avoid forcing a deep twist—gently ease your body into the rotation while maintaining the correct posture.

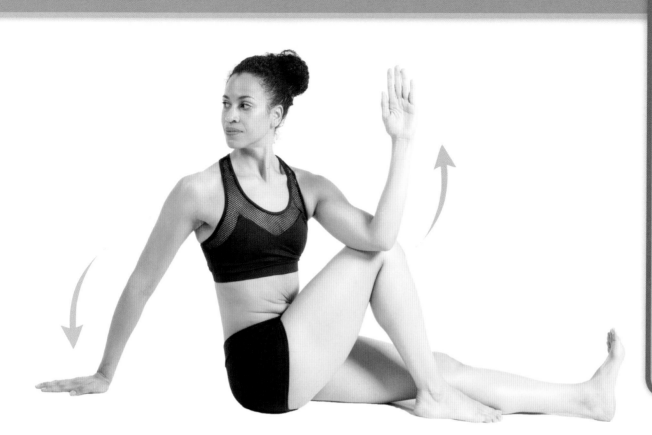

FACT FILE

SANSKRIT
• Marichyasana III

TARGETS
• Spine
• Hips
• Abdominals

BENEFITS
• Stimulates
  digestion
• Strengthens and
  stretches spine
• Opens hips
• Removes toxins
  from internal
  organs

CAUTIONS
• High or low
  blood pressure
• Back issues
• Knee issues

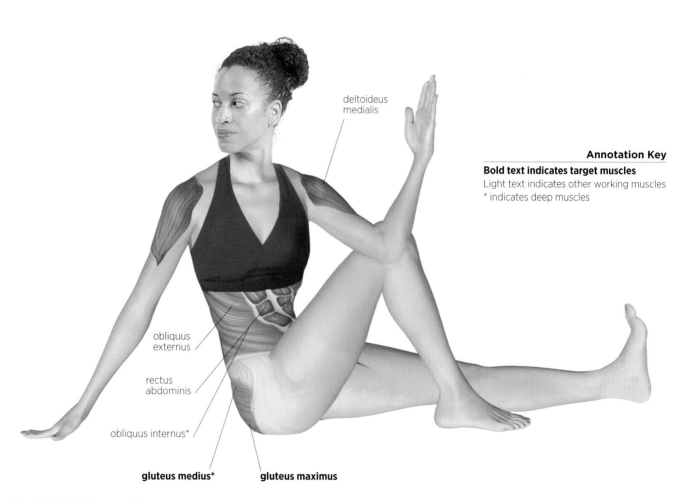

deltoideus
medialis

Annotation Key

Bold text indicates target muscles
Light text indicates other working muscles
* indicates deep muscles

obliquus
externus

rectus
abdominis

obliquus internus*

gluteus medius*   **gluteus maximus**

Bharadvaja's Twist I

Named after Bharadvaja, one of the seven great Hindu sages, this seated twist helps keep your spine limber. It also massages your internal organs.

HOW TO DO IT

- Sit in Staff Pose (pages 218–19). Shift your weight onto your right buttock, and bend your knees to your left, allowing your right thigh to rest on the floor. With your heels pointed toward your left hip, your left thigh should rest on top of your right calf, and your left ankle should sit on top of your right foot.

- Inhale and lift up from your spine. Exhale and twist to your right, looking over your right shoulder. Place your left hand near your right knee, and your right hand on the floor beside your right hip. With each exhale, deepen the twist while keeping your torso upright and your shoulders pressed back.

- Bend your right elbow to reach across your back. Hook your right hand beneath the bend in your left elbow.

- Hold for the recommended breaths, and then gently untwist as you exhale, and repeat on the opposite side.

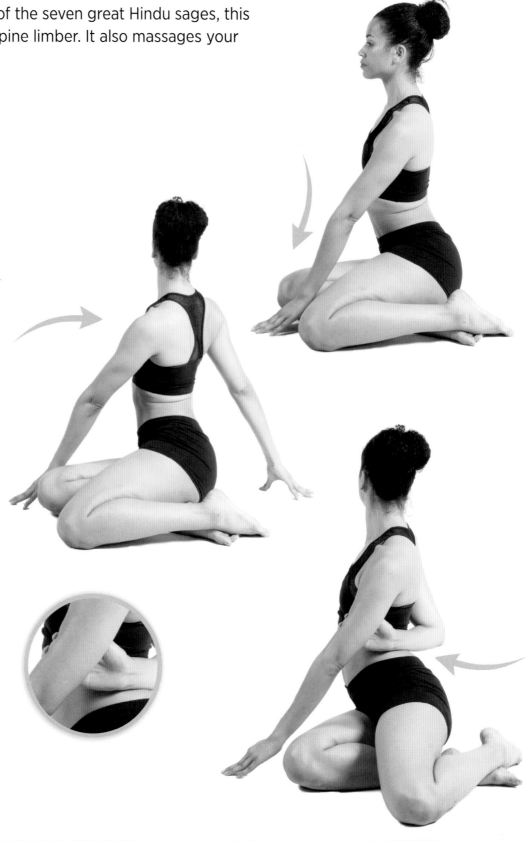

TARGETS
• Spine
• Shoulders
• Hips

BENEFITS
• Stretches spine, shoulders, and hips
• Stimulates digestion
• Relieves stress
• Relieves lower backache, neck pain, and sciatica

CAUTIONS
• Knee issues
• Shoulder issues
• Diarrhea
• Headache
• High or low blood pressure
• Menstruation

Annotation Key

Bold text indicates target muscles
Light text indicates other working muscles
* indicates deep muscles

DO IT RIGHT
• Press both sit bones into the floor while twisting.
• Avoid popping out your rib cage.
• Avoid dropping your head.

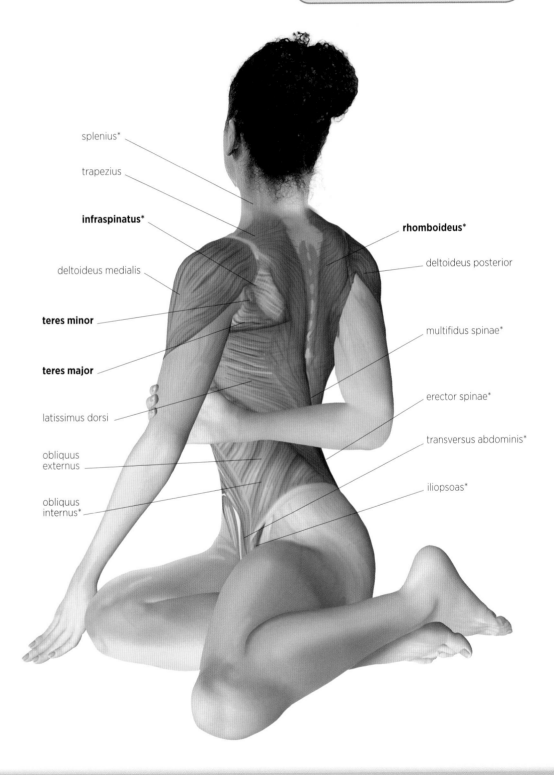

splenius*

trapezius

infraspinatus*

deltoideus medialis

teres minor

teres major

latissimus dorsi

obliquus externus

obliquus internus*

rhomboideus*

deltoideus posterior

multifidus spinae*

erector spinae*

transversus abdominis*

iliopsoas*

Bharadvaja's Twist II

This impressive-looking binding pose combines Hero Pose and Half Lotus Pose. It will stretch your abdominals, knees, ankles, and feet while increasing shoulder and spine mobility.

HOW TO DO IT

- Sit in Staff Pose (pages 218–19), and then draw your left leg underneath you as if in Hero Pose (pages 224–25).

- Lean forward, exhale, and place your right foot at the crease of your left hip as you would in Half Lotus Pose (page 231). Place your left hand on the outside of your right knee.

- Exhale deeply, swing your right arm around behind your back, and grip your right foot.

- Hold for the recommended breaths, and then gently untwist as you exhale, and repeat on the opposite side.

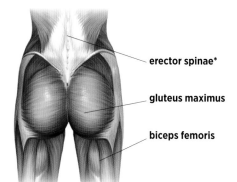

erector spinae*

gluteus maximus

biceps femoris

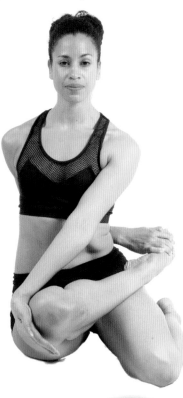

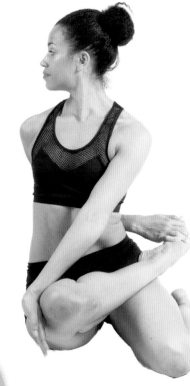

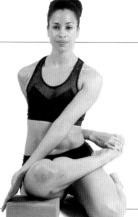

FACT FILE

SANSKRIT
- Bharadvajasana II

TARGETS
- Spine
- Shoulders
- Hips

BENEFITS
- Stretches spine, shoulders, and hips
- Stimulates digestion
- Relieves stress
- Relieves lower backache, neck pain, and sciatica

CAUTIONS
- Diarrhea
- Headache
- High or low blood pressure
- Insomnia
- Menstruation

Annotation Key

Bold text indicates target muscles
Light text indicates other working muscles
* indicates deep muscles

DO IT RIGHT

- Press both sit bones into the floor while twisting.
- Avoid popping out your rib cage.
- Avoid dropping your head.

MODIFICATION

EASIER: If your knee doesn't rest comfortably on the floor, tuck a yoga block or thickly folded blanket beneath it.

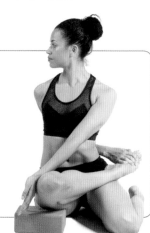

Half Lotus Pose

The Lotus Poses have come to symbolize the discipline of yoga. The Half Lotus Pose is a great way for new practitioners to develop the lower-body flexibility needed to achieve the more advanced version.

FACT FILE

SANSKRIT
• Ardha Padmasana

TARGETS
• Hips
• Knees
• Ankles

BENEFITS
• Opens hips
• Stretches the pelvis, leg, and ankle muscles

CAUTIONS
• Knee issues
• Hip issues

HOW TO DO IT

• Sit in Staff Pose (pages 218–19), and then bend your left knee and open it to the side. Allow your hip to open, and lower your left thigh to the floor.

• Lean forward slightly, and grab your left shin with your hands. Place your left foot on top of your right thigh, with your heel nestled against your groin. Make sure that the rotation is coming from your hips.

• Carefully position your right foot beneath your left thigh. Draw your knees closer together. Push into the floor with your groin, keeping both sit bones firmly in place.

• Extend upward through your spine, and place the backs of your hands on each knee, forming an "O" with your index fingers and thumbs.

DO IT RIGHT

• Maintain a deep, even breath throughout the pose.
• Alternate legs. We all have a dominant side; allow your less dominant side to stretch as well.

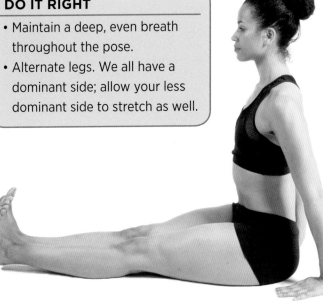

MODIFICATION

HARDER: Grasp a weighted Swiss ball as you perform the exercise. Keep your arms extended and the ball stable throughout the exercise.

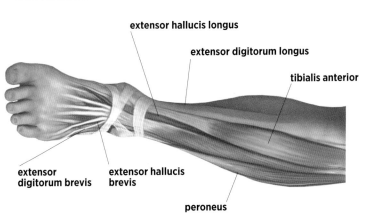

extensor hallucis longus

extensor digitorum longus

tibialis anterior

extensor digitorum brevis

extensor hallucis brevis

peroneus

Fire Log Pose

This intermediate pose is a deep hip opener that also stretches the buttocks. Make sure to practice this pose near the end of your session, when you are warmed up and your hips are nicely loosened.

HOW TO DO IT

• Begin by sitting in Staff Pose (pages 218–19).

• Bend your right knee, and place your right ankle over your straight left knee. Bend your left leg under, and place your left ankle beneath your right knee, stacking your ankle over or under your knee so that your shins are parallel to each other. Flex both feet and press out through your heels to keep both knees in alignment.

• You may find that this is enough of a hip stretch for you, especially if your right knee is lifting high off your left ankle. You can stay here and feel your hips opening. To deepen the stretch, inhale and lengthen your torso, then exhale and fold forward from your hips. Hold for the recommended breaths, then repeat on the opposite side.

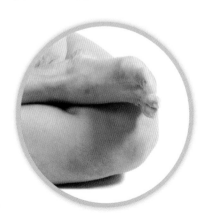

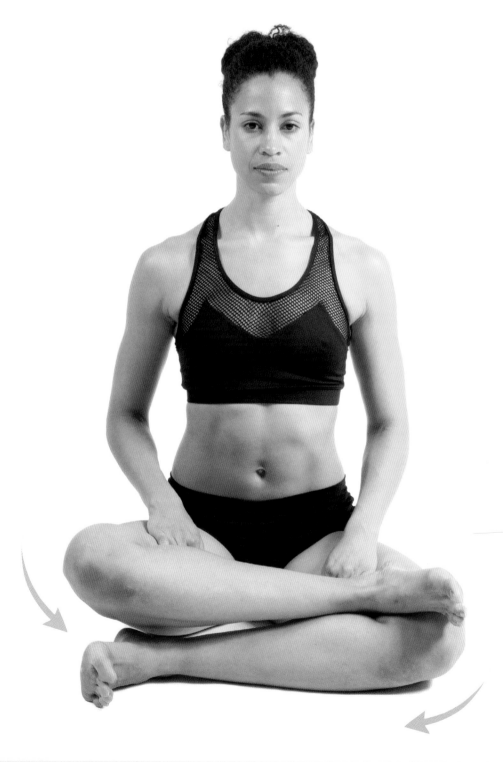

FACT FILE

SANSKRIT
- Agnistambhasana

TARGETS
- Knees
- Abdominals
- Hips

BENEFITS
- Deeply stretches outer hips and groin
- Increases knee flexibility

CAUTIONS
- Groin issues
- Knee issues

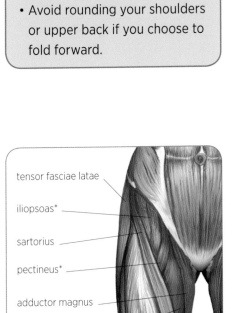

tensor fasciae latae

iliopsoas*

sartorius

pectineus*

adductor magnus

adductor longus

gracilis

vastus lateralis

Annotation Key
Bold text indicates target muscles
Light text indicates other working muscles
* indicates deep muscles

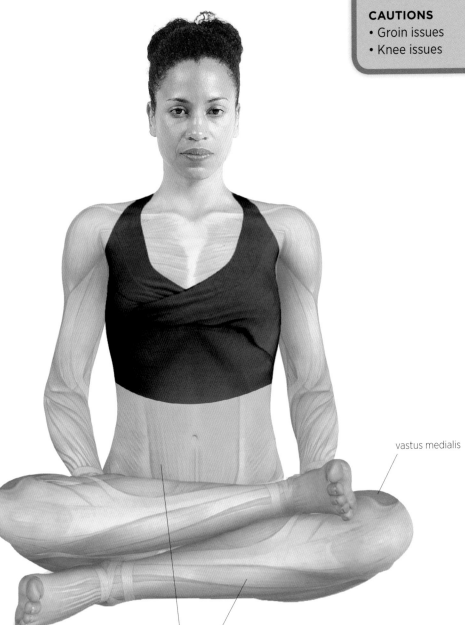

vastus medialis

transversus abdominis*

tibialis anterior

Cow Face Pose

Cow Face Pose takes diligent practice to perfect. It is difficult to assume all the components of Cow Face Pose correctly at the same time. Focus on achieving the proper alignment of your arms and then your legs until you can accomplish this posture with ease.

HOW TO DO IT

• Begin in Staff Pose (pages 218–19), with your legs extended in front of you. Bend your right knee, and then cross your right leg over your left, positioning your legs so that they cross at the inner thighs.

• Bend your left leg to stack your thighs one on top of the other. Draw your shins and heels slightly forward.

• Reach your right arm out to the side, parallel to the floor. Tilt your hand to face the ceiling, externally rotate your arm, and reach toward your ear. Bend your elbow so that it points toward the ceiling as your fingers point down your spine.

• Reach your left arm out to the side, parallel to the floor, internally rotating it. Allow your hand to face behind you with your thumb pointing downward. Bend your arm, pointing your elbow toward the floor, and bring your hand behind your back, palm away from your body and fingers pointing up your spine.

• Bring your hands toward each other, and clasp them together. Hold for the recommended breaths, and then repeat on the opposite side.

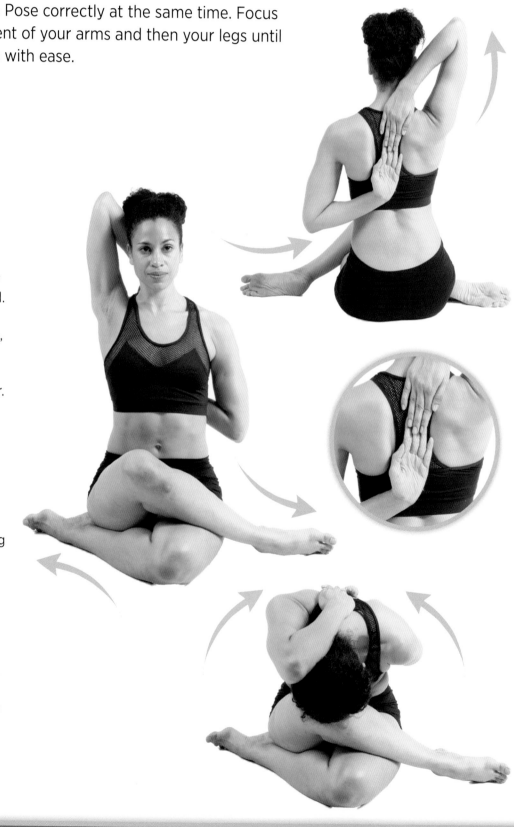

TARGETS
• Legs
• Hips
• Arms
• Chest

BENEFITS
• Stretches ankles, hips, thighs, triceps, and upper back
• Opens shoulders and chest

CAUTIONS
• Knee pain
• Shoulder issues

Annotation Key

Bold text indicates target muscles
Light text indicates other working muscles
* indicates deep muscles

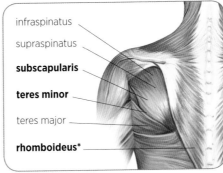

infraspinatus
supraspinatus
subscapularis
teres minor
teres major
rhomboideus*

DO IT RIGHT

• Position your feet so that both are the same distance from your hips.
• If your hips are uneven when you are sitting on the floor, sit on top of a block or a blanket.
• If you can't quite clasp your hands, try using a strap.
• Draw your elbows in opposite directions as you hold the pose.
• Keep your head and gaze forward.
• Avoid asking someone to help bring your hands together; this can strain your shoulders or rotator cuffs.

MODIFICATION

HARDER: Lengthen your spine, and lift your top elbow and your chest as you fold forward. Keep your legs in place and your hips facing forward as you hold for the recommended breaths.

triceps brachii
deltoideus medialis
deltoideus posterior
latissimus dorsi
erector spinae*
multifidus spinae*

Revolved Cow Face Pose

This pose provides a deep stretch of the hips and is helpful for relieving chronic knee pain. The Cow Face Poses actually do resemble a cow: the bent, crossed knees form the lips.

HOW TO DO IT
- Begin in Staff Pose (pages 218–19).

- Stack your right knee over your left knee, and bring your lower legs out to the sides with the soles of both your feet facing out.

- Bring your right hand around your abdomen, and rest it on your left side.

- Gently twist to the left, and reach back with your left hand to grasp your left foot.

- Hold for the recommended breaths, and then repeat on the opposite side.

FACT FILE

SANSKRIT
- Parivrtta Gomukhasana

TARGETS
- Hips
- Knees
- Shoulders

BENEFITS
- Stretches arms, wrists, and hips
- Improves shoulder flexibility

CAUTION
- Shoulder injury
- Knee issues

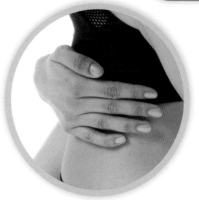

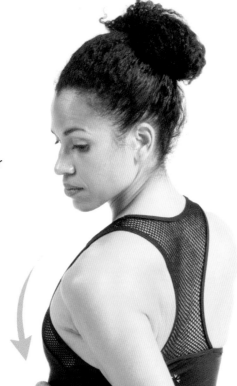

DO IT RIGHT
- Position your feet so that they are the same distance from your hips.
- Make sure to lengthen your spine as you twist.
- Avoid swiveling your head around to look over your shoulder.

Revolved Cow Face Side Bend

Revolved Cow Face Side Bend focuses on stretching your spine, hips, and shoulders and stimulating your internal organs. By gazing upward, you will open your chest and heart and feel the energy release from your fingertips.

HOW TO DO IT

- Begin by sitting in Staff Pose (pages 218–19).

- Stack your right knee over your left knee, and draw your feet back near your hips.

- Lengthen your spine, tilting your shoulders down, and extend your left arm out over your right thigh.

- Reach your right arm overhead, and turn your gaze toward the ceiling.

- Form the Gyan Mudra with both hands, by bringing the thumbs and index fingers together.

- Hold for the recommended breaths, and then repeat on the opposite side.

FACT FILE

SANSKRIT
- None

TARGETS
- Shoulders
- Spine
- Knees

BENEFITS
- Stretches arms, sides, hamstrings, and back
- Strengthens the abdomen
- Increases hip flexibility

CAUTIONS
- Knee pain
- Neck issues

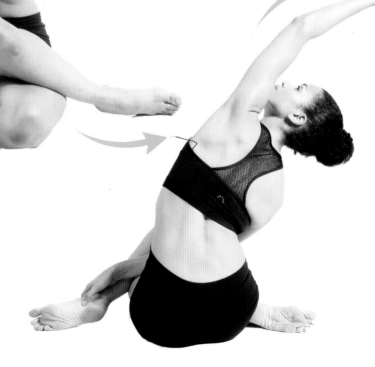

DO IT RIGHT
- Make sure to keep your feet the same distance from your hips.
- Avoid dropping your head too far back.

MODIFICATION

EASIER: Begin in Staff Pose. Stack your right knee over your left. Bend your torso to the right, and reach your right hand back to your left foot. Extend your left hand overhead toward the ceiling. Hold for the recommended breaths, and then repeat on the opposite side.

Mermaid Pose

This pose focuses on your chest and back, yet provides a complete stretch that engages much of your upper body. It also strengthens your lateral obliques, the muscles that shape your waistline, helping to eliminate the excess bulges known as "love handles" at your hips and any "spare tire" around your midsection.

HOW TO DO IT

- Sit to one side with your knees bent and one leg folded over the other.

- Place your right hand on your ankles. Inhale, reaching your left arm toward the ceiling.

- Exhale, reaching your left arm in the direction of your ankles. Pull your navel into your spine, and rotate your torso slightly backward.

- Inhale, return to the starting position, and then repeat on the opposite side.

DO IT RIGHT

- Make sure to find a comfortable position before starting so that your torso can move freely.
- Reach your arm far behind your body to open your chest and reach a maximum stretch.
- If you experience knee pain in the initial position, sit on a pillow or straighten your top leg out to your side.

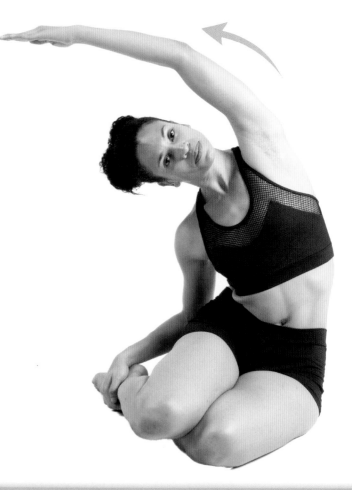

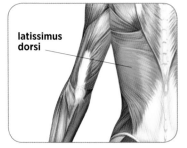

latissimus dorsi

FACT FILE

SANSKRIT
• None

TARGETS
• Core muscles
• Back
• Upper arms

BENEFITS
• Stretches arms and torso
• Opens chest
• Releases tight back muscles

CAUTIONS
• Intense back pain
• Hip pain
• Knee pain

rectus abdominis

obliquus externus

obliquus internus*

transversus abdominis*

Half Lord of the Fishes Pose

Half Lord of the Fishes Pose is a deeper variation of Marichi's, or Sage's, Pose (pages 226–27). This seated spinal twist, ideal for stretching your back, helps open your hips and shoulders.

HOW TO DO IT

- Sit in Staff Pose (pages 218–19), with your legs extended in front of you. Bend your right knee, and place your right foot on the outside of your left thigh, resting flat on the floor. Your left knee should point straight up toward the ceiling.

- Shift your weight slightly to the right as you bend your left leg inward and bring your heel close to your right hip.

- Extend your right hand on the floor behind your left hip, fingers pointing back. Inhale and lift your left arm to find length on the left side of your body.

- Exhale and twist your upper body to the right, and bring your left elbow to the outside of your right knee. Ground down evenly through both sit bones.

- To deepen the twist, find resistance between your raised arm and your bent leg. If desired, turn your gaze over your right shoulder, and raise your left hand, palm turned away from your body. Hold for the recommended breaths, and then repeat on the opposite side.

DO IT RIGHT

- Sit up tall and lengthen your spine as you twist.
- Distribute your weight evenly between both sit bones; if your hips feel uneven, try sitting on a block or a blanket.
- Broaden your collarbones as you draw your shoulder blades together.
- Avoid twisting your neck into an uncomfortable position.

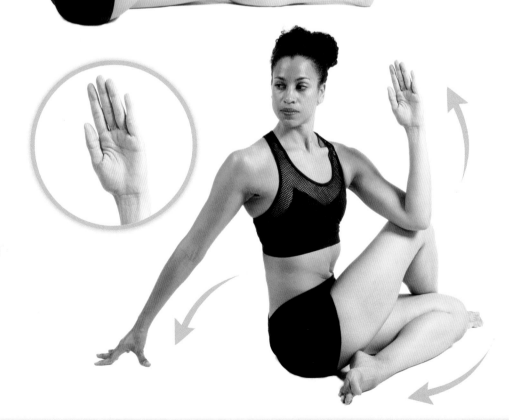

SANSKRIT
• Ardha
  Matsyendrasana

TARGETS
• Upper body

BENEFITS
• Stretches spine,
  shoulders, hips,
  and neck
• Detoxifies
• Aids digestion

CAUTIONS
• Spine injury

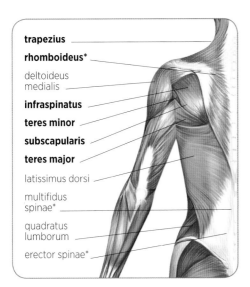

trapezius
rhomboideus*
deltoideus
medialis
infraspinatus
teres minor
subscapularis
teres major
latissimus dorsi
multifidus
spinae*
quadratus
lumborum
erector spinae*

MODIFICATION

HARDER: Weave your left forearm
back beneath your raised right knee,
then draw your left arm behind
your back toward your left hip, until
your hands meet. Clasp your hands
together in this bound position.

iliopsoas*
iliacus*
tensor
fasciae latae
pectineus*
adductor
longus

Annotation Key

Bold text indicates target muscles
Light text indicates other working muscles
* indicates deep muscles

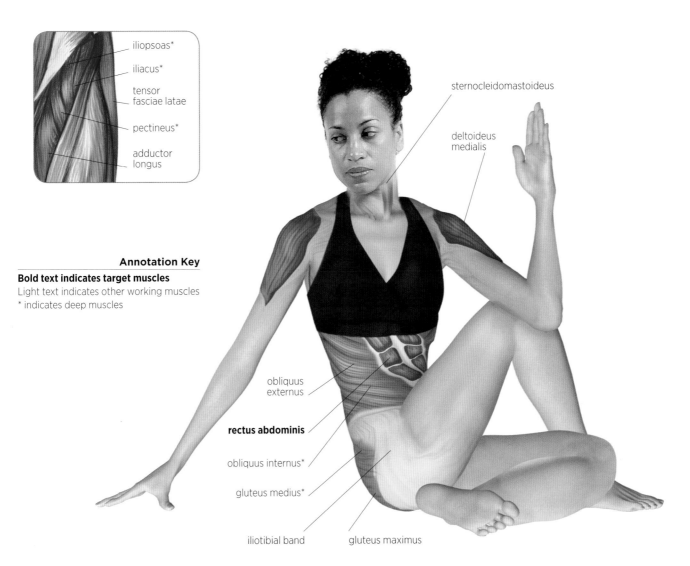

sternocleidomastoideus
deltoideus
medialis
obliquus
externus
rectus abdominis
obliquus internus*
gluteus medius*
iliotibial band
gluteus maximus

Boat Pose

Boat Pose can help you develop incredible core strength and stability. It is often considered the gateway core yoga pose because it grounds the midline while firing it up. With repeated practice, you will increasingly feel your deep abdominal muscles and hip flexors working.

HOW TO DO IT

• Begin in Staff Pose (pages 218–19). Bend both knees and place your feet on the floor as you grasp your hands around the outsides of your thighs.

• Shift your weight so you are balanced between the tripod of your sit bones and your tailbone. Lift your feet off the floor in line with your knees so that your shins are parallel to the floor. Extend your arms forward and parallel to the floor, with your palms facing inward toward your knees. Take a moment to find your balance.

• Slowly straighten your legs so that they form a 45-degree angle, with your toes lifted very slightly higher than your head.

• Internally rotate your thighs as you firm your outer hips to find stability. Squeeze your legs together as if they were a single unit. Reach out through your fingers and toes as you lift your sternum to broaden across your collarbones. Lengthen your spine and engage your stomach muscles as you hold for the recommended breaths.

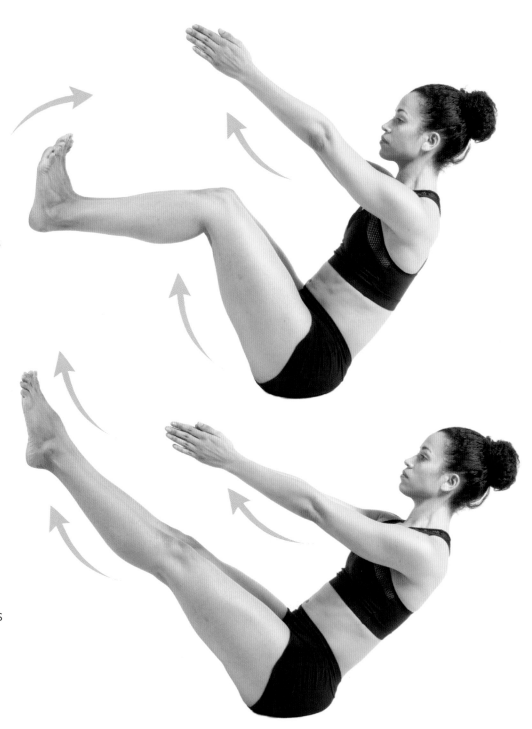

SANSKRIT
- Paripurna Navasana

TARGETS
- Spine
- Abdominals
- Hips

BENEFITS
- Strengthens stomach, back, and hip flexors
- Develops stability
- Aids digestion

CAUTIONS
- Pregnancy
- Groin injury

DO IT RIGHT

- Pull your belly button in toward your spine.
- Maintain the position of your legs, keeping them active and strong.
- Draw your sacrum into your body to help keep your spine long and straight.
- Avoid letting your legs drop downward or letting your stomach bulge out.
- Avoid rounding your lower back.

MODIFICATION

EASIER: You can hold the pose after the second step, keeping your legs bent as your feet stay in line with your knees and your shins stay parallel to the floor.

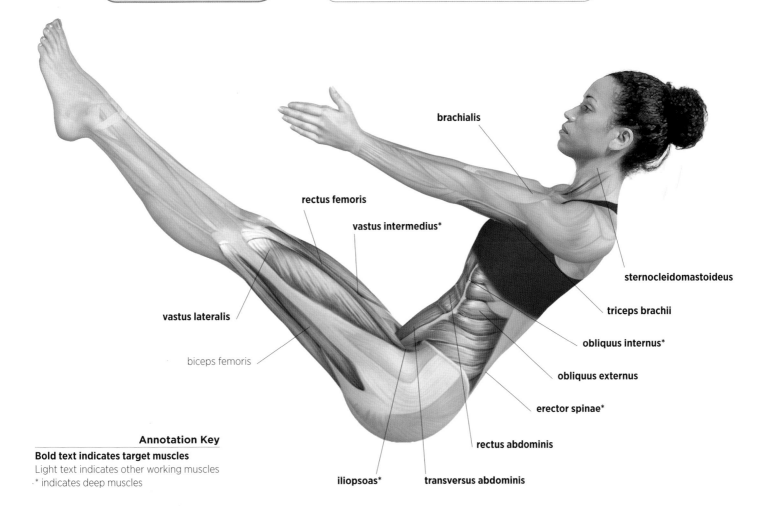

brachialis

rectus femoris

vastus intermedius*

vastus lateralis

biceps femoris

sternocleidomastoideus

triceps brachii

obliquus internus*

obliquus externus

erector spinae*

rectus abdominis

iliopsoas*

transversus abdominis

Annotation Key

Bold text indicates target muscles
Light text indicates other working muscles
* indicates deep muscles

Revolved Supported Boat Pose

Like all Boat Poses, this pose focuses on toning the deep core muscles and strengthening the hip flexors as well as improving stability and balance.

HOW TO DO IT
• Sit in Staff Pose (pages 218–19).

• Lift your legs to a 45-degree angle and straighten them, toes outstretched, as you rotate your upper body to your left. Extend your left hand behind your left hip, and place your right hand between your thighs. Both palms should be flat on the floor.

• Cross your right foot over your left and flex your left foot upward. Hold for the recommended breaths, and then repeat on the opposite side.

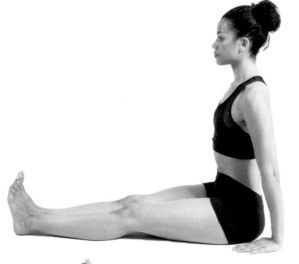

FACT FILE
SANSKRIT
• Parivrtta Salamba Navasana

TARGETS
• Abdominals
• Hip flexors

BENEFITS
• Builds core strength
• Opens hips
• Improves stability
• Cultivates self-awareness

CAUTION
• Pregnancy or groin injury
• Neck issues

Annotation Key
Bold text indicates target muscles
Light text indicates other working muscles
* indicates deep muscles

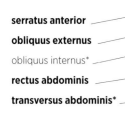

serratus anterior

obliquus externus

obliquus internus*

rectus abdominis

transversus abdominis*

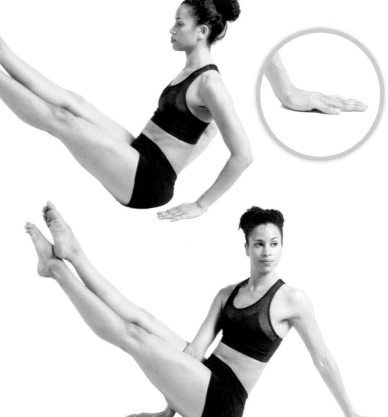

DO IT RIGHT
• Be sure to keep your legs as straight as possible.
• Elongate your spine as you twist your torso.
• Avoid over-rotating your head; your face should be in line with your rear shoulder.

Revolved Boat Pose with Prayer Hands

Adding the Anjali Mudra to Boat Pose creates a sense of peace and unity. Pressing your palms together unifies the right and left sides of your brain, and pressing the thumbs to the chest opens your heart.

HOW TO DO IT

- Begin in Staff Pose (pages 218–19), with legs forward and hands at your sides.

- Bend your knees and lift your feet, so your shins are parallel to the floor.

- Lean back slightly, and press your palms together at your chest. Cross your right foot over your left.

- Twist your torso to the left, and turn your gaze downward. Hold for the recommended breaths, and then repeat on the opposite side.

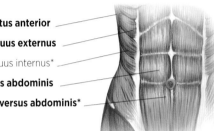
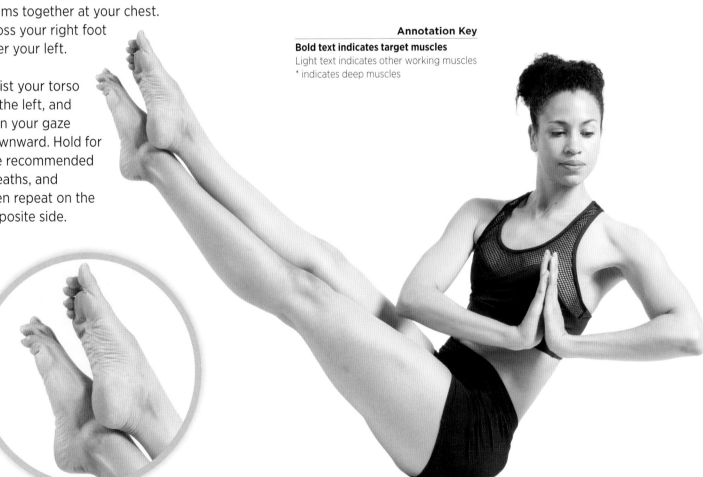

FACT FILE

SANSKRIT
- Parivrtta Navasana Namaskar

TARGETS
- Abdominals
- Hips

BENEFITS
- Stretches hamstrings
- Strengthens abdomen
- Increases hip flexibility

CAUTIONS
- Groin issues
- Lower-back pain

Revolved Head-to-Knee Pose

As you practice the Revolved Head-to-Knee Pose, which is the counterpose to Head-to-Knee Forward Bend (pages 142–43), you will begin to feel a deep stretch along your sides.

HOW TO DO IT

- Sit up tall in Staff Pose (pages 218-19). Bend your left knee while bringing your left foot in close to your groin. Place your left sole against your inner right thigh.

- Widen the pose by bringing your right foot farther to your right—as you externally rotate your hip—and sliding your left leg farther left.

- Place your right forearm on the inside of your right shin and grasp your foot.

- Raise your left arm toward the ceiling, and then outwardly rotate it as you bring it down over your left ear. Bend sideways to your right, reaching for the outside of your right foot with your left hand.

- Nestle your right shoulder toward the inside of your right leg, and slightly bend both elbows away from each other. Use this resistance to twist the right side of your torso toward the ceiling. Hold for the recommended breaths, and then repeat on the opposite side.

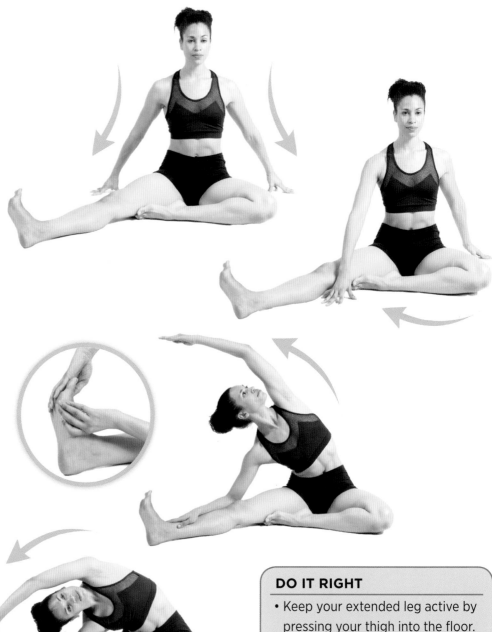

DO IT RIGHT
- Keep your extended leg active by pressing your thigh into the floor.
- Avoid rounding or hunching your shoulders.

SANSKRIT
• Parivrtta Janu
  Sirsasana

TARGETS
• Shoulders and
  sides
• Hips
• Hamstrings

BENEFITS
• Stretches core
  and spine
• Opens hips
  and groin

CAUTIONS
• Knee issues
• Lower-back
  issues

Annotation Key

Bold text indicates target muscles
Light text indicates other working muscles
* indicates deep muscles

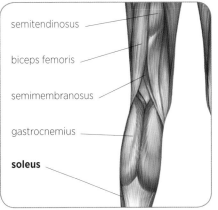

semitendinosus

biceps femoris

semimembranosus

gastrocnemius

soleus

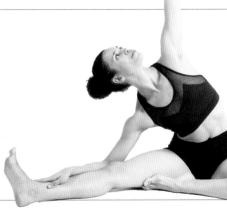

trapezius

infraspinatus

rhomboideus

latissimus dorsi

erector spinae*

gluteus medius*

MODIFICATION

EASIER: Instead of leaning
your body all the way to
the side, place one hand
on your shin and extend
your other hand up beside
your ear while bending
slightly to the side.

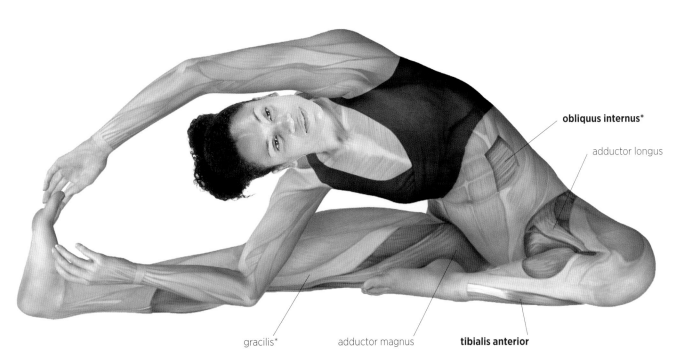

obliquus internus*

adductor longus

gracilis*

adductor magnus

tibialis anterior

Lotus Pose

Full Lotus Pose is a highly effective hip opener commonly used during meditation. You can work up to this cross-legged sitting asana—in which your legs resemble the open petals of the lotus flower—by starting with Half Lotus Pose (page 231) until you feel comfortable in the advanced position.

HOW TO DO IT

- Begin in Staff Pose (pages 218–19), and then bend your knees into Easy Pose (pages 220–21). Use your hands to lift your right foot and shin up, drawing the right heel in toward your left hip and resting your foot on your left thigh. (You can skip the next step, keeping your legs in this position and proceeding through the final two steps, to complete Half Lotus Pose, or Ardha Padmasana.)

- With your hands, position your left foot on top of your right thigh so that both feet are resting on opposite thighs. Hook your ankles as far as possible up your thighs, drawing them toward your hips. Flex your feet to help keep your knees and ankles in alignment.

- Balance on your sit bones and press them evenly into the floor. Externally rotate your hips, feeling your inner knees opening away from each other. Find a neutral pelvis, drawing your tailbone toward the floor. Draw your stomach in toward your spine.

- Sit up tall, lengthening your torso and broadening across your collarbones to lift your sternum and open your chest. Allow your arms to draw open, and position hands either facing up, in a gesture of receiving, or facing down, in a gesture of grounding. Close your eyes as you hold for the recommended breaths, and then repeat on the opposite side.

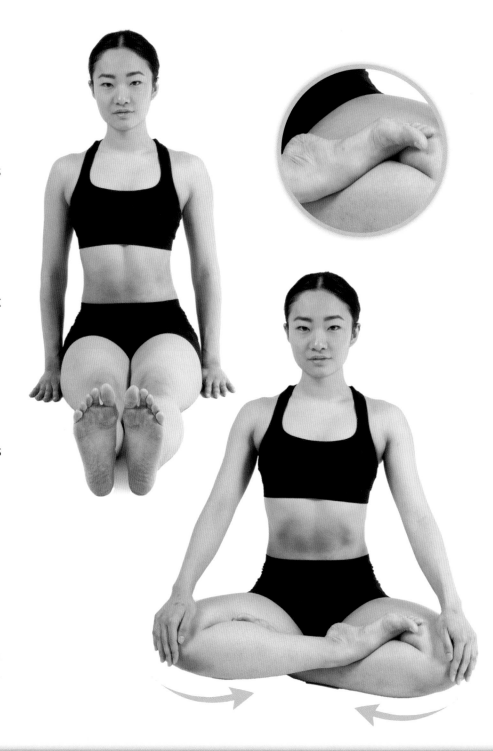

FACT FILE

SANSKRIT
- Padmasana

TARGETS
- Hips
- Glutes
- Legs

BENEFITS
- Stretches lower body, knees, ankles, and buttocks
- Opens hips and groin
- Stimulates digestion
- Calms mind and body

CAUTIONS
- Ankle injuries
- Hip issues
- Knee issues

DO IT RIGHT

- Keep your back and upper body straight; if you have trouble sitting straight, place a folded blanket beneath your hips to raise them above your knees.
- Lengthen your torso.
- Avoid straining your knees; if you're not quite ready to perform the pose, gradually ease into it with practice.
- Do not overextend your outer ankles.
- Avoid leaning or tilting your upper body to one side.

Annotation Key

Bold text indicates target muscles
Light text indicates other working muscles
* indicates deep muscles

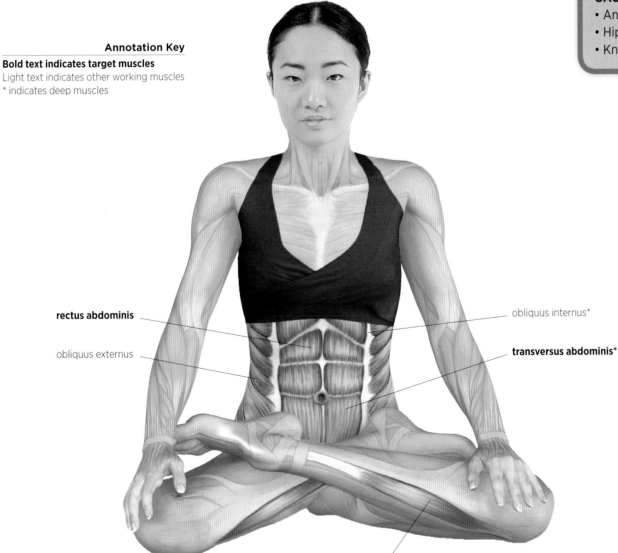

rectus abdominis

obliquus externus

obliquus internus*

transversus abdominis*

tibialis anterior

Big Toe Pose

Big Toe Pose not only stretches the entire back of the body but gradually loosens even the tightest of hamstrings. This posture also challenges your sense of balance, improving your focus and concentration.

HOW TO DO IT

- Sit with knees bent.

- Lean back slightly and lift your legs, so your shins are parallel to the floor.

- Reach between your legs, and grab your big toes with either hand.

- Find your balance, and straighten your legs. Hold for the recommended breaths.

DO IT RIGHT

- Keep you head and neck in a neutral position.
- Avoid rocking back and forth while in the pose.

FACT FILE

SANSKRIT
- Padangusthasana

TARGETS
- Hamstrings
- Spine
- Shoulders

BENEFITS
- Strengthens thighs and ankles
- Stretches back and legs
- Opens hips, shoulders, and arms
- Improves balance and focus

CAUTIONS
- Lower-back issues
- Ankle injuries

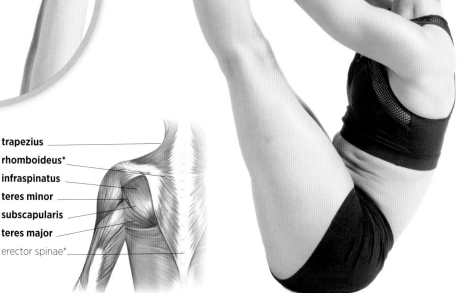

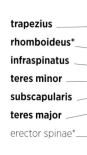

Annotation Key

Bold text indicates target muscles
Light text indicates other working muscles
* indicates deep muscles

trapezius

rhomboideus*

infraspinatus

teres minor

subscapularis

teres major

erector spinae*

Double Compass Pose

The advanced Double Compass Pose is demanding on the shoulders, hips, and hamstrings, and also requires a great degree of balance, flexibility, and coordination.

HOW TO DO IT

- Sit with your knees bent, your feet raised off the mat, and your shins parallel to the floor.

- Extend your arms forward, and cross your left hand over your right.

- Grasp each ankle with the opposite hand.

- Straighten your right arm and left leg.

- Pull your left elbow back, straighten your right leg, and bring your right knee to your right shoulder. Hold for the recommended breaths, and then repeat on the opposite side.

DO IT RIGHT

- Be sure to elongate the side with your arm raised.
- Your raised arm should be positioned alongside your ear.
- Avoid rounding your lower back.

FACT FILE

SANSKRIT
- Parivrtta Surya Yantrasana

TARGETS
- Hips
- Abdominals
- Upper legs

BENEFITS
- Stretches hamstrings and spine
- Strengthens abdomen
- Increases hip flexibility
- Stimulates internal organs

CAUTIONS
- Groin injuries
- Lower-back issues

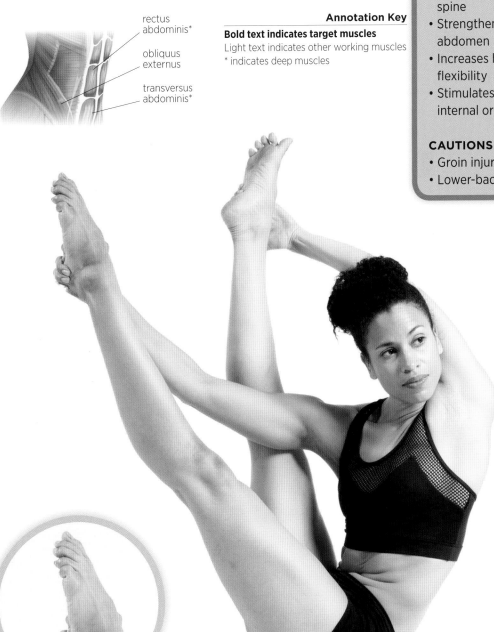

rectus abdominis*

obliquus externus

transversus abdominis*

Annotation Key

Bold text indicates target muscles
Light text indicates other working muscles
* indicates deep muscles

Monkey Pose

Monkey Pose is one of the more challenging advanced asanas. And it can't be rushed—be aware that it will take time, patience, and practice for you to build up to performing the full split.

HOW TO DO IT

• Kneel on the floor, with your back straight, your hips open, and your arms at your sides. Step your left foot forward to come into Low Lunge (pages 62–63), and place your fingertips on the floor on either side of your foot.

• Extend your left leg forward, flexing the foot so that your heel is on the floor and your toes point back toward you. It helps to pause in this position, taking several breaths as you stretch your hamstrings.

• Slide your left heel forward, keeping your left leg straight. Continue to slide forward until your right leg is also straight. Keep your hips square by visualizing that you are drawing your right hip crease back and your left hip forward.

• Inhale and raise your arms straight above your head, shoulder-width apart. Arch your back slightly, and reach your fingers toward the ceiling. Hold for the recommended number of breaths, and then repeat on the opposite side.

DO IT RIGHT

• Always ease your way into the split. Working on a smooth floor at first can help.
• As you descend, push into the floor with your front heel and the top of your back foot.
• Avoid allowing the hip of your back leg to turn outward.
• Do not force yourself into the full pose when you are not yet ready.

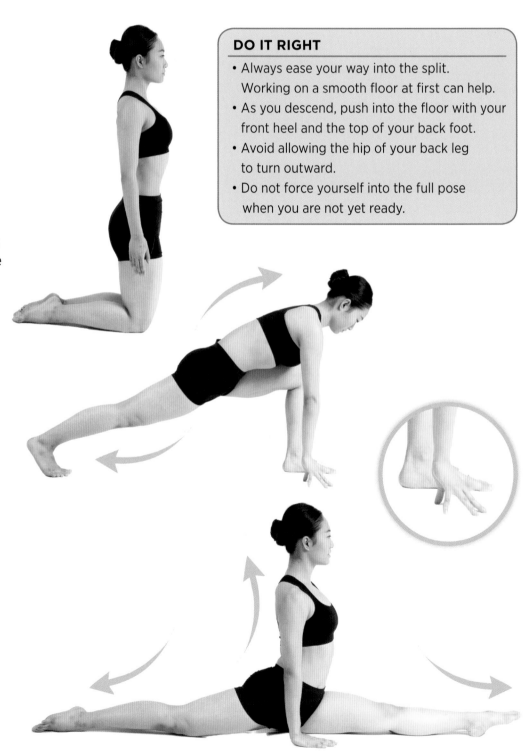

TARGETS
- Abdominals and obliques
- Glutes
- Legs

BENEFITS
- Stretches hamstrings, groin, thighs, and hips
- Opens lower body
- Improves overall flexibility

CAUTIONS
- Groin issues
- Hamstring issues

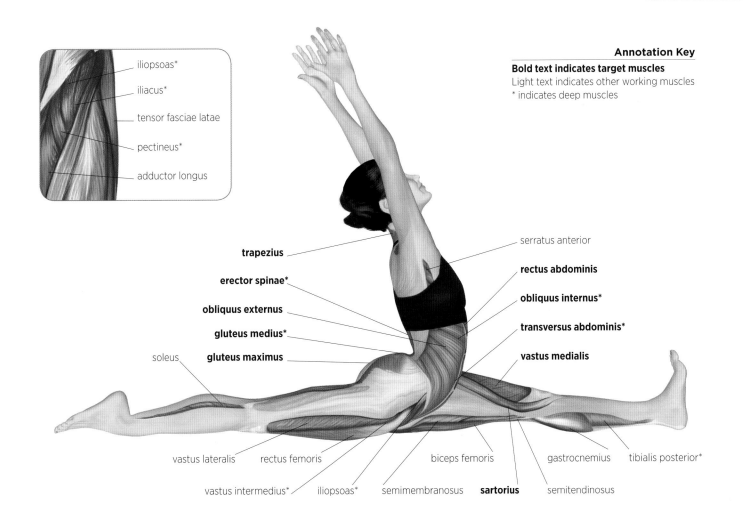

iliopsoas*
iliacus*
tensor fasciae latae
pectineus*
adductor longus

Annotation Key

Bold text indicates target muscles
Light text indicates other working muscles
* indicates deep muscles

serratus anterior
rectus abdominis
obliquus internus*
transversus abdominis*
vastus medialis

trapezius
erector spinae*
obliquus externus
gluteus medius*
soleus
gluteus maximus

vastus lateralis
rectus femoris
biceps femoris
gastrocnemius
tibialis posterior*

vastus intermedius*
iliopsoas*
semimembranosus
sartorius
semitendinosus

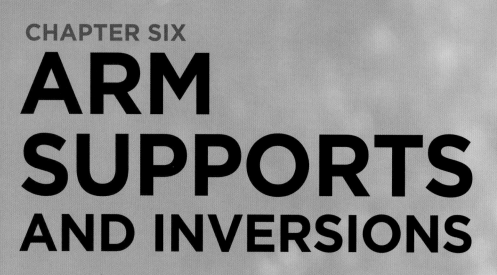

CHAPTER SIX

ARM SUPPORTS AND INVERSIONS

Yoga arm supports or arm balances are effective for strengthening your arms, wrists, hands, shoulders, core, and back. Balance poses, including inversions, require engaging your abdominals to support and stabilize your body. Inversions reverse the effects of gravity, and by keeping your heart above your head for a time, you can clear your sinuses and lungs and stimulate your digestive tract. Inversion poses also offer psychological benefits, such as alleviating depression and anxiety.

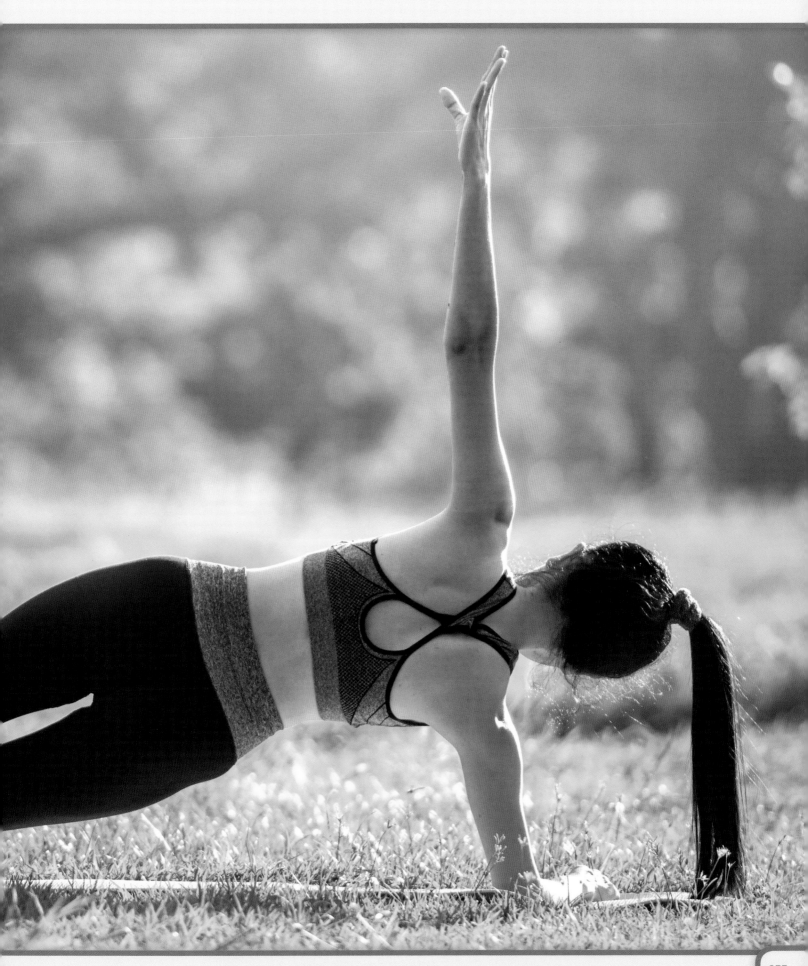

Scapular Range of Motion

This exercise is a great way to prepare your upper body for the demands of arm supports and inversion poses. This shoulder-rolling sequence helps strengthen your neck, shoulders, and upper back. It also improves your flexibility and range of motion.

HOW TO DO IT

• Sit or stand upright, keeping your neck, shoulders, and torso in a relaxed, neutral position. With your chin level, look straight ahead.

• Rest your arms at your sides, and bend your elbows slightly. Turn your palms faceup.

• Roll your shoulders forward, concentrating on separating your shoulder blades from your spine.

• Roll your shoulders slightly upward and back, squeezing your shoulder blades together.

• Roll your shoulders farther back and downward.

• Lower your shoulders while continuing to squeeze your shoulder blades together.

• Return to the starting position, and perform the recommended repetitions.

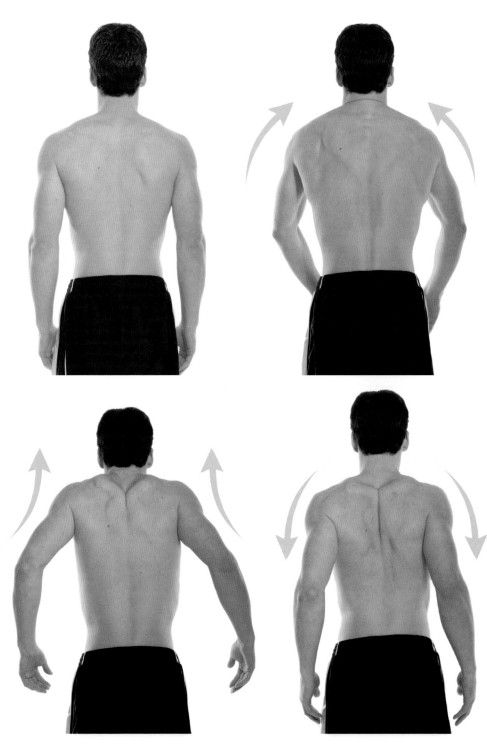

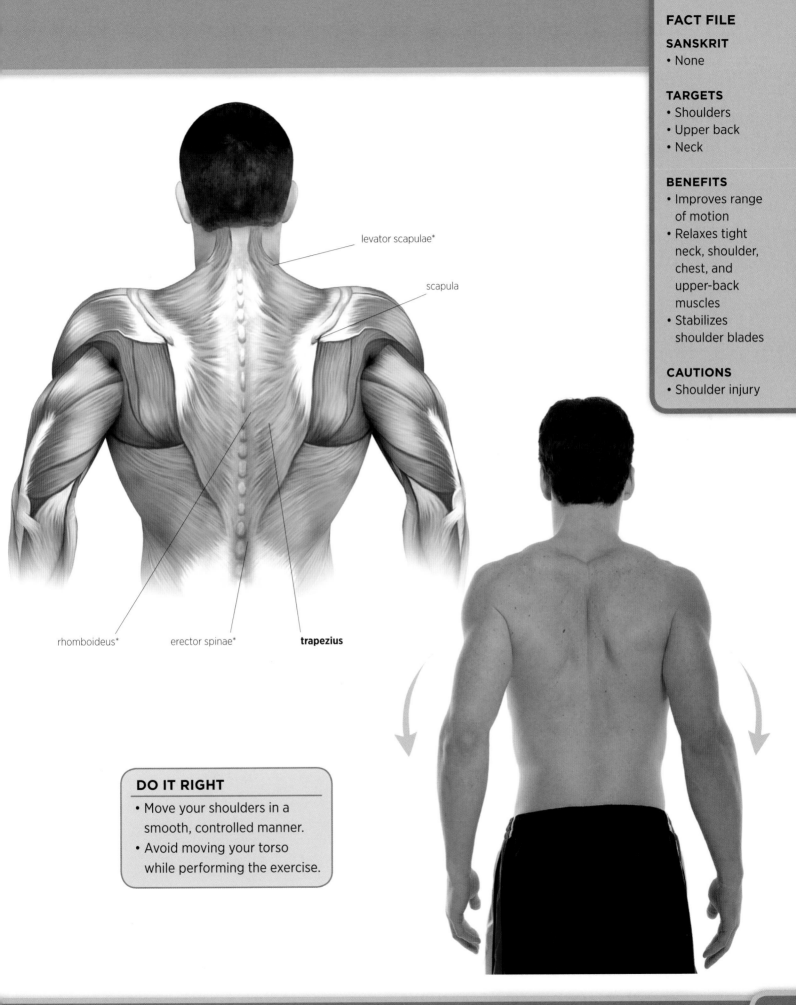

levator scapulae*

scapula

rhomboideus*   erector spinae*   **trapezius**

FACT FILE

SANSKRIT
• None

TARGETS
• Shoulders
• Upper back
• Neck

BENEFITS
• Improves range
  of motion
• Relaxes tight
  neck, shoulder,
  chest, and
  upper-back
  muscles
• Stabilizes
  shoulder blades

CAUTIONS
• Shoulder injury

DO IT RIGHT
• Move your shoulders in a
  smooth, controlled manner.
• Avoid moving your torso
  while performing the exercise.

Lifting Up

This exercise helps prepare you for arm supports and inversions. It not only improves upper-body strength but also engages your abdominals and legs.

HOW TO DO IT

• Begin in Easy Pose (pages 220–21). Spread your shoulder blades, and then pull them downward. Practice activating and relaxing your shoulders.

• Place your hands flat on the floor, fingers facing forward, with elbows straight. Spread your shoulder blades, then pull your shoulders down so that your rib cage lifts up.

• Press your shoulders down and lift your hips. Lower your hips, and return to a neutral position.

• Push down with your hands, and lift your hips, leaving your feet on the floor. Lower your hips, and return to a neutral position.

• To lift your feet, try lifting one knee, then your foot, then your other knee and foot. Lower your hips, and return to a neutral position.

• Perform the sequence for the recommended repetitions.

DO IT RIGHT

• Move in a smooth, controlled manner.
• Avoid rolling your shoulders forward— direct them down and apart.

FACT FILE

SANSKRIT
• None

TARGETS
• Shoulders
• Abdominals
• Legs

BENEFITS
• Stretches hamstrings
• Strengthens abdomen
• Increases hip flexibility

CAUTIONS
• Groin injury

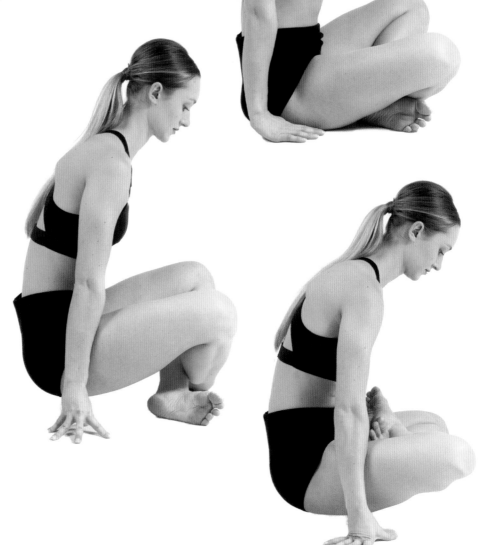

Turtle Neck

This exercise helps strengthen the muscles in your neck, which are typically engaged during arm supports and inversions.

HOW TO DO IT

- Sit or stand with your neck, shoulders, and torso straight. Keeping your chin level, look straight ahead.

- Move your chin in as if you were a turtle going back into your shell, until you feel a stretch in the back of your neck. Hold for the recommended breaths.

- Extend your head forward, this time as if you were a turtle coming out of your shell. Hold for the recommended breaths.

- Return to the starting position, and perform the recommended repetitions.

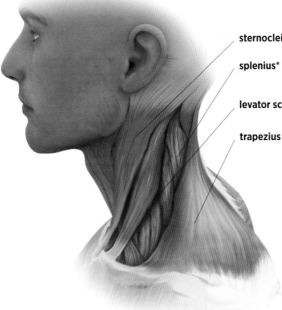

sternocleidomastoideus

splenius*

levator scapulae*

trapezius

FACT FILE

SANSKRIT
- None

TARGETS
- Neck

BENEFITS
- Improves range of motion
- Corrects forward head protrusion

CAUTIONS
- Pain or numbness along your arms or hands

DO IT RIGHT

- Move in a smooth, controlled manner.
- Avoid lifting your chin as you move your head back.

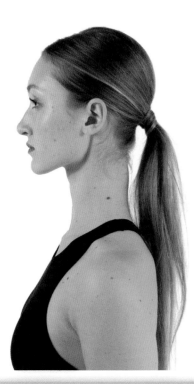
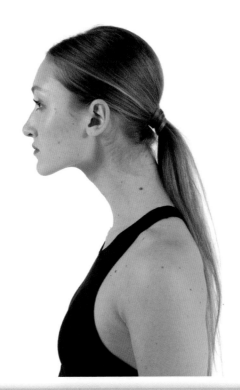
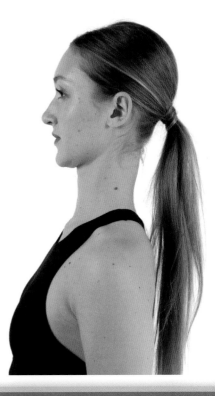

Plank Pose

A classic across disciplines, Plank Pose strengthens and tones the arms, abdominals, and wrists. It plays a part in many yoga sequences and is also a good precursor to more challenging arm balances.

HOW TO DO IT

• From Downward-Facing Dog (pages 268–69), inhale and shift your weight forward so that your shoulders are in line with your wrists. At the same time, come onto the balls of your feet, with your toes spread out and your heels reaching back.

• Keep your arms straight and parallel to each other, externally rotating your outer upper arms so that your inner elbows draw forward.

• As you hold the pose, soften between your shoulder blades as you broaden across your collarbones to lift your sternum. Internally rotate your inner thighs, keeping your thighs firm. Lengthen your tailbone down toward your heels. Hold for the recommended breaths.

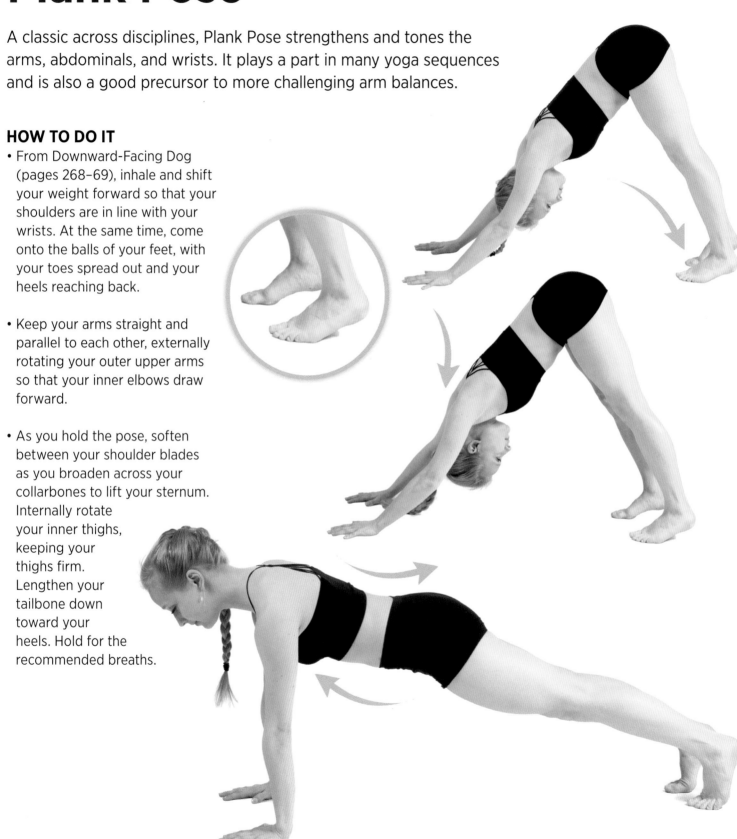

DO IT RIGHT

- Make sure your wrist creases are parallel to the front of your mat.
- Spread your fingers wide, and ground down through every knuckle.
- Use your breath to get you through holding the pose.
- Avoid lifting your fingers off the floor.
- Avoid rounding your upper back.

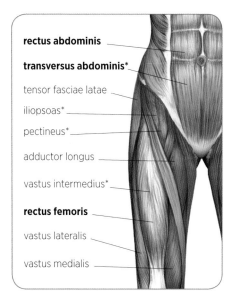

rectus abdominis

transversus abdominis*

tensor fasciae latae

iliopsoas*

pectineus*

adductor longus

vastus intermedius*

rectus femoris

vastus lateralis

vastus medialis

FACT FILE

SANSKRIT
- Phalakasana
- Also Adho Mukha Dandasana, Santolasana, or Kumbhakasana

TARGETS
- Spine
- Chest
- Neck

BENEFITS
- Strengthens arm and core muscles
- Develops core stability
- Prepares the body for other arm balances

CAUTIONS
- Wrist injuries
- Elbow injuries
- Shoulder issues

Annotation Key

Bold text indicates target muscles
Light text indicates other working muscles
* indicates deep muscles

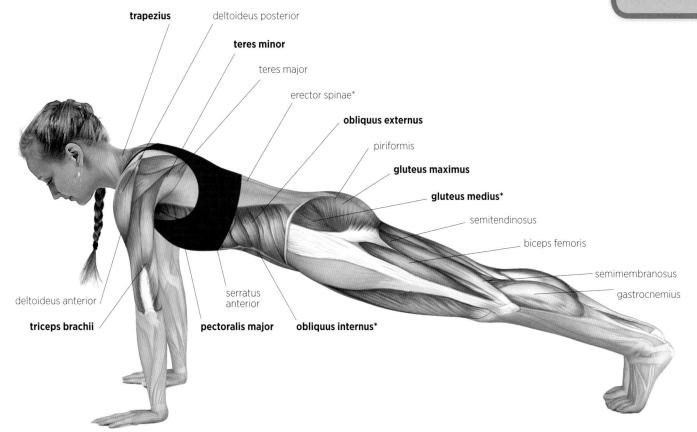

trapezius

deltoideus posterior

teres minor

teres major

erector spinae*

obliquus externus

piriformis

gluteus maximus

gluteus medius*

semitendinosus

biceps femoris

semimembranosus

gastrocnemius

deltoideus anterior

serratus anterior

triceps brachii

pectoralis major

obliquus internus*

Four-Limbed Staff Pose

Sometimes called Four-Limbed Staff Pose, Chaturanga is a yoga essential. Part of many yoga flows, it challenges your core strength and stability. It is also an effective strengthener for the arms, legs, and shoulders.

HOW TO DO IT

• Begin in Plank Pose (pages 260–61), with your hands planted on the floor shoulder-width apart, your arms straight, and your body lifted off the mat to form a straight line. Your feet should be parallel, with your heels lifted.

• Exhale as you bend your elbows over your wrists, and lower yourself down so that your shoulders are in line with your elbows. As you lower your body, ground your palms and fingers into the floor.

• Hold the pose, rotating your inner thighs and drawing your tailbone downward so that you do not sink into your lower back. Lift your thighs away from the floor. Draw your shoulder blades together as you lift the heads of your shoulders away from the floor. Hold for the recommended breaths.

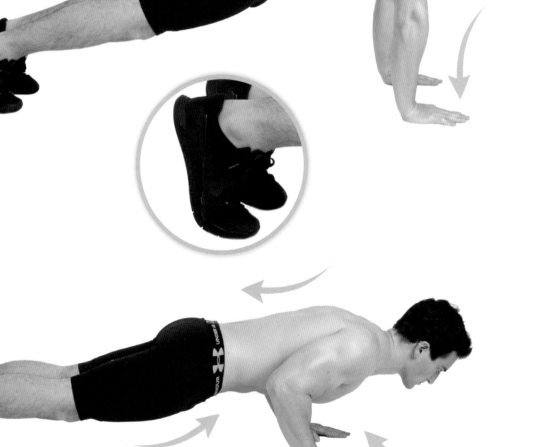

SANSKRIT
• Chaturanga
  Dandasana

TARGETS
• Abdominals
• Pectorals
• Shoulders

BENEFITS
• Improves
  balance
• Strengthens
  abdomen,
  arms, legs,
  and wrists

CAUTIONS
• Elbow issues
• Shoulder
  issues
• Wrist issues

DO IT RIGHT

• Keep the back of your neck long by gazing slightly beyond the edge of your mat.
• Avoid bending your elbows so much that your chest collapses and your shoulders round forward.
• Avoid dropping your hips lower than your shoulders.
• Tighten your glutes and tuck in your abs to maintain core stability; keep your legs taut and extended.

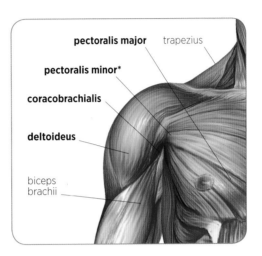

pectoralis major trapezius

pectoralis minor*

coracobrachialis

deltoideus

biceps
brachii

Annotation Key
Bold text indicates target muscles
Light text indicates other working muscles
* indicates deep muscles

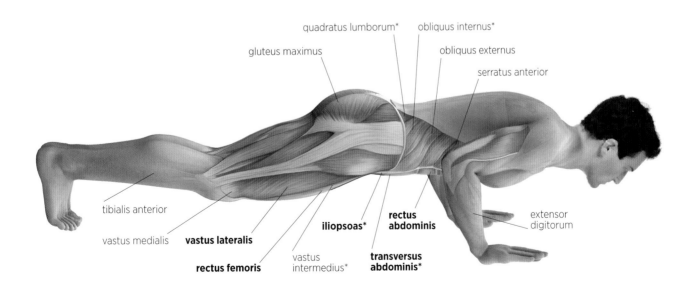

quadratus lumborum* obliquus internus*

gluteus maximus obliquus externus

serratus anterior

tibialis anterior

vastus medialis **vastus lateralis**

rectus femoris vastus
intermedius*

iliopsoas* **rectus
abdominis**

**transversus
abdominis***

extensor
digitorum

Forearm Side Plank Pose

Forearm Side Plank Pose, also known as Pose Dedicated to the Sage Vasistha, not only stabilizes your spine, but is also an effective shoulder, abdominal, and lower-back strengthener. Like other versions of Plank Pose, it improves both strength and stability, which can help prevent injuries.

HOW TO DO IT

• Lie on your left side with your legs straight and parallel to each other. Keep your feet flexed.

• Bend your left arm to form a 90-degree angle, with the knuckles of your hand facing forward. Place your right hand on your waist or hip.

• Pressing your forearm down into the floor, raise your torso and hips until your body is in a long, straight line. Raise your right arm toward the ceiling, with your fingers reaching upward.

• Hold for the recommended breaths, and then repeat on the opposite side.

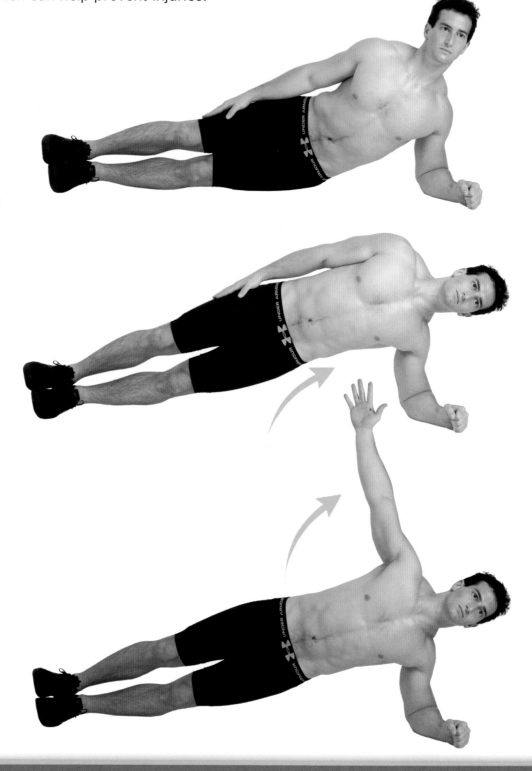

DO IT RIGHT

• Make sure to keep your hips in line with your shoulders.
• Keep your back straight.
• Avoid allowing your back to sway.
• Avoid leaning forward.

FACT FILE

SANSKRIT
• Vasisthasana

TARGETS
• Shoulders
• Abdominals
• Lower back

BENEFITS
• Strengthens core
• Stabilizes upper body

CAUTIONS
• Shoulder issues
• Lower-back issues
• Wrist issues

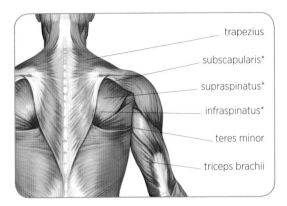

erector spinae*

gluteus maximus

semitendinosus

biceps femoris

semimembranosus

gastrocnemius

trapezius

subscapularis*

supraspinatus*

infraspinatus*

teres minor

triceps brachii

Annotation Key

Bold text indicates target muscles
Light text indicates other working muscles
* indicates deep muscles

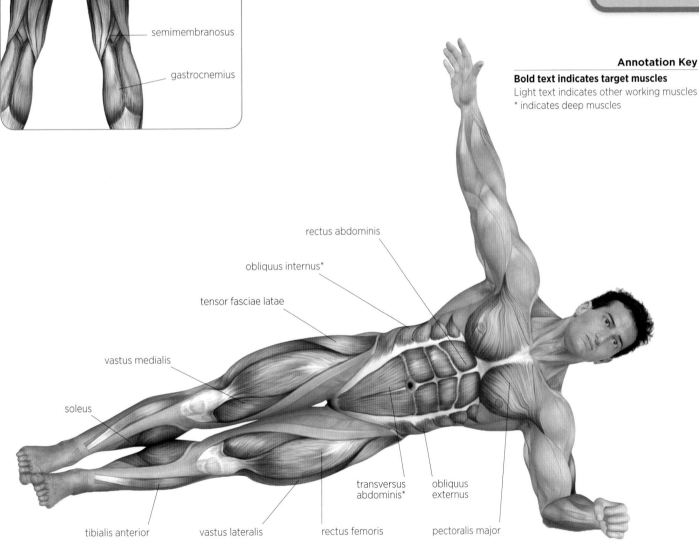

rectus abdominis

obliquus internus*

tensor fasciae latae

vastus medialis

soleus

tibialis anterior

vastus lateralis

rectus femoris

transversus abdominis*

obliquus externus

pectoralis major

Side Plank Pose

Multipurpose Side Plank Pose is valuable for strengthening your wrists, arms, legs, and abdominals. It also develops your balance in preparation for more advanced balancing poses. Its challenge lies in maintaining alignment in your spine and legs as gravity works against you.

HOW TO DO IT

• Begin in Plank Pose (pages 260–61), and then shift your weight onto the outside of your right foot and onto your straightened right arm. Shift your left shoulder up and back.

• Stack your left foot onto your right foot, pressing your legs together as you straighten them. Keep both feet flexed.

• Exhale, raise your left arm toward the ceiling, and turn your head to gaze at your fingertips. Hold for the recommended breaths, release back into Plank Pose, and repeat on the opposite side.

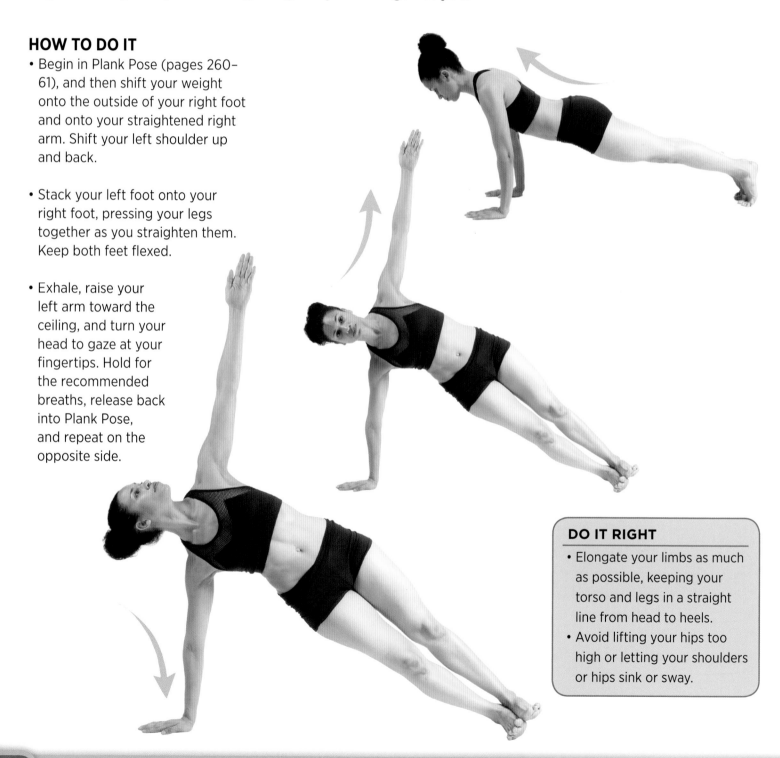

DO IT RIGHT

• Elongate your limbs as much as possible, keeping your torso and legs in a straight line from head to heels.
• Avoid lifting your hips too high or letting your shoulders or hips sink or sway.

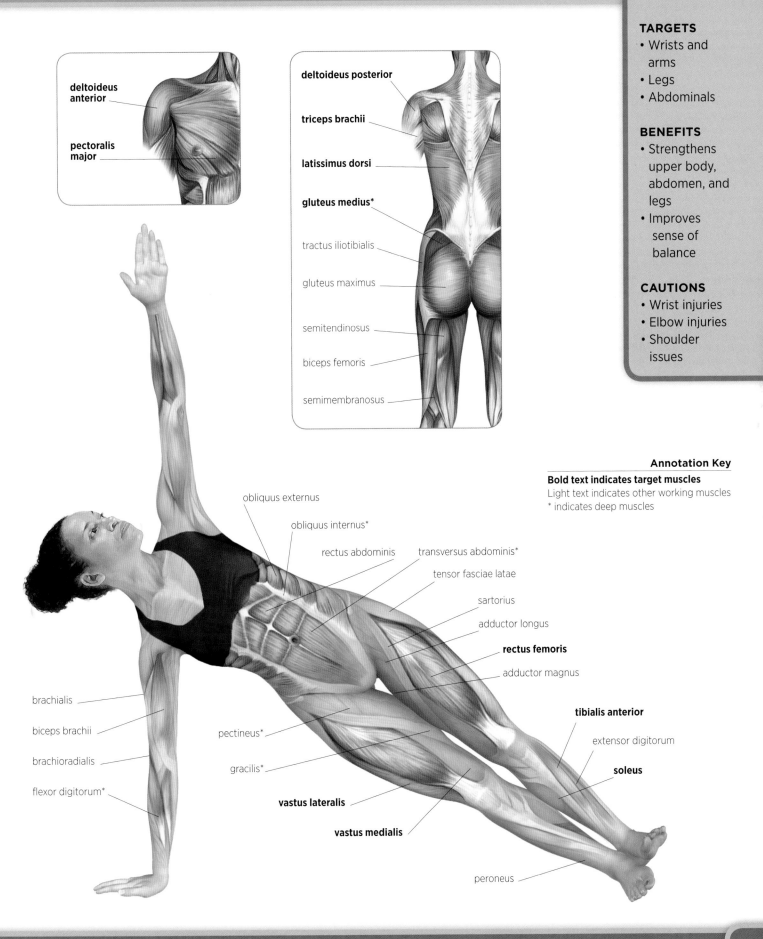

SANSKRIT
- Vasisthasana

TARGETS
- Wrists and arms
- Legs
- Abdominals

BENEFITS
- Strengthens upper body, abdomen, and legs
- Improves sense of balance

CAUTIONS
- Wrist injuries
- Elbow injuries
- Shoulder issues

deltoideus anterior

pectoralis major

deltoideus posterior

triceps brachii

latissimus dorsi

gluteus medius*

tractus iliotibialis

gluteus maximus

semitendinosus

biceps femoris

semimembranosus

Annotation Key
Bold text indicates target muscles
Light text indicates other working muscles
* indicates deep muscles

obliquus externus

obliquus internus*

rectus abdominis

transversus abdominis*

tensor fasciae latae

sartorius

adductor longus

rectus femoris

adductor magnus

tibialis anterior

extensor digitorum

soleus

brachialis

biceps brachii

brachioradialis

flexor digitorum*

pectineus*

gracilis*

vastus lateralis

vastus medialis

peroneus

Downward-Facing Dog

This well-known asana is among the most frequently performed yoga poses—one you'll come into time and again. "Down Dog," as it is often called, stretches and strengthens the entire body.

HOW TO DO IT

• Begin on all fours, with your hands planted directly below your shoulders and your knees aligned beneath your hips.

• Tuck your toes under, and "walk" your hands forward about a palm's distance in front of your shoulders. With your hands and toes firmly planted, lift your hips up as you straighten your legs and draw your heels toward the floor.

• Press your chest toward your thighs, and bring your head between your arms. Lengthen up through your tailbone and keep your thighs slightly internally rotated, finding a neutral pelvis. Gaze between your feet or toward your navel. Hold for the recommended breaths.

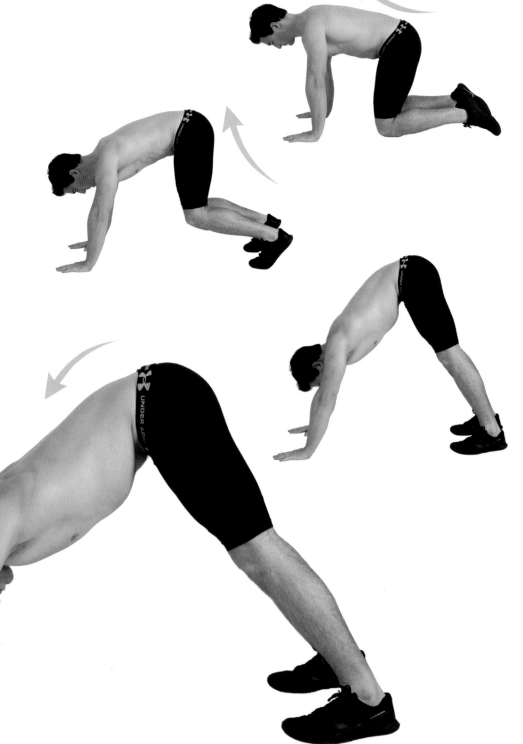

SANSKRIT
- Adho Mukha Svanasana

TARGETS
- Shoulders and arms
- Hamstrings
- Calves

BENEFITS
- Strengthens arms and legs
- Stretches spine, hamstrings, calves, and arches of feet
- Aids digestion
- Helps relieve menstrual cramps
- Helps relieve headaches

CAUTIONS
- Low blood pressure
- Shoulder issues
- Hamstring issues
- Carpal tunnel syndrome

DO IT RIGHT

- Engage your entire hand fully into the floor at all times to avoid excess strain on your wrist joint.
- Keep your head in line with your spine.
- Keep your back flat and your chest elevated.
- Avoid holding your breath: relax your jaw slightly and breathe normally.

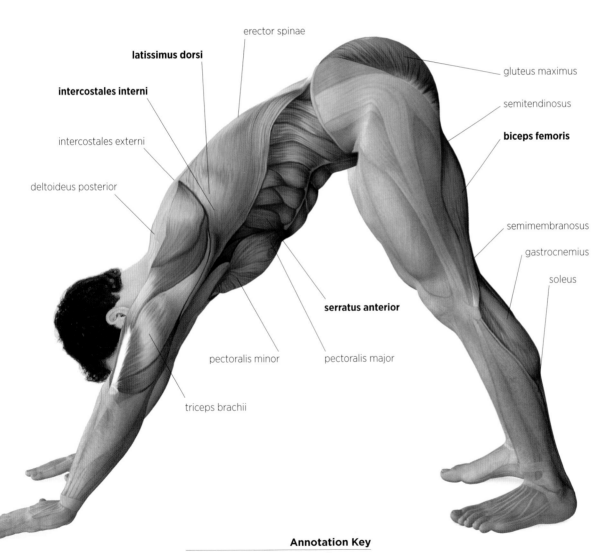

erector spinae

latissimus dorsi

intercostales interni

intercostales externi

deltoideus posterior

gluteus maximus

semitendinosus

biceps femoris

semimembranosus

gastrocnemius

soleus

serratus anterior

pectoralis minor

pectoralis major

triceps brachii

Annotation Key

Bold text indicates target muscles
Light text indicates other working muscles
* indicates deep muscles

Dolphin Pose

Dolphin Pose is known to strengthen both your upper and lower body—your shoulders, arms, abdominals, and spine, as well as your thighs and calves. This energizing posture also helps you improve your balance.

HOW TO DO IT

• Kneel on the floor with your hips lifted off your heels.

• Bend forward and place your hands on the mat in front of you; lower your elbows to the floor, keeping them tucked in at your sides and aligned with your shoulders.

• Straighten your legs as you lift your sit bones toward the ceiling. Tuck your tailbone toward your pubis, and squeeze your legs together.

• Push through your forearms, and extend the stretch through your shoulders. Keep your head and chest lifted off the mat.

• Hold for the recommended breaths.

FACT FILE

SANSKRIT
• Ardha Pincha Mayurasana

TARGETS
• Abdominals
• Glutes
• Back
• Hamstrings

BENEFITS
• Strengthens and tones abdomen
• Engages arms, legs, and spine
• Improves balance
• Invigorates and energizes by increasing blood flow to the brain

CAUTIONS
• Back injuries
• Neck injuries
• Headache
• High blood pressure

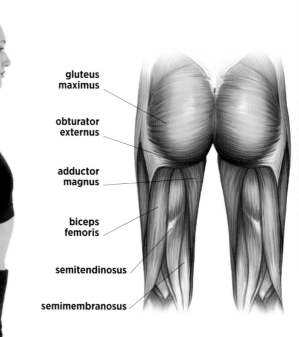

gluteus maximus

obturator externus

adductor magnus

biceps femoris

semitendinosus

semimembranosus

Annotation Key
Bold text indicates target muscles
Light text indicates other working muscles
* indicates deep muscles

DO IT RIGHT

• While holding Dolphin Pose, keep your back straight. If you cannot straighten your legs without sagging or rounding your spine, keep your knees slightly bent.
• Avoid raising your heels off the mat.

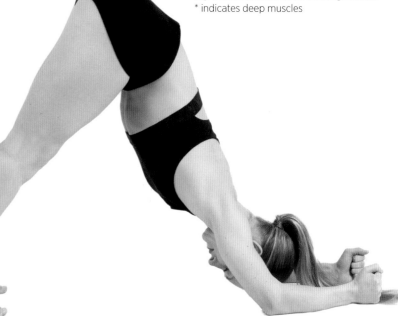

Dolphin Plank Pose

Like all plank poses, this modification strengthens your abdominals and benefits your shoulders, upper arms, and obliques. The isometric hold also helps to build lean muscle.

HOW TO DO IT

- Begin on all fours, with your toes curled forward and facing the front of your mat.

- Plant your forearms on the floor, shoulder-width apart and parallel to each other. Raise your knees off the mat and extend your legs until they are in line with your arms. Do not let your hips or buttocks sink too low or rise too high. Your body should form a straight line from your shoulders to your heels.

- Hold this position for the recommended breaths.

Annotation Key

Bold text indicates target muscles

Light text indicates other working muscles

* indicates deep muscles

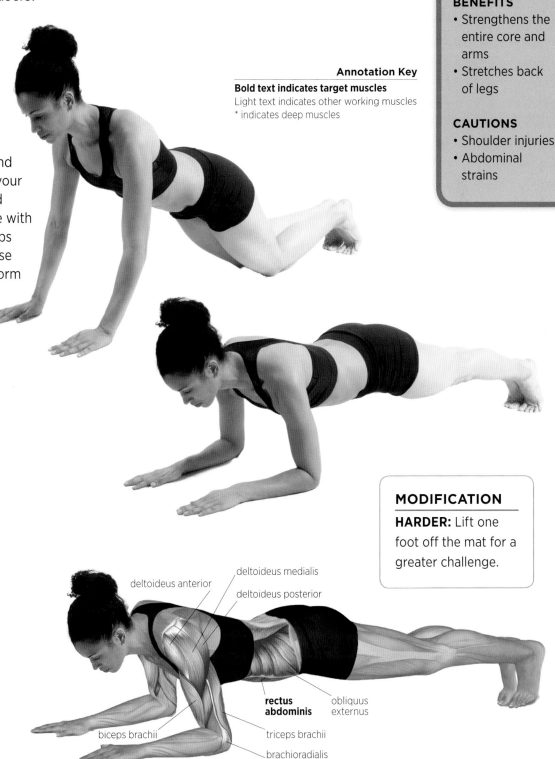

deltoideus medialis

deltoideus anterior

deltoideus posterior

rectus abdominis

obliquus externus

biceps brachii

triceps brachii

brachioradialis

DO IT RIGHT

- Keep your abdominal muscles tight and your body in a straight line.
- Keep your shoulder blades and collarbone wide. This prepares you for other balance poses, such as Crow Pose.
- Avoid bridging too high, since this can take stress off your working muscles.

MODIFICATION

HARDER: Lift one foot off the mat for a greater challenge.

FACT FILE

SANSKRIT

- Makara Adho Mukha Svanasana

TARGETS

- Abdominals
- Shoulders
- Obliques

BENEFITS

- Strengthens the entire core and arms
- Stretches back of legs

CAUTIONS

- Shoulder injuries
- Abdominal strains

Dolphin Plank with Arm Reach

This more challenging variation of Plank Pose (pages 260–61) is effective in strengthening your forearms, upper arms, shoulders, and back. It also improves your stamina and posture by building up the muscles that support your spine. Swimmers, gymnasts, and dancers can all benefit from this pose.

HOW TO DO IT

- Begin on all fours with your toes curled forward and facing the front of your mat.

- Plant your forearms on the floor parallel to each other. Raise your knees off the mat and lengthen your legs until they are in line with your arms. Your body should form a straight line from your shoulders to your heels.

- Maintaining proper plank form, slowly raise your right arm off the mat and extend it away from your shoulder, fingers outstretched.

- Hold for the recommended breaths, release the pose, and then repeat on the opposite side.

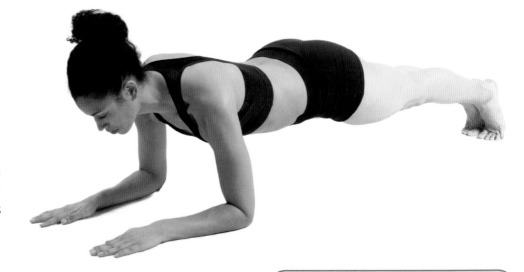

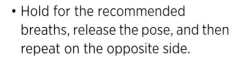

DO IT RIGHT

- Keep your abdominal muscles tight and your body in a straight line.
- Your neck should be in a neutral position, not extended or crunched.
- Avoid letting your hips or buttocks sink too low or rise too high.

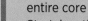

FACT FILE

SANSKRIT
• None

TARGETS
• Abdominals
• Thighs
• Shoulders

BENEFITS
• Strengthens the entire core
• Stretches the hamstrings
• Opens the chest and shoulders
• Improves posture

CAUTIONS
• Groin injuries
• Shoulder issues
• Ankle injuries

Annotation Key

Bold text indicates target muscles
Light text indicates other working muscles
* indicates deep muscles

MODIFICATION

EASIER: Instead of extending your arm out to your sides, raise only your forearm a few inches off the mat. You can also make the pose less taxing by bending your knees.

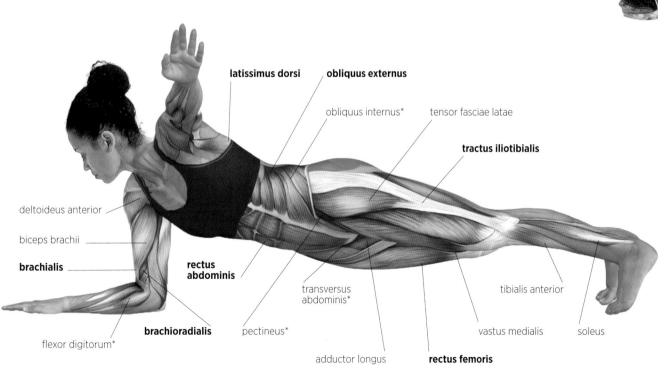

latissimus dorsi · obliquus externus · obliquus internus* · tensor fasciae latae · **tractus iliotibialis** · deltoideus anterior · biceps brachii · **brachialis** · **rectus abdominis** · transversus abdominis* · tibialis anterior · **brachioradialis** · pectineus* · vastus medialis · soleus · flexor digitorum* · adductor longus · **rectus femoris**

One-Legged Plank

The intermediate One-Legged Plank can be challenging to line up and maintain. Muscle length, strength, and movement flow are all worked thoroughly during this pose.

HOW TO DO IT

• Start in Plank Pose (pages 260–61), with the front of your body facing the mat in one long line. Position your arms directly under your shoulders with your fingers pointing forward. Extend your legs parallel and hip-width apart, with your weight on the balls of your feet.

• Inhale to prepare, and press your shoulder blades down your back for stabilization.

• Exhale as you push back on your heels and lift your left leg to hip height, keeping your left foot flexed. Hold for the recommended breaths.

• Inhale, lower your leg, and repeat on the opposite side. Perform the recommended repetitions.

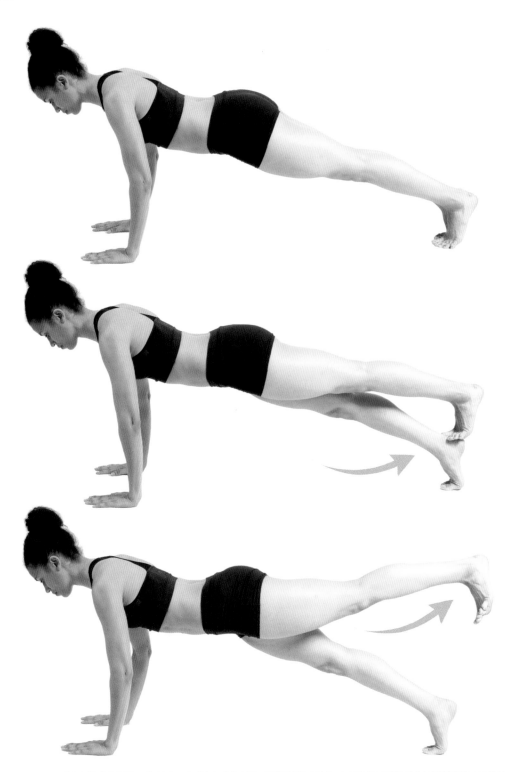

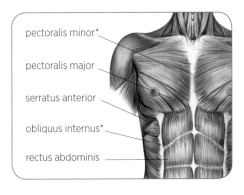

pectoralis minor*

pectoralis major

serratus anterior

obliquus internus*

rectus abdominis

DO IT RIGHT

- Maintain your pelvis and abdomen at the same height throughout the pose.
- Remain open across the front of your chest.
- Keep your major muscles engaged.
- Avoid raising your shoulders toward your ears.
- Do not arch your neck or allow your head to hang.
- Avoid twisting your hips as you move your leg.

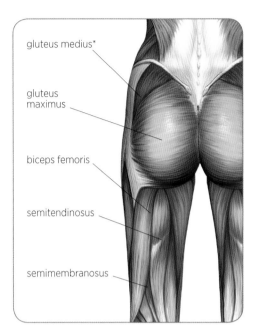

gluteus medius*

gluteus maximus

biceps femoris

semitendinosus

semimembranosus

FACT FILE

SANSKRIT
- Eka Pada Phalakasana

TARGETS
- Shoulders
- Abdominals
- Obliques
- Glutes

BENEFITS
- Stretches Achilles tendon
- Strengthens upper limbs and shoulder girdle
- Stabilizes major muscles

CAUTIONS
- Elbow issues
- Toe joint stiffness
- Wrist weakness

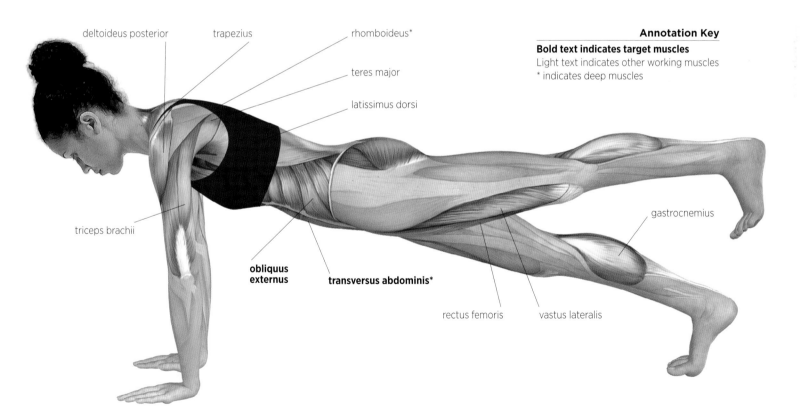

deltoideus posterior

trapezius

rhomboideus*

teres major

latissimus dorsi

triceps brachii

obliquus externus

transversus abdominis*

rectus femoris

vastus lateralis

gastrocnemius

Annotation Key

Bold text indicates target muscles
Light text indicates other working muscles
* indicates deep muscles

Bird Dog Pose

Bird Dog Pose, which resembles a dog pointing at a game bird, stabilizes your upper and lower back as well as your shoulders. The Bird Dog may look simple, but it really challenges your sense of balance and coordination. As an isometric exercise, you contract and hold specific muscles in a static position. This offers the added benefit of stabilizing the associated joints.

HOW TO DO IT

- Squat down and place your hands on the mat, making sure that they are aligned under your shoulders, with your fingers facing the front of the mat.

- Extend your legs parallel and hip-width apart, with your weight on the balls of your feet, so that your body forms one long line from your shoulders to your heels.

- Extend your left arm forward and parallel to the floor, while lifting your right leg and extending it behind you.

- Hold for the recommended breaths, and then repeat on the opposite side.

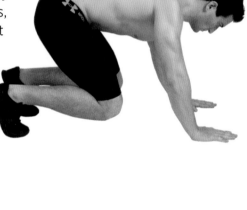

DO IT RIGHT

- Be sure to raise both the extended arm and leg high enough so that they are parallel to the floor.
- Engage your abdominals by drawing your navel toward your spine.
- You may wobble a bit at first—it will take you a few tries to get your balance.
- Avoid allowing your lower back to sag.

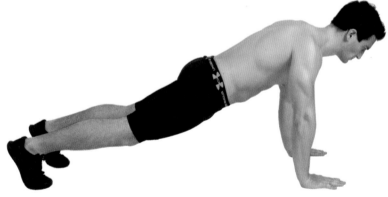

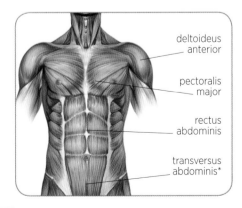

deltoideus anterior

pectoralis major

rectus abdominis

transversus abdominis*

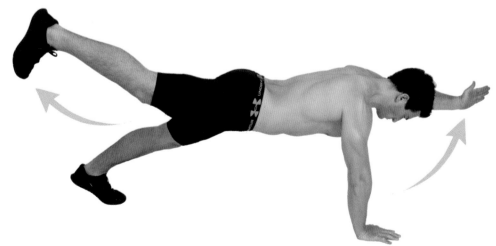

SANSKRIT
• Parsva Balasana

TARGETS
• Upper arms
• Core
• Glutes
• Hamstrings

BENEFITS
• Stabilizes upper and lower back
• Stabilizes shoulders
• Strengthens abdomen and obliques
• Improves balance and coordination

CAUTIONS
• Shoulder issues
• Wrist injuries
• Lower-back injuries

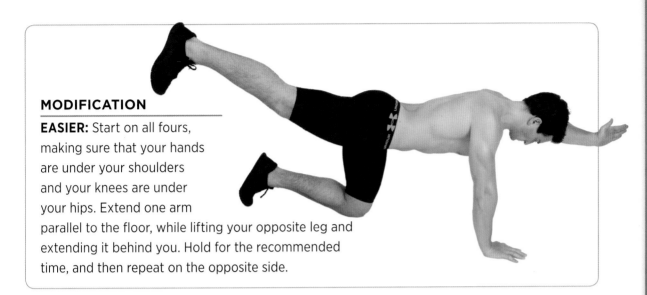

MODIFICATION

EASIER: Start on all fours, making sure that your hands are under your shoulders and your knees are under your hips. Extend one arm parallel to the floor, while lifting your opposite leg and extending it behind you. Hold for the recommended time, and then repeat on the opposite side.

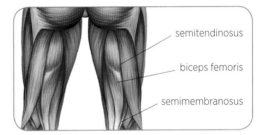

trapezius
subscapularis*
supraspinatus*
infraspinatus*
teres minor
rhomboideus*
erector spinae*

semitendinosus
biceps femoris
semimembranosus

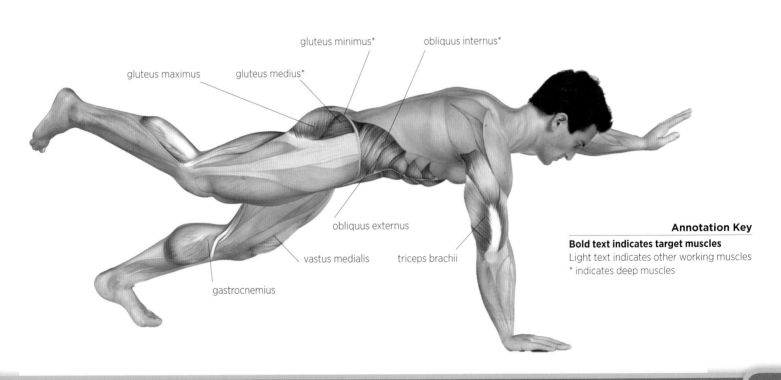

gluteus minimus*
obliquus internus*
gluteus maximus
gluteus medius*
obliquus externus
vastus medialis
triceps brachii
gastrocnemius

Annotation Key
Bold text indicates target muscles
Light text indicates other working muscles
* indicates deep muscles

Plow Pose

Plow Pose stretches the entire back of your body, from your shoulders to your heels. It can also provide a rejuvenating experience—nourishing the spine, calming and restoring the sympathetic nervous system, improving memory, and relieving stress.

HOW TO DO IT

- Lie on your back with your knees bent. Your arms should be at your sides, with your palms placed flat on the mat.

- Tighten your abdominals and extend your legs straight up toward the ceiling.

- Inhale, press your arms into the mat, and tuck your tailbone toward your pubis. Begin to roll your back off the mat, lifting up your buttocks and hips and extending your legs over your head. Your torso should now be perpendicular to the floor.

- Exhale and continue to extend your legs beyond your head. Squeeze your legs together and bend at your waist until your toes touch the floor. Keep pressing your palms into the mat, pushing through your arms to maintain the lift in your hips.

- Hold for the recommended breaths, and then slowly return to the starting position.

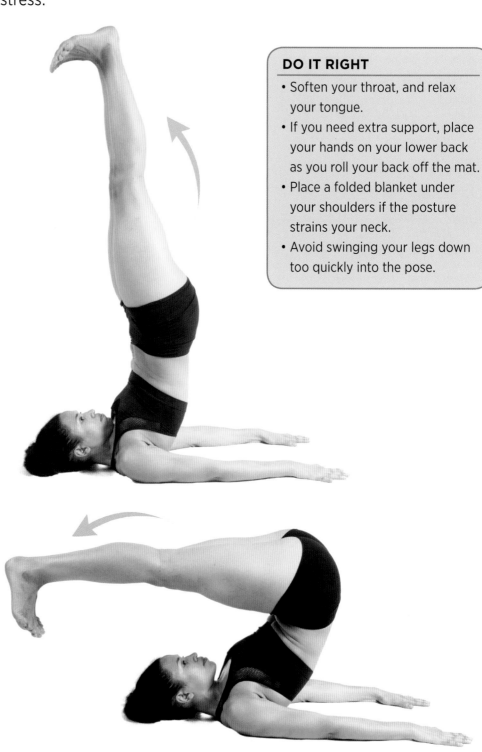

DO IT RIGHT

- Soften your throat, and relax your tongue.
- If you need extra support, place your hands on your lower back as you roll your back off the mat.
- Place a folded blanket under your shoulders if the posture strains your neck.
- Avoid swinging your legs down too quickly into the pose.

FACT FILE

SANSKRIT
• Halasana

TARGETS
• Spine
• Core
• Hamstrings

BENEFITS
• Stretches spine and legs
• Relieves stress and restores energy
• Relieves backache and headache
• Stimulates digestion

CAUTIONS
• High blood pressure
• Neck issues
• Pregnancy

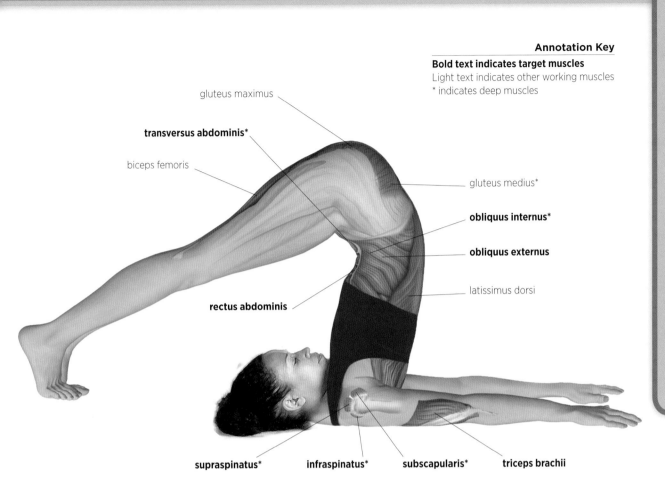

Annotation Key

Bold text indicates target muscles
Light text indicates other working muscles
* indicates deep muscles

gluteus maximus

transversus abdominis*

biceps femoris

gluteus medius*

obliquus internus*

obliquus externus

latissimus dorsi

rectus abdominis

supraspinatus* **infraspinatus*** **subscapularis*** **triceps brachii**

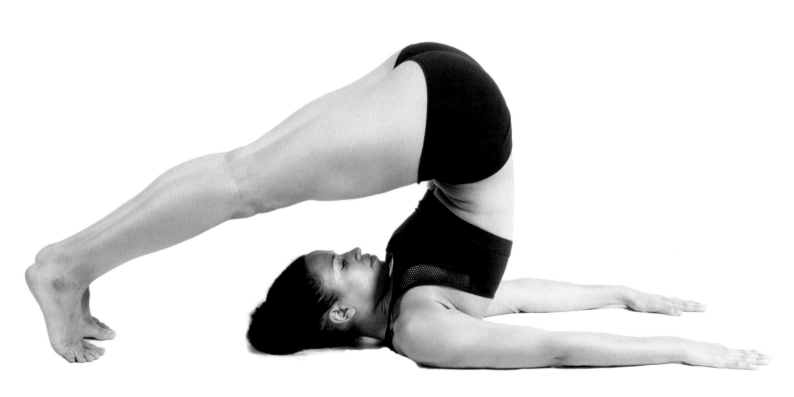

Reverse Tabletop Pose

Reverse Tabletop Pose, also called Half Upward Plank Pose, provides a great counterpose after performing forward bends, but it also has many benefits of its own. It stretches the front of your body and your shoulders, and strengthens your arms, wrists, and legs. This energizing chest opener also improves your posture.

HOW TO DO IT

- Begin in Staff Pose (pages 218–19), sitting with your legs straight in front of you. Place your palms flat on the mat at your hips, with your fingers pointing toward your feet.

- Bend your knees and place your feet flat on the mat. Leave some space between your hips and feet, so that when you come up into position, your knees are perpendicular to the floor.

- Pressing firmly into your hands and feet, inhale and squeeze your buttocks and thighs as you lift your hips up to knee height.

- Straighten your arms, and check that your thighs and torso are parallel to the floor.

- Your wrists should be directly beneath your shoulders. Draw your shoulder blades together, and open your chest. Keep your neck neutral, or gently begin to drop your head if this feels comfortable. Try to relax your buttocks, and hold the pose only with the strength of your legs.

- Hold for the recommended breaths, then release your hips back to the mat, and straighten your legs.

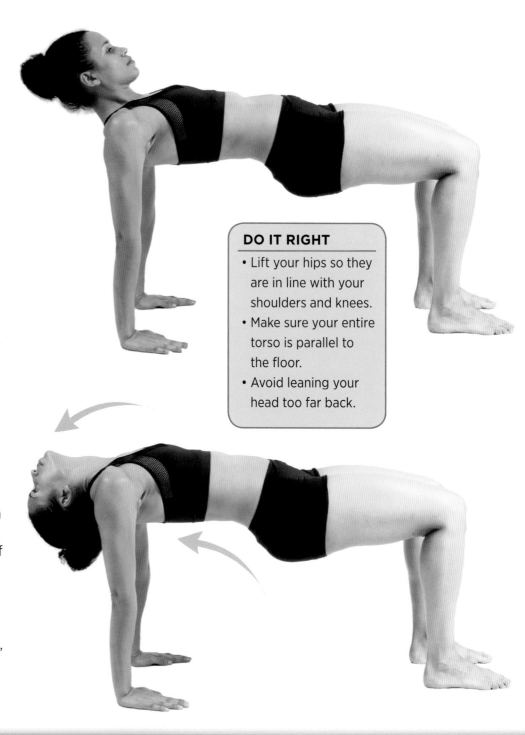

DO IT RIGHT

- Lift your hips so they are in line with your shoulders and knees.
- Make sure your entire torso is parallel to the floor.
- Avoid leaning your head too far back.

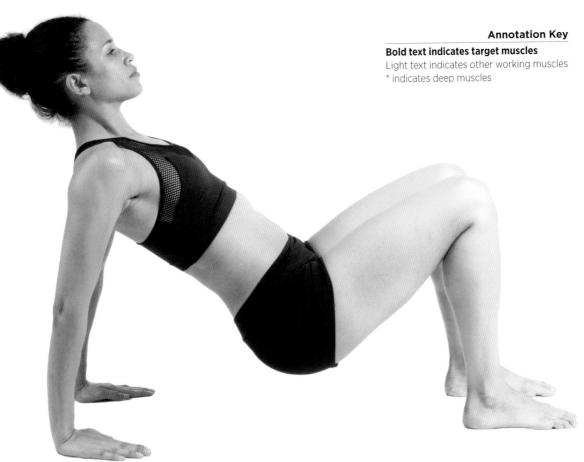

FACT FILE

SANSKRIT
• Ardha Purvottanasana

TARGETS
• Thighs
• Glutes
• Chest
• Shoulders

BENEFITS
• Opens chest
• Stretches quads and hamstrings
• Strengthens glutes and upper back

CAUTIONS
• Lower-back issues
• Wrist injuries

Annotation Key

Bold text indicates target muscles
Light text indicates other working muscles
* indicates deep muscles

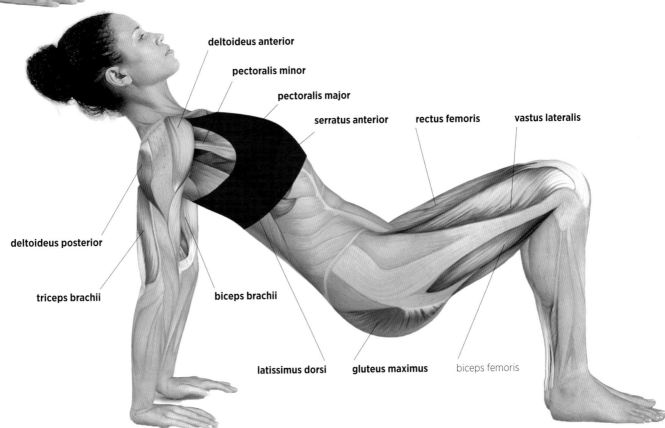

deltoideus anterior

pectoralis minor

pectoralis major

serratus anterior

rectus femoris

vastus lateralis

deltoideus posterior

triceps brachii

biceps brachii

latissimus dorsi

gluteus maximus

biceps femoris

Upward Plank Pose

This pose has much to offer: it builds up the muscles of your arms, legs, and spine and stretches your chest, abdominals, ankles, and feet. Upward Plank Pose also helps hone your sense of balance.

HOW TO DO IT

- Sit in Staff Pose (pages 218–19), with your legs extended in front of you and your hands on the floor at your sides.

- Bring your hands several inches behind your hips, and rotate your palms so that your fingertips point forward, keeping your hands shoulder-width apart.

- Bend your knees and place your fleet flat on the floor, turning your big toes slightly inward and placing your heels at least a foot away from your buttocks.

- Exhale and press down with your hands and feet, lifting your hips until your back and thighs are parallel to the floor. Keep your shoulders directly above your wrists.

- Without lowering your hips, straighten your legs one at a time.

- Lift your chest, and bring your shoulder blades together while pushing your hips higher, creating a slight arch in your back. Do not squeeze your buttocks to create the lift.

- Slowly elongate your neck, and let it drop back gently. Hold for the recommended breaths, and then return to Staff Pose.

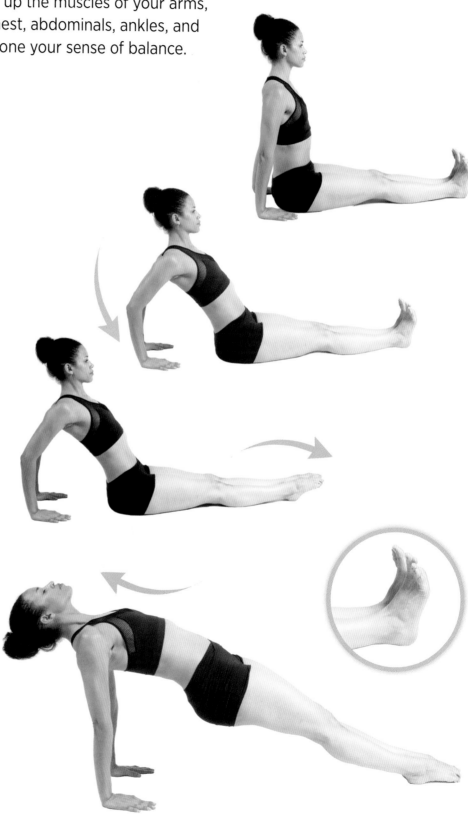

DO IT RIGHT

- Be careful not to overextend your back; instead, use your hamstrings and shoulders to open your hips and chest.
- If you have weak hamstrings, widen your legs while holding your hips elevated.
- Deepen the extension of your upper back by breathing steadily.

FACT FILE

SANSKRIT
- Purvottanasana

TARGETS
- Spine
- Arms and wrists
- Hamstrings

BENEFITS
- Strengthens the spine, arms, and hamstrings
- Extends the hips and chest

CAUTIONS
- Wrist injuries
- Elbow injuries
- Shoulder issues
- Neck issues

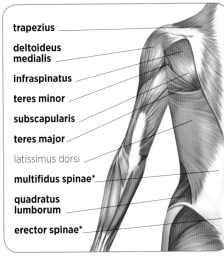

trapezius
deltoideus medialis
infraspinatus
teres minor
subscapularis
teres major
latissimus dorsi
multifidus spinae*
quadratus lumborum
erector spinae*

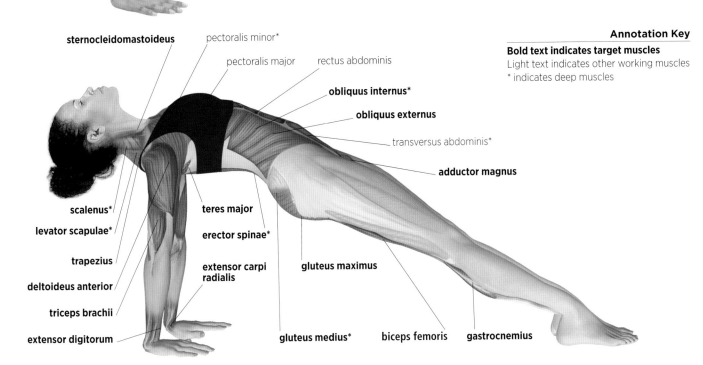

Annotation Key

Bold text indicates target muscles
Light text indicates other working muscles
* indicates deep muscles

sternocleidomastoideus
pectoralis minor*
pectoralis major
rectus abdominis
obliquus internus*
obliquus externus
transversus abdominis*
adductor magnus
scalenus*
levator scapulae*
teres major
erector spinae*
trapezius
extensor carpi radialis
gluteus maximus
deltoideus anterior
triceps brachii
extensor digitorum
gluteus medius*
biceps femoris
gastrocnemius

Upward Plank with Lifted Leg

Like other plank poses, this variation works many parts of the body—your shoulders, abdominals, sides, hips, glutes, thighs, and lower legs. It also helps improve your balance.

HOW TO DO IT

• Sit with your legs parallel and extended in front of you. Place your hands on the floor behind you, with your fingers pointed toward your feet.

• Press up through your arms and lift up your chest, squeezing your buttocks and lifting your hips while pressing your heels into the floor. Continue lifting your pelvis until your body forms a long straight line from your shoulders to your feet.

• Without allowing your pelvis to drop, raise your right leg to about shoulder height.

• Hold for the recommended breaths, slowly lower your foot to the mat, and repeat on the opposite side. Perform the recommended repetitions.

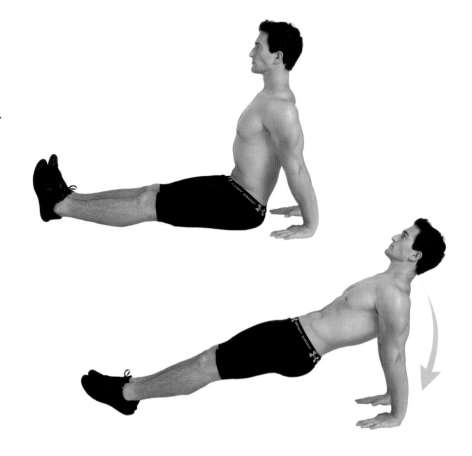

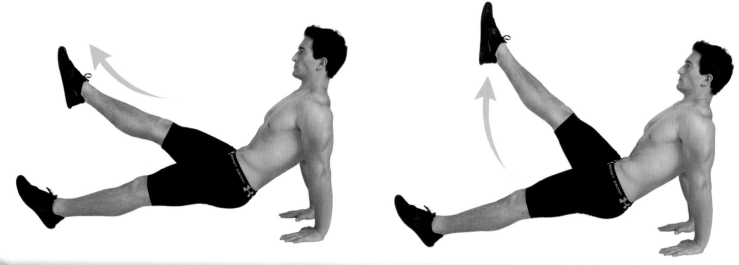

SANSKRIT
• None

TARGETS
• Hip extensor
  muscles
• Core stabilizers
• Arms
• Legs

BENEFITS
• Strengthens
  shins and calves
• Stretches
  quadriceps and
  hamstrings
• Targets
  abdomen and
  obliques

CAUTIONS
• Wrist pain
• Knee pain
• Shoulder injuries
• Shooting pains
  down leg

DO IT RIGHT

• Your pelvis should remain
  elevated throughout the
  exercise.
• Avoid allowing your
  shoulders to sink into their
  sockets. If your legs do
  not feel strong enough
  to support your body,
  slightly bend your knees.

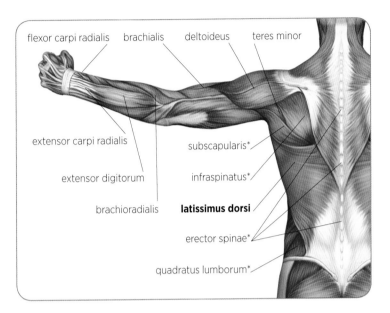

flexor carpi radialis
brachialis
deltoideus
teres minor
extensor carpi radialis
subscapularis*
extensor digitorum
infraspinatus*
brachioradialis
latissimus dorsi
erector spinae*
quadratus lumborum*

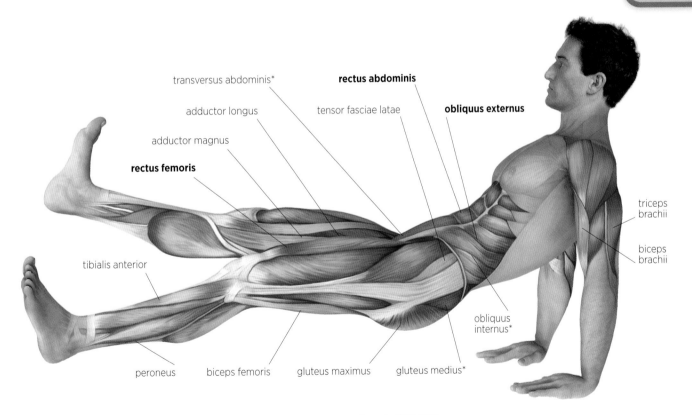

transversus abdominis*
rectus abdominis
adductor longus
tensor fasciae latae
obliquus externus
adductor magnus
rectus femoris
triceps
brachii
tibialis anterior
biceps
brachii
obliquus
internus*
peroneus
biceps femoris
gluteus maximus
gluteus medius*

Annotation Key

Bold text indicates target muscles
Light text indicates other working muscles
* indicates deep muscles

Supported Shoulderstand

Shoulderstand has been variously called the "queen" and the "mother" of all asanas, and as such, it has many variations. They all stretch your shoulders, neck, and upper spine and help improve your balance. This Supported Shoulderstand is an inverted asana found in hatha yoga.

HOW TO DO IT

• Lie on your back, with your knees bent and arms at your sides.

• Tighten your abdominal muscles, and lift your feet off the mat. Exhale, press your arms into the floor, and raise your legs higher so that your buttocks come off the floor.

• Continue lifting your legs, bringing your knees toward your face, as you roll your back off the mat from your hips to your shoulders. With your upper arms firmly planted on the floor, bend your elbows, and place your hands against your lower back. Draw your elbows in closer to your sides.

• Inhale, tuck your tailbone toward your pubis, and straighten your legs back toward your head. Your torso should be perpendicular to the floor.

• With your next inhalation, extend your legs up toward the ceiling, opening your hips as you lift. Squeeze your buttocks, and press down with your elbows to create a straight, elongated line from your chest to your toes.

• Hold for the recommended breaths. Bend your knees and hips, and then return to the starting position.

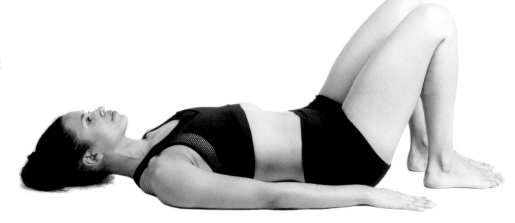

DO IT RIGHT

• Be sure to soften your throat, and relax your tongue.
• If you can't lift your pelvis, practice a few feet away from a wall and walk your feet up the wall until you can place your hands on your back.
• Place folded blankets below your shoulders if the posture strains your neck.
• Avoid bending at your hips once you are in the posture, because it puts added pressure on your neck and spine.
• Avoid splaying your elbows.

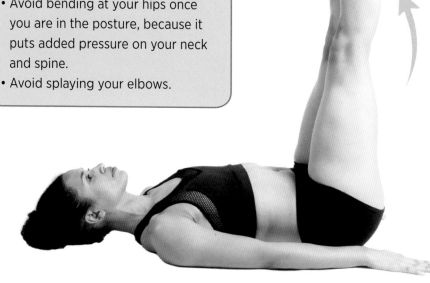

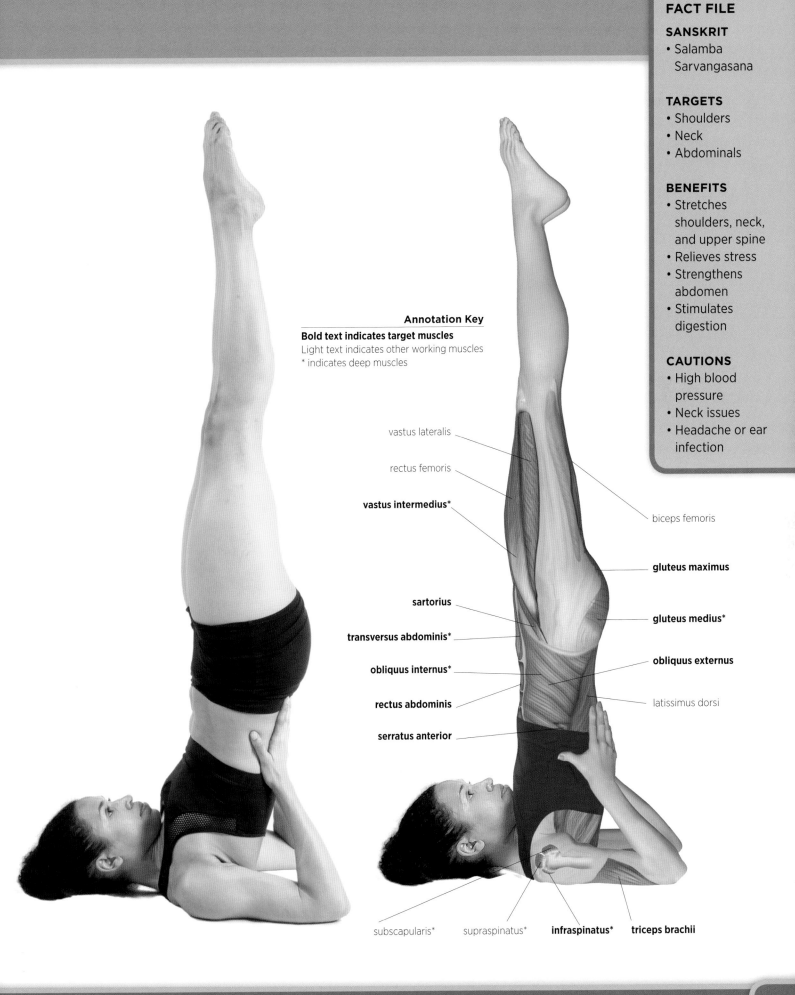

SANSKRIT
• Salamba Sarvangasana

TARGETS
• Shoulders
• Neck
• Abdominals

BENEFITS
• Stretches shoulders, neck, and upper spine
• Relieves stress
• Strengthens abdomen
• Stimulates digestion

CAUTIONS
• High blood pressure
• Neck issues
• Headache or ear infection

Annotation Key

Bold text indicates target muscles
Light text indicates other working muscles
* indicates deep muscles

vastus lateralis

rectus femoris

vastus intermedius*

biceps femoris

gluteus maximus

sartorius

gluteus medius*

transversus abdominis*

obliquus externus

obliquus internus*

latissimus dorsi

rectus abdominis

serratus anterior

subscapularis*   supraspinatus*   **infraspinatus***   **triceps brachii**

One-Legged Side Plank Prep

Side planks are excellent poses for stabilizing your spine and building up core strength. This One-Legged Side Plank Prep really engages your abdominal obliques as well as your back, shoulders, and arms. It also develops a strong sense of balance.

HOW TO DO IT

• Begin in Plank Pose (pages 260–61), with your wrists directly under your shoulders. Turn your hands out until your index fingers are parallel to each other. Press down through the knuckles of your index fingers. Separate your shoulder blades, and slide them down your back.

• Shift your weight onto your extended left arm and your left foot, keeping your legs together at your ankles.

• Raise your right arm straight up from your shoulder, fingers extended toward the ceiling, and lift your right leg until it is parallel to the floor.

• Hold for the recommended breaths, return to the starting position, and then repeat on the opposite side.

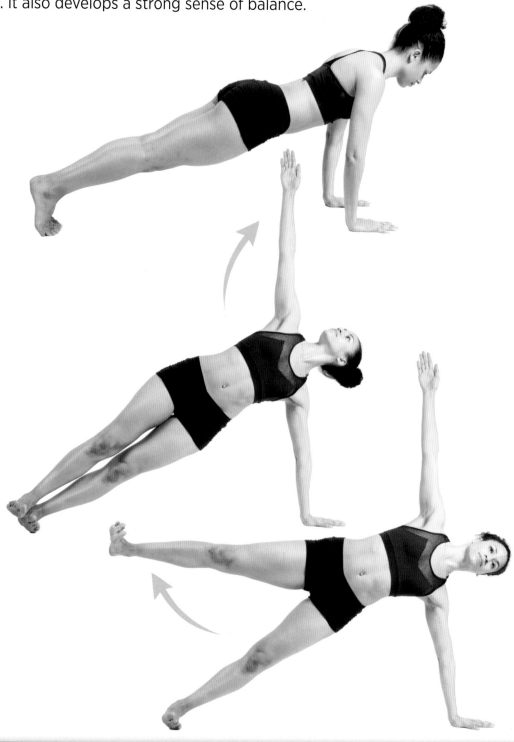

SANSKRIT
• Eka Pada
  Vasisthasana

TARGETS
• Legs and hips
• Shoulders
• Abdominals

BENEFITS
• Stretches
  hamstrings
• Strengthens
  abdomen
• Increases hip
  flexibility

CAUTIONS
• Groin injuries
• Back issues
• Ankle injuries

DO IT RIGHT

• Lift your hips high to take the weight off your upper body.
• Maintain stability in your shoulders by pressing your lower arm into the floor.
• Keep body movement to a minimum.
• Press through your fingers if your wrists start to hurt from the pressure.
• Avoid allowing your body weight to sink into your wrists or shoulders.

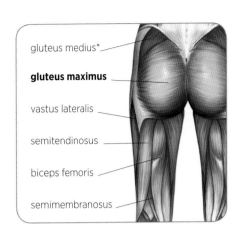

gluteus medius*
gluteus maximus
vastus lateralis
semitendinosus
biceps femoris
semimembranosus

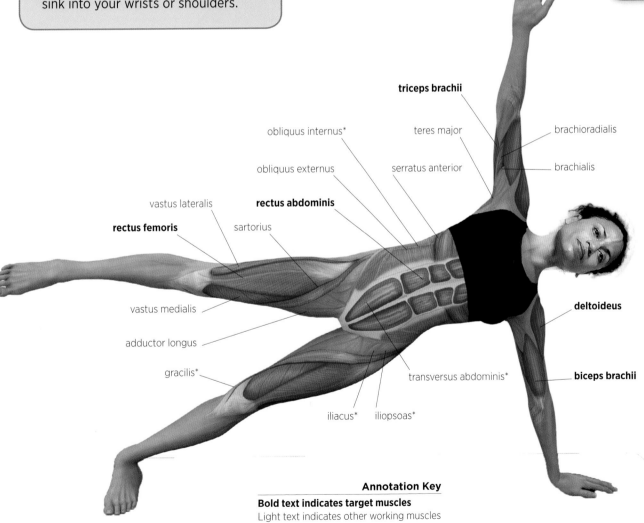

triceps brachii
obliquus internus*
teres major
brachioradialis
obliquus externus
serratus anterior
brachialis
vastus lateralis
rectus abdominis
rectus femoris
sartorius
deltoideus
vastus medialis
adductor longus
gracilis*
transversus abdominis*
biceps brachii
iliacus* iliopsoas*

Annotation Key
Bold text indicates target muscles
Light text indicates other working muscles
* indicates deep muscles

One-Legged Side Plank Pose

This extended arm support pose stretches your spine and hips, while opening your shoulders and chest. Doing it properly requires a strong sense of balance and a great deal of flexibility.

HOW TO DO IT

- Begin in Side Plank Pose (pages 266–67), balancing on your left side.

- While resting on the outer edge of your left foot, externally rotate your right hip in order to bend your right leg, and then grasp your big toe with your fingers while keeping your left side in a straight diagonal line.

- Straighten your right leg until it is perpendicular to the floor, while grasping your right toe. Gaze forward.

- Hold for the recommended breaths, and then repeat on the opposite side.

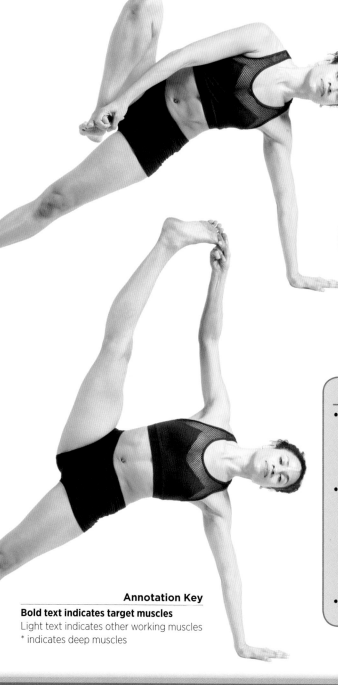

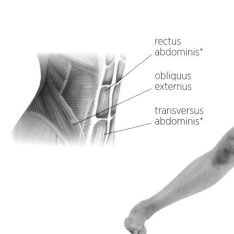

rectus abdominis*

obliquus externus

transversus abdominis*

Annotation Key
Bold text indicates target muscles
Light text indicates other working muscles
* indicates deep muscles

FACT FILE

SANSKRIT
- Eka Pada Vasisthasana

TARGETS
- Abdominals
- Arms and wrists
- Thighs

BENEFITS
- Opens shoulders and chest
- Stretches hips and hamstrings
- Improves balance

CAUTIONS
- Groin injuries
- Shoulder issues

DO IT RIGHT

- Look down at first to maintain balance, then gaze up if your neck feels comfortable.
- To hold the pose, continue to externally rotate your upper right arm, draw in the sides of your waist, and lift your navel in and up.
- Avoid arching your back.

Side Plank with Tree Legs

If you think your Side Plank could use a little more precision, this variation will help you hone it. It stretches your shoulders and thighs, and strengthens your arms and abdominals.

HOW TO DO IT

- Begin in Side Plank Pose (pages 266–67), with your left hand on the mat and your right arm raised toward the ceiling, fingers outstretched.

- Bend your right knee, and slide your right foot up the inside of your left leg.

- Attempt to get your right foot up to your inner left thigh. If it does not come up that high, place it on your left calf. Avoid placing it directly on the side of your knee.

- Your right foot will exert some pressure on your left leg, making it even more important to keep lifting your hips so they don't end up on the floor.

- Hold for the recommended breaths, return to the starting position, and then repeat on the opposite side.

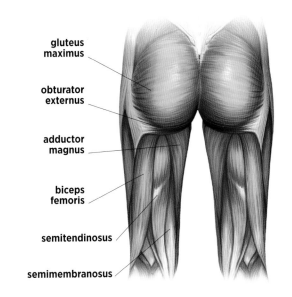

gluteus maximus

obturator externus

adductor magnus

biceps femoris

semitendinosus

semimembranosus

FACT FILE

SANSKRIT
- Vasisthasana

TARGETS
- Core
- Legs
- Shoulders

BENEFITS
- Engages abdomen and obliques
- Strengthens shoulders, arms, and wrists
- Improves balance and concentration

CAUTIONS
- Wrist injuries
- Ankle injuries
- Shoulder issues

DO IT RIGHT

- Keep your torso and lower leg diagonally aligned.
- Avoid letting your head roll back; keep your gaze forward.

Celibate's Pose

This demanding pose requires arm and shoulder strength as well as a powerful core. In Sanskrit, the name of this empowering pose means "having control over your senses and your lower limbs."

HOW TO DO IT

• Sit in Staff Pose (pages 218–19), with your legs together and outstretched.

• Place your palms on the floor beside your hips, with your elbows straight and your fingers facing the front of the mat.

• Adjust your hand position slightly forward, until you find your center of gravity.

• Inhale and push down with your arms, simultaneously using your abdominals to lift your hips, legs, and feet from the mat. Your legs should be horizontal and straight, and your spine slightly curved.

• Hold for the recommended breaths, then slowly lower your hips and legs to the mat.

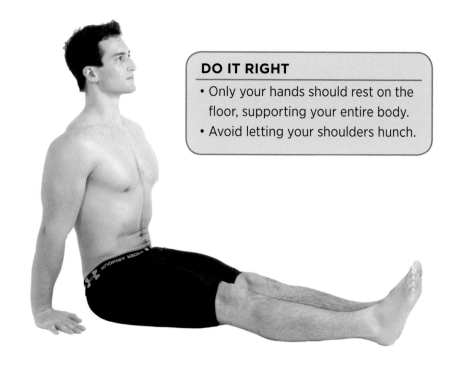

DO IT RIGHT
• Only your hands should rest on the floor, supporting your entire body.
• Avoid letting your shoulders hunch.

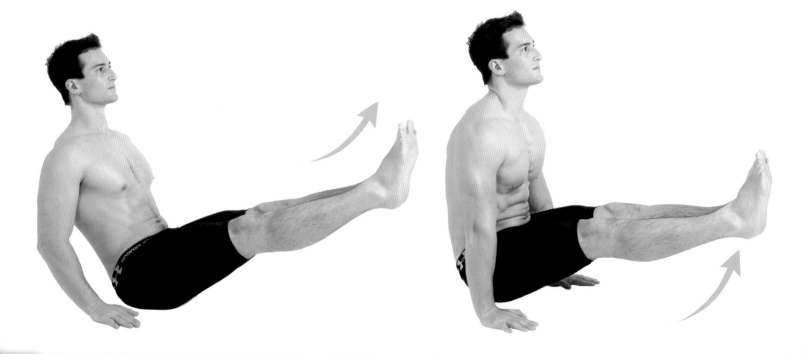

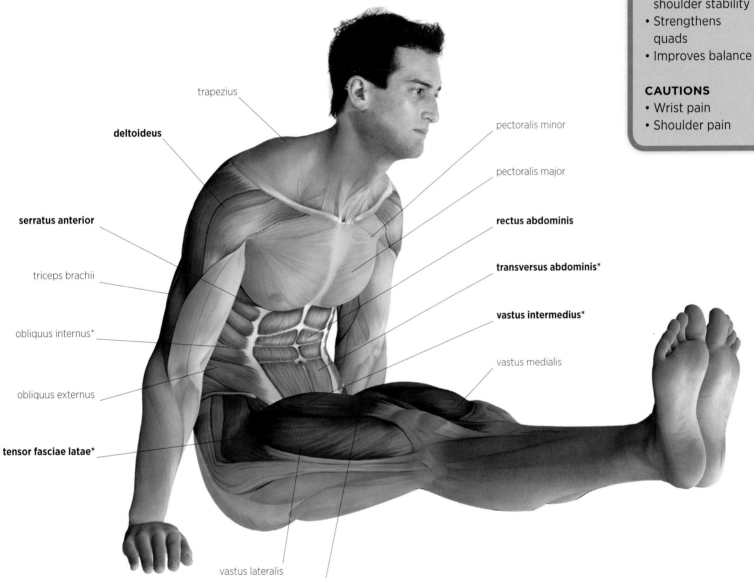

FACT FILE

SANSKRIT
• Brahmacharyasana

TARGETS
• Abdominals
• Shoulders
• Thighs

BENEFITS
• Increases core, pelvic, and shoulder stability
• Strengthens quads
• Improves balance

CAUTIONS
• Wrist pain
• Shoulder pain

trapezius

deltoideus

serratus anterior

triceps brachii

obliquus internus*

obliquus externus

tensor fasciae latae*

vastus lateralis

rectus femoris

pectoralis minor

pectoralis major

rectus abdominis

transversus abdominis*

vastus intermedius*

vastus medialis

Annotation Key

Bold text indicates target muscles
Light text indicates other working muscles
* indicates deep muscles

Crow Pose

A graceful asana, Crow Pose strengthens and tones your upper body and serves as an introduction to even more advanced arm balances. Crow Pose is often confused with Crane Pose (pages 296–97). The key difference between the two is in your arms: bend your elbows to perform Crow, and keep them straight to perform Crane.

HOW TO DO IT

- Begin in Garland Pose (pages 48–49), squatting with your feet and knees more than hip-width apart.

- Lean your torso forward, and place your hands in front of you on the mat, facing slightly inward, fingers spread.

- Bend your elbows, and rest your knees against your upper arms.

- Lifting up on the balls of your feet and leaning forward with your torso, bring your thighs toward your chest and your shins to your upper arms. Round your back as you feel your weight transfer to your wrists. Hold for the recommended breaths.

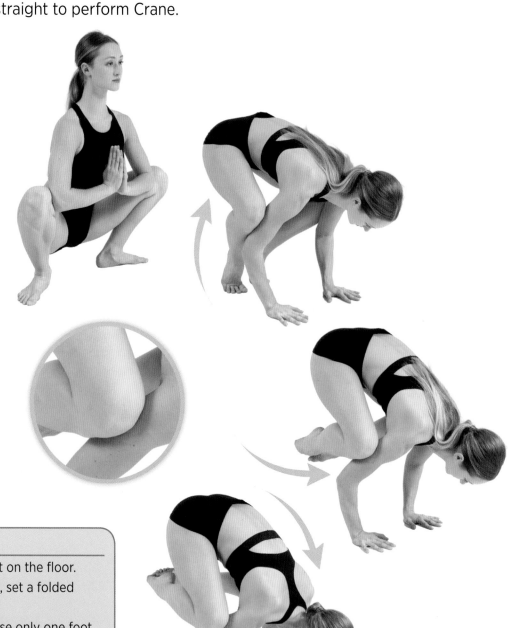

DO IT RIGHT

- To maintain balance, gaze at a spot on the floor.
- If you are afraid of tipping forward, set a folded blanket or cushion in front of you.
- Avoid "jumping" into the pose—raise only one foot at a time.
- Do not lower your head; keep it in a neutral position.

FACT FILE

SANSKRIT
- Kakasana

TARGETS
- Arms
- Shoulders
- Abdominals

BENEFITS
- Strengthens and tones arms and abdomen
- Strengthens wrists
- Improves balance

CAUTIONS
- Wrist injuries

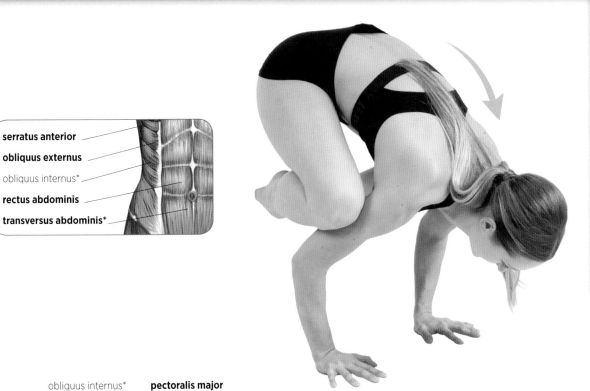

serratus anterior
obliquus externus
obliquus internus*
rectus abdominis
transversus abdominis*

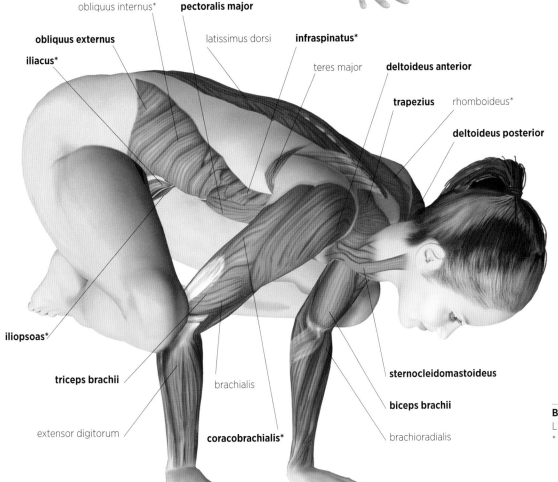

obliquus internus*
obliquus externus
iliacus*
pectoralis major
latissimus dorsi
infraspinatus*
teres major
deltoideus anterior
trapezius
rhomboideus*
deltoideus posterior
iliopsoas*
triceps brachii
brachialis
sternocleidomastoideus
biceps brachii
extensor digitorum
coracobrachialis*
brachioradialis

Annotation Key

Bold text indicates target muscles
Light text indicates other working muscles
* indicates deep muscles

Crane Pose

An asana for the adventurous, Crane Pose is an exciting arm balance. As you perform this pose, you will encounter the fear of falling, which you will eventually overcome.

HOW TO DO IT

• Begin in Garland Pose (pages 48–49), squatting with your feet and knees more than hip-width apart.

• Stretch your arms forward, bend your elbows, and then plant your hands on the floor. Rest the backs of your upper arms on your shins.

• Tuck your inner thighs against the sides of your torso and your shins into your armpits. Slide your upper arms down as low as you can onto your shins. Lift up onto the balls of your feet, and lean forward so that your weight is resting on the backs of your upper arms.

• Exhale and lean even farther forward until your feet leave the floor, so that your torso and legs now balance on the backs of your upper arms.

• Squeeze your legs against your arms, and firmly press your inner hands into the floor. Inhale, and then straighten your elbows. Hold for the recommended breaths.

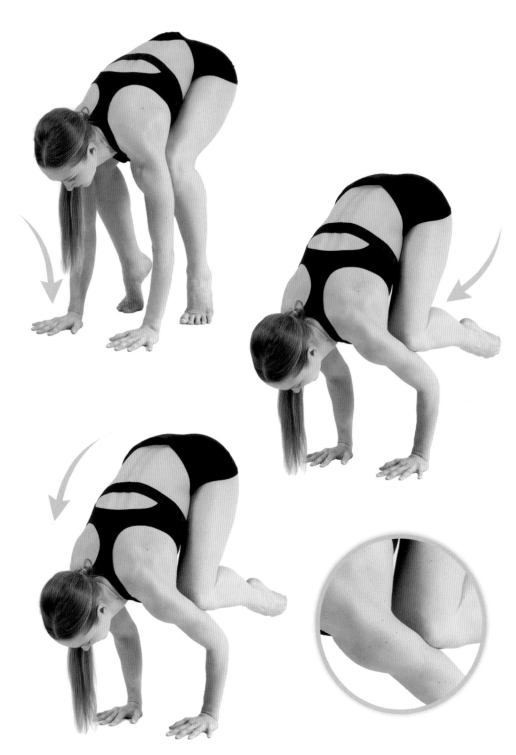

TARGETS
- Arms
- Shoulders
- Abdominals

BENEFITS
- Strengthens and tones arms and abdomen
- Strengthens wrists
- Improves balance

CAUTIONS
- Wrist injuries

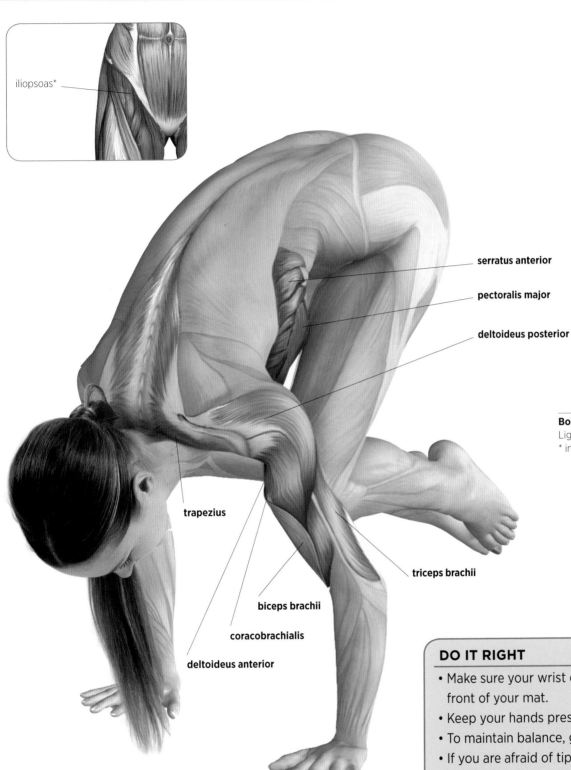

iliopsoas*

serratus anterior

pectoralis major

deltoideus posterior

trapezius

triceps brachii

biceps brachii

coracobrachialis

deltoideus anterior

Annotation Key

Bold text indicates target muscles
Light text indicates other working muscles
* indicates deep muscles

DO IT RIGHT
- Make sure your wrist creases are parallel to the front of your mat.
- Keep your hands pressed into the floor.
- To maintain balance, gaze at a spot on the floor.
- If you are afraid of tipping forward, set a folded blanket or cushion in front of you.
- Avoid dropping your head; this might cause you to tip forward.
- Avoid lifting or twisting your neck to the point where it feels strained.

Side Crane Pose

This more advanced version of Crane Pose (pages 296–97) strengthens both the upper body and the core. Poses like Side Crane remind us that yoga takes practice. Be patient—and have fun!

HOW TO DO IT

- Begin in Prayer Pose (pages 34–35), with your palms together at the middle of your chest. Keeping your legs together, perform a deep squat until your buttocks are just above your heels.

- Bring your arms across your body to your right side, touching your left elbow to the outside of your right thigh as your palms flatten on the floor. Exhale as you deepen the twist by pulling your right shoulder back.

- Position the outside of your right thigh on your left upper arm. Lean to the right until your hands are shoulder-width apart. Your hips and shoulders should maintain a deep twist.

- Slowly lift your pelvis as you shift your weight toward your hands, using your bent left arm as a support for your right thigh. Continue shifting to the right, drawing your abdominals in toward your spine. With your feet together, raise your bent legs completely off the floor, exhaling.

- Hold for the recommended breaths, and then exhale as you bring your feet to the floor. Repeat on the opposite side.

DO IT RIGHT

- To maintain balance, gaze at a spot on the floor.
- If you are afraid of tipping forward, set a folded blanket or cushion in front of you.
- Focus on twisting deeply as you enter the pose.
- Avoid "jumping" into the pose; ease your legs off the floor.

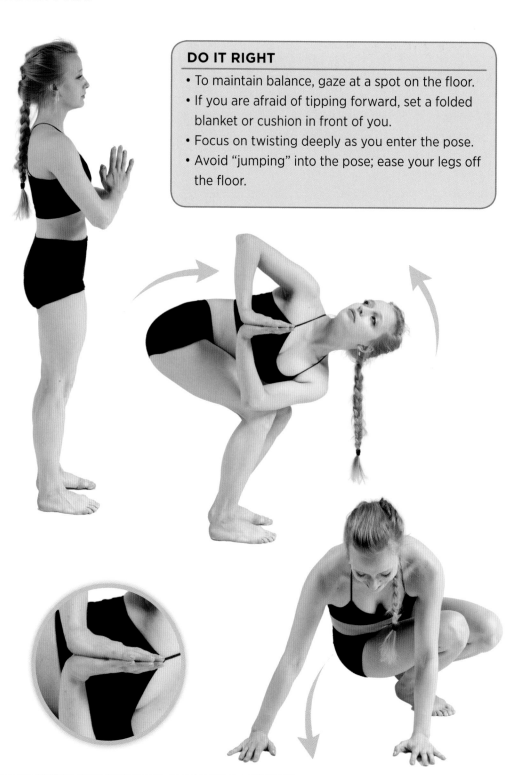

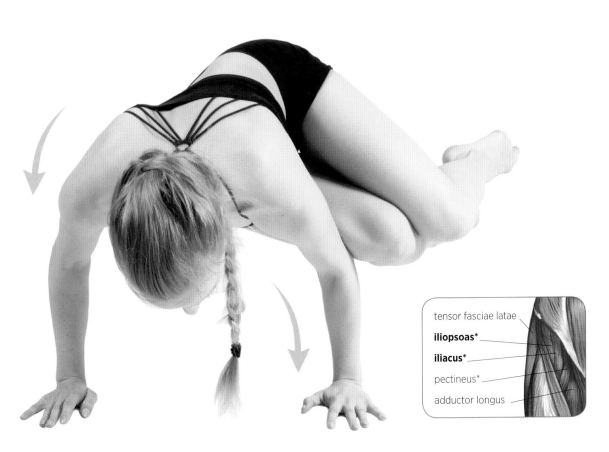

tensor fasciae latae
iliopsoas*
iliacus*
pectineus*
adductor longus

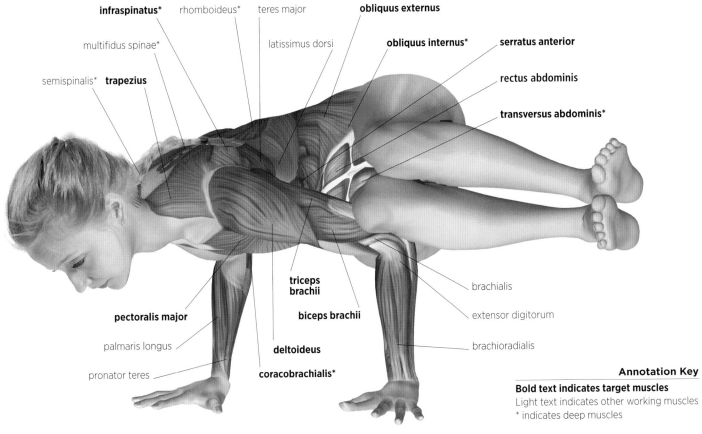

infraspinatus*   rhomboideus*   teres major   **obliquus externus**

multifidus spinae*   latissimus dorsi   **obliquus internus***   **serratus anterior**

semispinalis*   **trapezius**   **rectus abdominis**

transversus abdominis*

triceps brachii   brachialis

pectoralis major   **biceps brachii**   extensor digitorum

palmaris longus   **deltoideus**   brachioradialis

pronator teres   **coracobrachialis***

Annotation Key

Bold text indicates target muscles
Light text indicates other working muscles
* indicates deep muscles

Eight-Angle Pose

This advanced pose works a number of muscle groups in your shoulders, arms, and torso—and even the back of your thighs and calves. Eight-Angle Pose can seem intimidating at first, but with patient practice, you will be able to carry out the full pose.

HOW TO DO IT

- Sit in Staff Pose (pages 218–19), with your legs extended in front of you and your hands on the floor at your sides.

- Raise your right leg so that your thigh is perpendicular to the floor. Use your arms to draw your right leg over your right shoulder so that the back of your knee rests on your shoulder.

- Lean your torso forward, and place your hands shoulder-width apart on the floor in front of you. Your right hand should be on the outside of your right hip.

- Shift your weight forward onto your hands, and press upward, lifting your chest. Straighten your left leg in front of you.

- Exhale and lower your torso until it is parallel to the floor. Draw your left leg toward the right. Bending both legs so that they lock at the ankles, hook your right ankle below the left.

- Bend your arms, and lower your chest toward the floor, squeezing your legs together and extending them to the right.

- Twist your torso to the left, and tuck your elbows in. Gaze forward.

- Hold for the recommended breaths, and then slowly straighten your arms, and lift your torso. Bend your knees, unhook your ankles, and return to a seated position on the floor. Repeat on the opposite side.

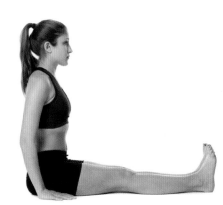

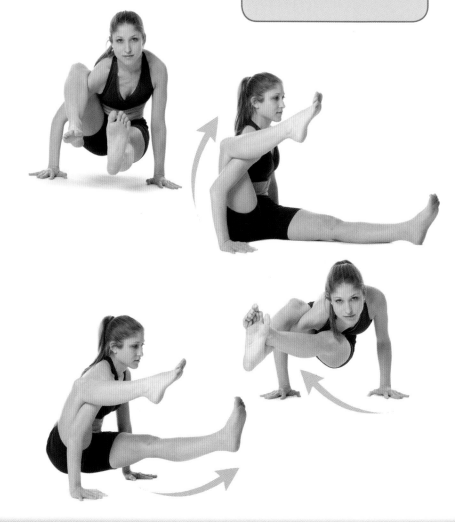

DO IT RIGHT

- Keep your legs symmetrical by twisting more from the spine than from your hips.
- If you struggle to keep your body lifted, use blocks for your hands in order to practice pressing your hips up as one leg rests on your shoulder.
- Avoid letting your upper hip rock backward; this will cause the bottom hip to drop.

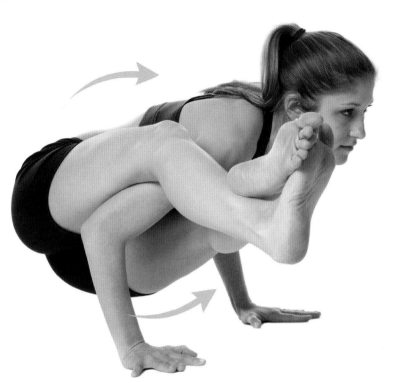
tensor fasciae latae
iliopsoas*
iliacus*
pectineus*
adductor longus

deltoideus medialis
teres minor
infraspinatus*
subscapularis
teres major
rhomboideus
latissimus dorsi
quadratus lumborum
erector spinae*

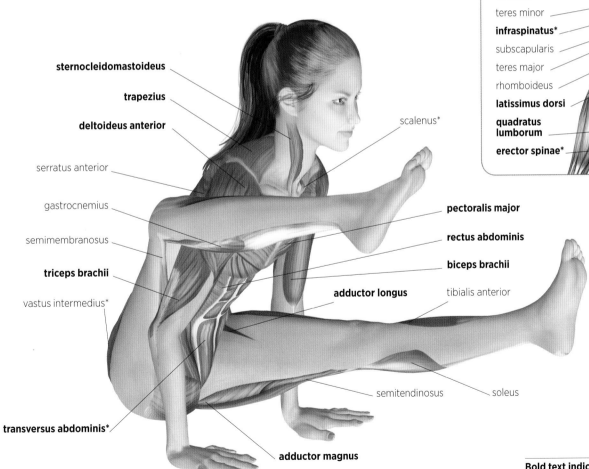

sternocleidomastoideus

trapezius

deltoideus anterior

serratus anterior

gastrocnemius

semimembranosus

triceps brachii

vastus intermedius*

transversus abdominis*

scalenus*

pectoralis major

rectus abdominis

biceps brachii

adductor longus

tibialis anterior

semitendinosus

soleus

adductor magnus

Annotation Key

Bold text indicates target muscles
Light text indicates other working muscles
* indicates deep muscles

Flying Pigeon Pose

This complicated inversion pose can be challenging even for yoga experts. With patience and practice, you can reap the rewards of this energizing pose, which opens your hips, strengthens your core, and develops your balance.

HOW TO DO IT

• Begin in Chair Pose (pages 54–55), pressing your palms together at the center of your chest. Raise your right foot and place your right ankle on your left thigh, flexing your foot. Breathe steadily.

• Bend your standing knee, lengthen your spine, and reach your arms toward the ceiling. Bring your fingertips to the floor in front of you. Keep your left foot flexed, and keep your hips level. Engage your lower abdominals.

• Start to shift your weight forward a little. Bend your elbows, creating a shelf for your right shin on your upper arms. Wrap your right foot around your left upper arm. Round your lower back, but move your chest forward as you shift forward.

• Stabilize your abdomen by drawing the left side of your abdomen toward your right side; this will help keep your pelvis from rolling open to your left as you extend your left leg behind you. Your raised leg should be in a straight line with your torso. Gaze at the floor in front of you.

• Hold for the recommended breaths, carefully return to the starting position, and repeat on the opposite side.

DO IT RIGHT
• Press downward with your hands and wrists to improve stability.
• Bring your bent knee as far up on your arm as possible.
• Avoid rounding your spine too greatly.

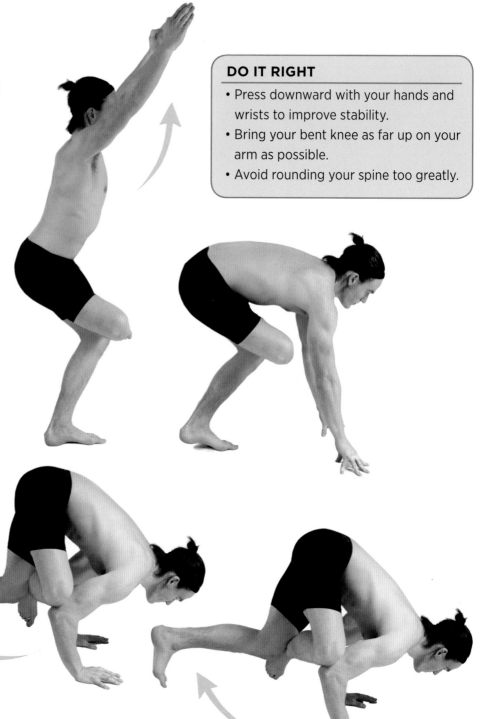

FACT FILE
SANSKRIT
• Eka Pada Galavasana

TARGETS
• Shoulders
• Hips
• Glutes

BENEFITS
• Opens hips and groin
• Strengthens shoulders and arms
• Improves balance

CAUTIONS
• Shoulder issues
• Groin injuries

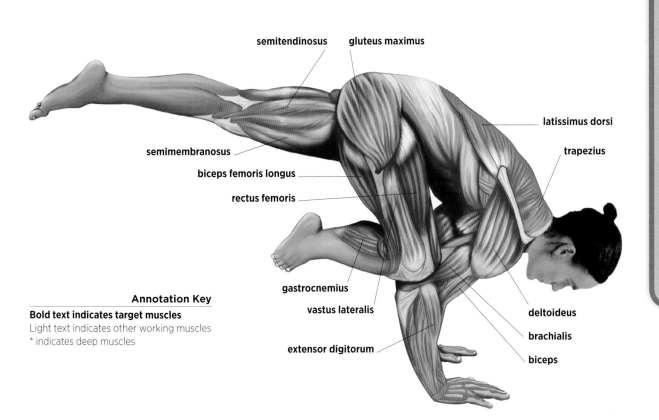

semitendinosus
gluteus maximus
latissimus dorsi
semimembranosus
trapezius
biceps femoris longus
rectus femoris
gastrocnemius
vastus lateralis
deltoideus
extensor digitorum
brachialis
biceps

Annotation Key

Bold text indicates target muscles
Light text indicates other working muscles
* indicates deep muscles

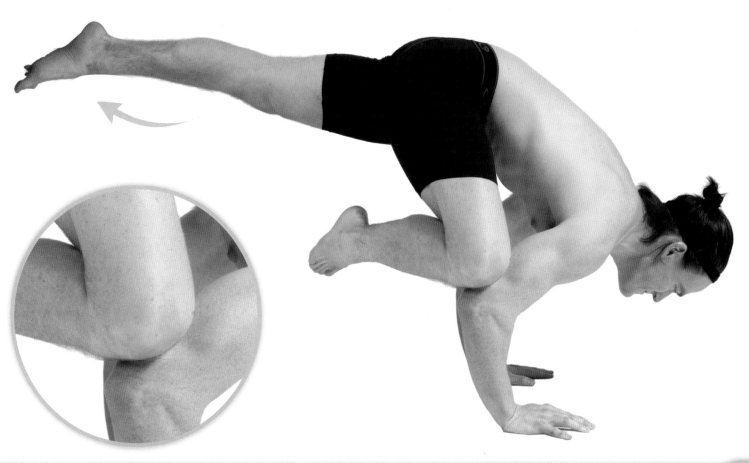

Supported Headstand

This advanced inversion pose, often called the "king of asanas," allows you to find clarity of mind while targeting your back, shoulders, and sides. If you are new to this pose, start by performing it against a wall. Once you feel more secure, you can balance on your own.

HOW TO DO IT

• Place your mat against a wall, if desired. Begin on all fours. Place your forearms on the floor, shoulder-width apart, externally rotating your outer upper arms and interlacing your fingers. Tuck your toes under and lift your hips upward. This position is called Dolphin Pose (page 270), which is great prep for Headstand.

• Maintaining your alignment, slightly release the grip of your fingers so that your palms are more open while your fingers stay interlaced. Place the top of your head on the floor and the back of your head on your hands. Find a solid foundation, with your forearms and outer wrists pressing down.

• Allowing your heels to lift off the floor, walk your feet toward your head until your hips are directly above your shoulders. At the same time, press your chest toward your thighs. This will help you lift up into the full pose and protect your neck from compression.

• Bend one knee and then the other into your chest. Begin to straighten both legs up toward the ceiling. Alternately, you can rest your feet against a wall before straightening your legs. Hold this pose for as long as you can maintain your form.

• Find a slight internal rotation in your thighs as you lengthen your tailbone up toward your heels. Reach the balls of your feet toward the ceiling to help activate the backs of your legs and your gluteal muscles.

• Hold for the recommended breaths, which should increase as you become more proficient. Release the pose by bending your knees into your chest and slowly lowering your legs to the mat.

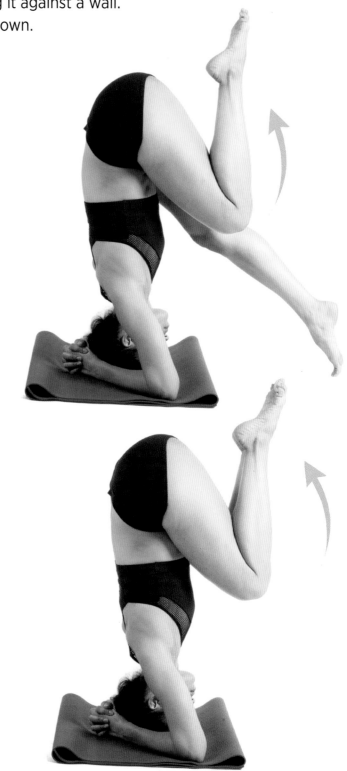

Annotation Key
Bold text indicates target muscles
Light text indicates other working muscles
* indicates deep muscles

FACT FILE
SANSKRIT
• Salamba
Sirsasana

TARGETS
• Legs
• Shoulders
• Sides

BENEFITS
• Strengthens
legs, arms, and
spine
• Calms mind and
body
• Relieves stress
• Increases
circulation
• Improves
digestion

CAUTIONS
• Back issues
• High blood
pressure
• Neck issues
• Glaucoma

DO IT RIGHT

• Press your forearms firmly
and evenly into the mat.
• Avoid placing your
forehead on the floor,
because this can cause
compression in your neck.

gluteus medius*

transversus abdominis*

latissimus dorsi

rectus abdominis

infraspinatus

trapezius

deltoideus medialis

triceps brachii

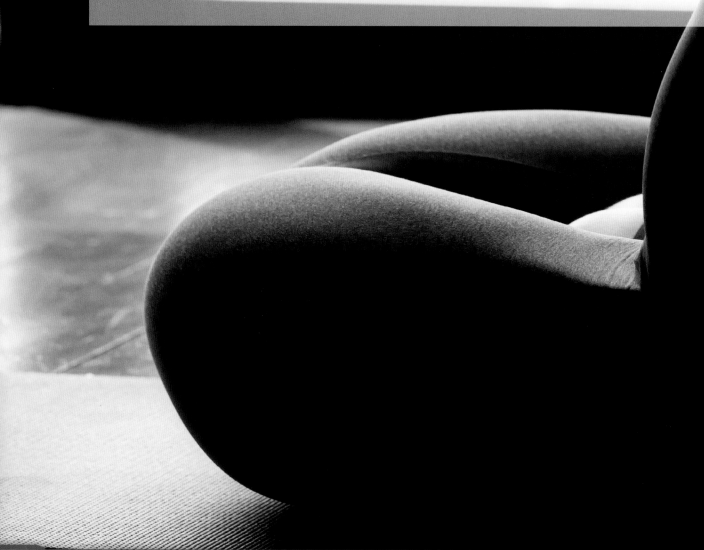

CHAPTER SEVEN

RECLINING AND RESTORATIVE POSES

Reclining poses not only relax and restore the body, but they also help you cool down at the end of a yoga session. In addition to calming the nervous system and easing tension, they allow your muscles to experience the positive effects of the positions you have just practiced. Do not rush to end these poses; savor them, and give them time to work their magic.

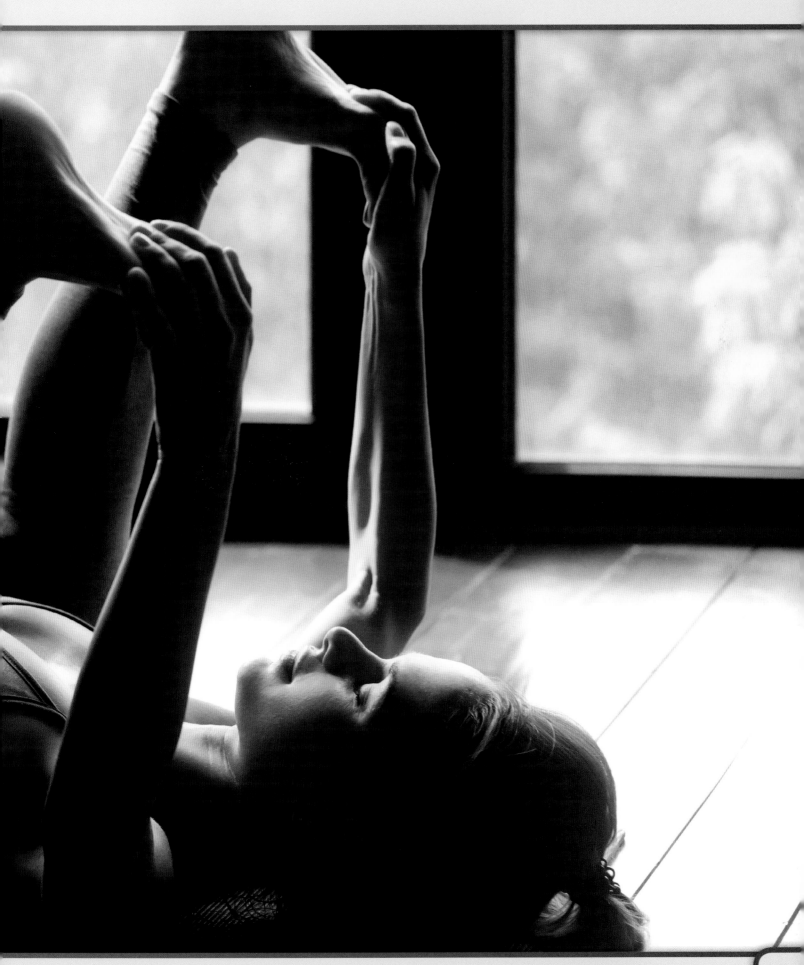

Corpse Pose

Corpse Pose may appear quite basic, but this pose can be highly challenging. Relaxing all your muscles requires total "surrender" to the pose and a quieting of both the body and mind.

HOW TO DO IT

• Lie on your back, and let your arms release outward from your sides far enough from your body for your armpits to have space. Relax your hands and turn your palms upward.

• Let your legs separate to about as wide as your mat so that your lower back starts to release. Allow your legs, feet, and ankles to relax completely. Draw your buttocks down toward your heels to create length in your lower back; to help with this, you can lift your hips slightly and use your hands to draw your buttocks down away from your waist before you completely relax.

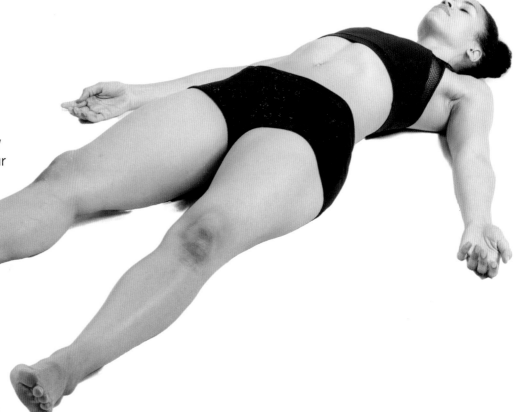

• Allow your eyes, jaw, tongue, and throat to soften. Release any controlled breath, and begin to breathe quietly. Remain in the position for the recommended time, or even longer if desired, before transitioning out of the pose.

FACT FILE

SANSKRIT
• Savasana

TARGETS
• Entire body

BENEFITS
• Encourages deep relaxation
• Calms mind and body
• Decreases depression
• Reduces anxiety, headache, and insomnia
• Helps treat high blood pressure

CAUTIONS
• Back issues

DO IT RIGHT

• If you feel any lower-back discomfort, place a rolled-up blanket underneath your knees.
• Make sure that your body isn't touching anything near your mat, such as your block, strap, or water bottle, that might distract you.
• Avoid keeping your eyes open or letting them wander around the room.
• Avoid positioning your body asymmetrically.
• If you are pregnant, do not lie on your back; instead, lie on your left side or elevate your spine using a block or other booster, and as you transition out of the pose, lie in a fetal position on the left side of the body to avoid compromising blood flow to your uterus.

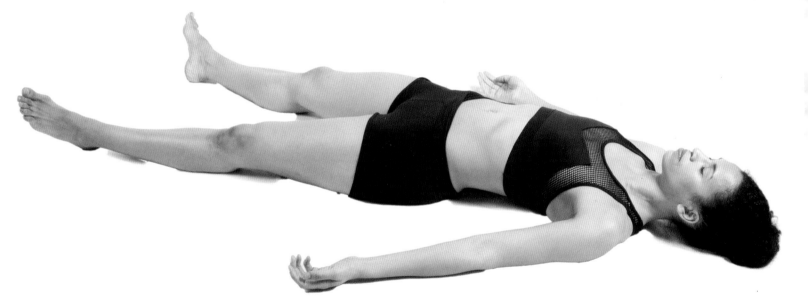

• To gradually transition out of the Corpse Pose, inhale and exhale deeply and then start to wiggle your fingers and toes, small movements that will bring awareness back to the rest of the body. Hug both knees into your chest, and then gently roll over onto your right side, taking pressure away from the heart. Pause for a moment in a fetal position, then slowly press yourself up until you are sitting in Easy Pose (pages 220–21), still keeping your eyes closed. Remain there for the recommended breaths (or minutes) before opening your eyes.

Knees-to-Chest Pose

The relaxing Knees-to-Chest Pose can help to alleviate lower-back pain by stretching your muscles and easing any tension you might carry there. It also relieves bloating, improves circulation, and rebalances your energy.

HOW TO DO IT

• Lie on your back with your legs extended. On an exhalation, bend both knees and raise them toward your chest. Grasp your shins with both hands.

• Draw your shoulders back and hug your knees closer into your chest. Lengthen your tailbone, elongating your spine.

• Hold for the recommended breaths, gently pulling your knees closer to your chest with each exhalation.

MODIFICATION

EASIER: Instead of bringing both knees to your chest, bring just one knee into your chest at a time. Keep your other leg outstretched, with the foot flexed.

SANSKRIT
• Apanasana

TARGETS
• Spine
• Gluteal region

BENEFITS
• Alleviates lower-back pain
• Opens hips
• Massages internal organs and aids digestion

CAUTIONS
• Knee issues
• Pregnancy

DO IT RIGHT
• Draw your stomach inward.
• Press down into the mat with your back and shoulders.
• Avoid straining your neck; if you have difficulty placing your head on the mat, try resting it on a folded blanket.

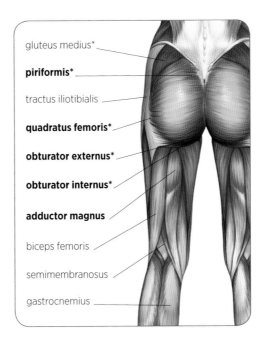

gluteus medius*
piriformis*
tractus iliotibialis
quadratus femoris*
obturator externus*
obturator internus*
adductor magnus
biceps femoris
semimembranosus
gastrocnemius

Annotation Key
Bold text indicates target muscles
Light text indicates other working muscles
* indicates deep muscles

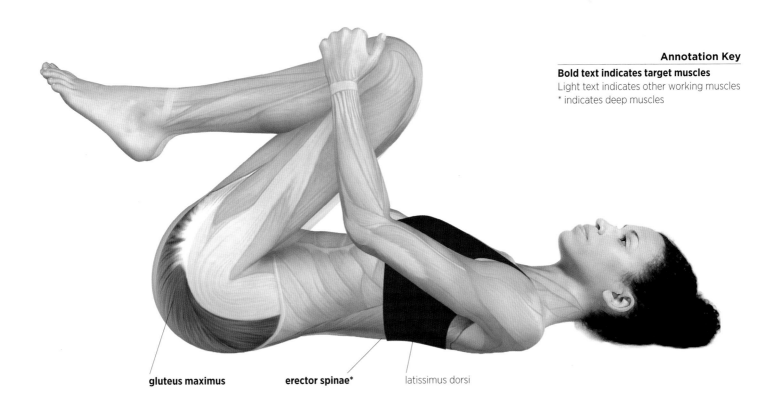

gluteus maximus

erector spinae*

latissimus dorsi

Reclining Pigeon Pose

Reclining Pigeon Pose, also known as Eye of the Needle, helps relieve tightness in your hips by lengthening your iliotibial (IT) band.

HOW TO DO IT

• Lie on your back with your legs extended.

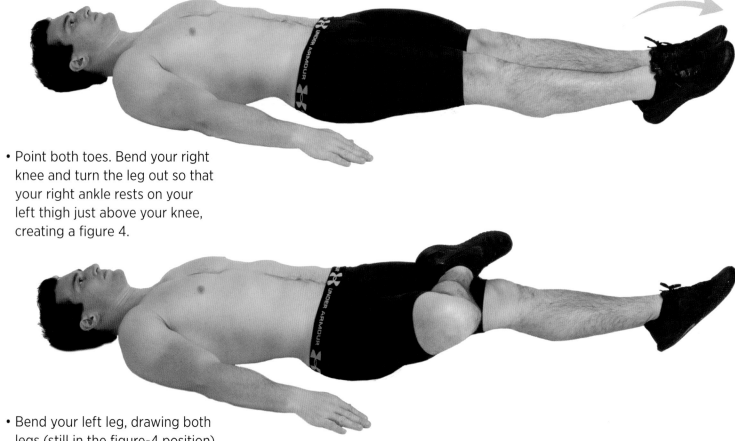

• Point both toes. Bend your right knee and turn the leg out so that your right ankle rests on your left thigh just above your knee, creating a figure 4.

• Bend your left leg, drawing both legs (still in the figure-4 position) in toward your chest as you grasp the back of your left thigh.

• Push your right elbow against your right inner thigh, turning out your right leg slightly to increase the intensity of the stretch.

• Hold for the recommended breaths, and then repeat on the opposite side.

> **DO IT RIGHT**
> • Keep your head and shoulder blades on the mat.
> • Avoid twisting your lower body; instead, keep your hips square.

SANSKRIT
• Sucirandhrasana

TARGETS
• Gluteal region

BENEFITS
• Opens hips
• Stretches glutes and thighs

CAUTIONS
• Groin injury
• Lower-back issues

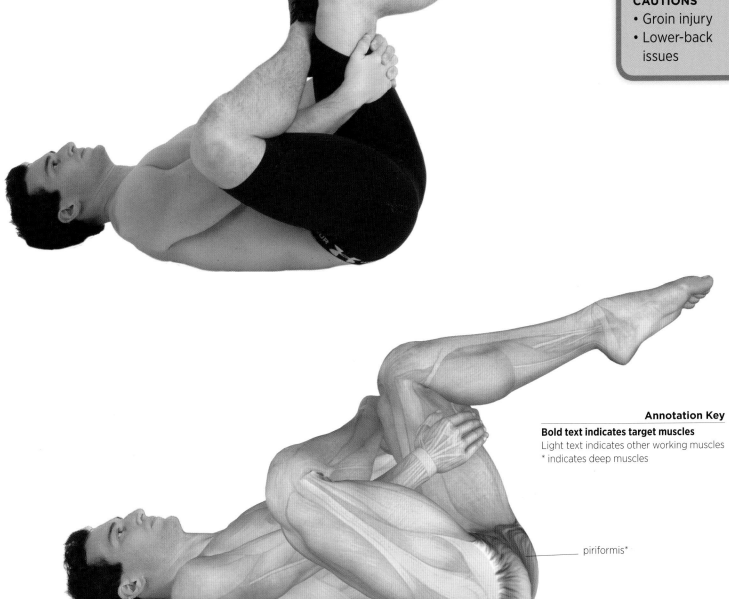

Annotation Key

Bold text indicates target muscles
Light text indicates other working muscles
* indicates deep muscles

piriformis*

gluteus maximus

gluteus minimus*

gluteus medius*

Happy Baby Pose

This pose, also known as Dead Bug Pose, may evoke giggles during yoga class, but it provides a serious stretch for your hamstrings and glutes, plus it effectively opens your hips.

HOW TO DO IT

• Lie on your back with your legs outstretched.

• Bend your knees up and in toward your chest, and grasp the outsides of your feet with your hands.

• Without releasing your grip on your feet, lower your knees toward the mat as you open your legs. Your thighs should be parallel to the floor.

• Hold for the recommended breaths before straightening your legs and easing them back down to the mat.

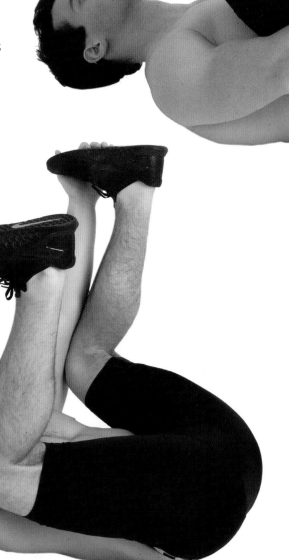

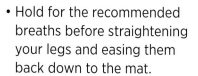

DO IT RIGHT

• Keep your elbows slightly bent.
• Draw your shoulders toward the mat.
• Tuck your pelvis forward slightly to engage your abdominals and keep your lower back anchored.
• Avoid lifting your head or shoulder blades off the mat.

SANSKRIT
• Ananda
  Balasana

TARGETS
• Gluteal region
• Hamstrings
• Lower back

BENEFITS
• Opens pelvic
  area
• Stretches
  hamstrings

CAUTIONS
• Groin injury
• Lower-back
  issues

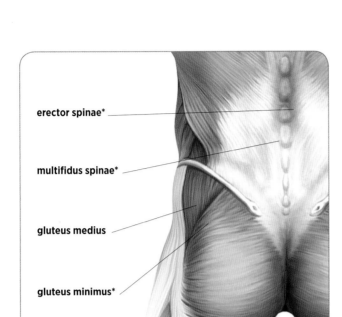

erector spinae*

multifidus spinae*

gluteus medius

gluteus minimus*

Annotation Key

Bold text indicates target muscles
Light text indicates other working muscles
* indicates deep muscles

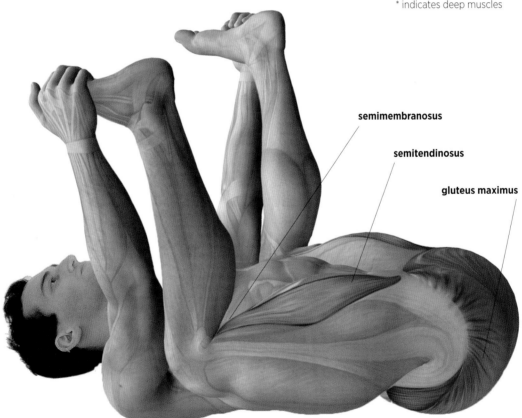

semimembranosus

semitendinosus

gluteus maximus

Reclining Spinal Twist

This twisting pose increases spinal mobility and helps relieve tension, while ridding your body of toxins.

HOW TO DO IT

- Lie on your back with both legs elongated and parallel and your arms outspread, palms faceup.

- Bend your right leg, placing the sole of your foot on the mat.

- Carefully lift your buttocks off the mat, tilting your torso 2 to 3 inches to your left, and cross your right leg over to your left side, with your knee bent at a right angle to your body.

- Hold for the recommended breaths, return to the starting position, and repeat on the opposite side.

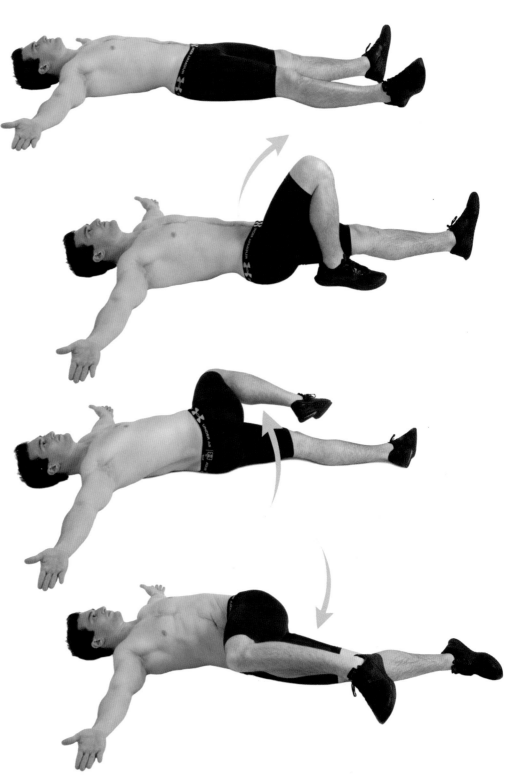

DO IT RIGHT

- Keep your elbows and wrists lower than your shoulders, protecting your rotator cuffs.
- Before you cross one leg over the other, ensure that your body is in a straight line from your head to your elongated pointed toe.
- Avoid lifting your shoulders; try to keep both shoulder blades in contact with the mat throughout the stretch.

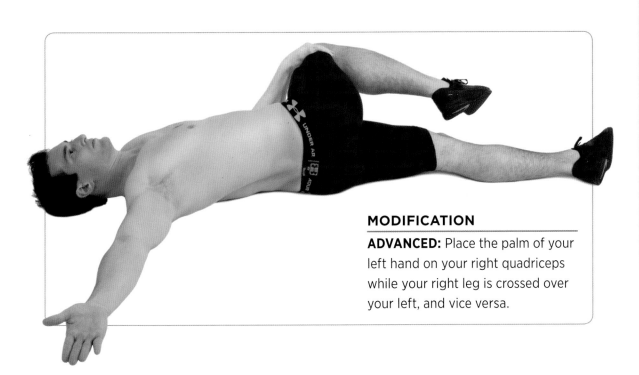

FACT FILE

SANSKRIT
- Supta Matsyendrasana

TARGETS
- Rotator muscles
- Gluteal region
- Chest

BENEFITS
- Lengthens spine
- Stretches outer hips, glutes, and lower back
- Massages internal organs

CAUTIONS
- Hip issues
- Lower-back injury

MODIFICATION

ADVANCED: Place the palm of your left hand on your right quadriceps while your right leg is crossed over your left, and vice versa.

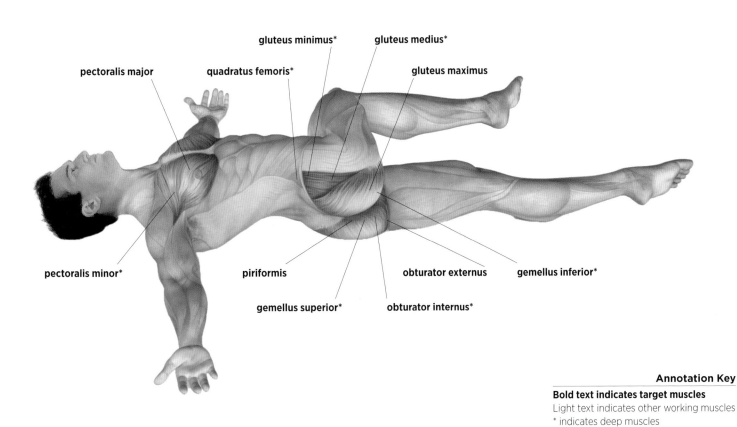

pectoralis major

gluteus minimus*

gluteus medius*

quadratus femoris*

gluteus maximus

pectoralis minor*

piriformis

obturator externus

gemellus inferior*

gemellus superior*

obturator internus*

Annotation Key

Bold text indicates target muscles
Light text indicates other working muscles
* indicates deep muscles

Double Knee Reclining Twist

This versatile pose allows you to twist away tension as you stretch your outer hips, IT band, back, abdominals, and obliques. It also lengthens, relaxes, and realigns your spine.

HOW TO DO IT

• Lie on a mat in Corpse Pose (pages 308–09). Bend your knees with your feet flat on the mat, and extend your arms straight out to the sides, palms faceup.

• Inhale and elongate your spine from your hips to the top of your neck. Lift your hips up slightly, and place them on the mat closer to your heels to lengthen and relax your spine further.

• Lift your feet off the mat, keeping your knees bent.

• Exhale and rotate your knees to the left, causing your hips and spine to twist. Keep your shoulder blades planted on the mat, and allow gravity to pull your left thigh to the mat with each exhalation. Turn your head to the right.

• Hold for the recommended breaths, and then repeat on the opposite side.

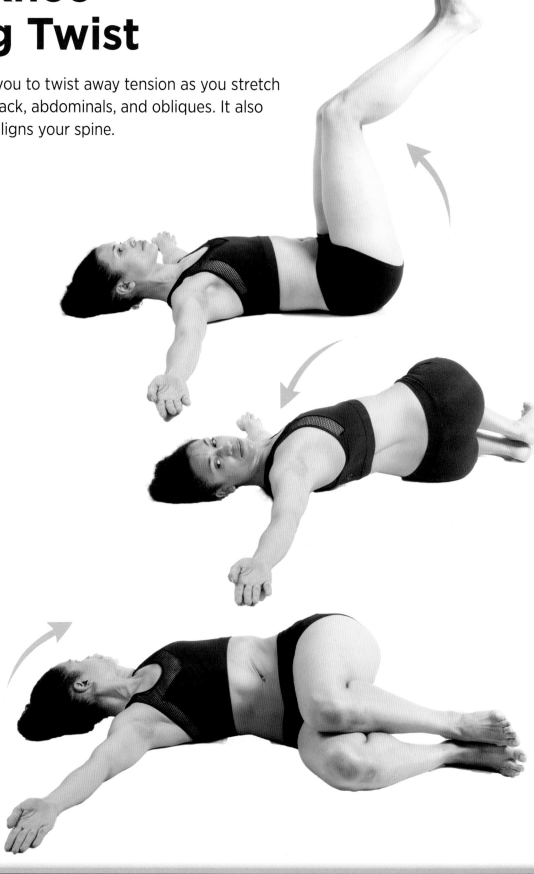

DO IT RIGHT

- Keep your chest open.
- If you struggle to bring your knees to the mat, place a folded blanket beneath them.
- Experiment with turning your head to both sides. This will change the sensation of the stretch.
- Relax—don't push—into the stretch. Let gravity help do the work.
- Avoid tensing your shoulders up near your ears.
- Do not allow your shoulder blades to lift off the mat. If your shoulder comes up, bend the arm of your lifted shoulder, and place your hand beneath your ribs for support.

FACT FILE

SANSKRIT
- Supta Matsyendrasana

TARGETS
- Spine
- Lower torso

BENEFITS
- Elongates spine
- Stretches core and lower body
- Restores equilibrium

CAUTIONS
- Lower-back injury
- Knee issues

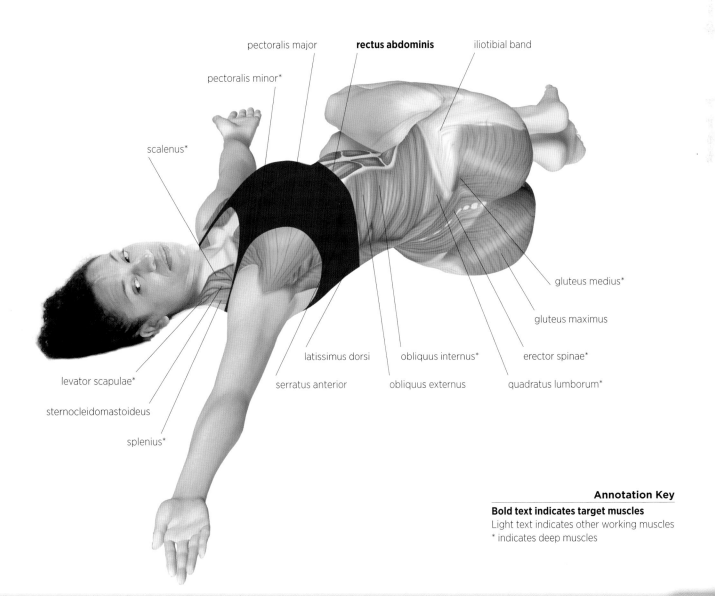

pectoralis major

rectus abdominis

iliotibial band

pectoralis minor*

scalenus*

gluteus medius*

gluteus maximus

levator scapulae*

latissimus dorsi

obliquus internus*

erector spinae*

sternocleidomastoideus

serratus anterior

obliquus externus

quadratus lumborum*

splenius*

Annotation Key
Bold text indicates target muscles
Light text indicates other working muscles
* indicates deep muscles

Reclining Hero Prep

This pose allows you to work up to the more challenging Reclining Hero Pose. Once you have mastered the basic pose, try the suggested modification that engages even more areas of your body.

- Kneel with your body upright, arms relaxed at your sides, and your buttocks resting lightly on your heels.

- Place your hands flat on the mat behind you, with your fingers pointing forward toward your body. Be sure to keep a slight bend in your elbows.

- Lean back slightly to increase the intensity of the stretch, so that your shoulders are above your wrists.

- Hold for the recommended breaths.

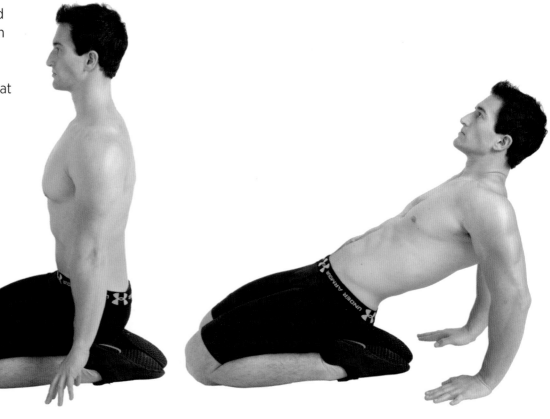

MODIFICATION

ADVANCED: Carefully bend your elbows until they rest on the mat. If more of a stretch is still required, lower down farther until your shoulder blades rest against the mat and your arms straighten beside your calves.

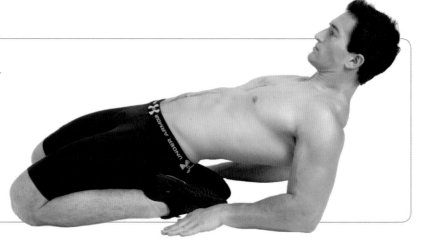

TARGETS
• Shins
• Quadriceps

BENEFITS
• Stretches
  quads and
  calves
• Opens knees

CAUTIONS
• Knee injury
• Lower-back
  issues

DO IT RIGHT

• Contract and engage your gluteal muscles to
  avoid a curve in your lumbar spine. If this pose
  is done correctly, you will have space between
  your heels and your glutes.
• Keep your head and neck in a neutral position.
• Do not raise your shoulders toward your ears.
• Avoid arching your back.

Annotation Key

Bold text indicates target muscles
Light text indicates other working muscles
* indicates deep muscles

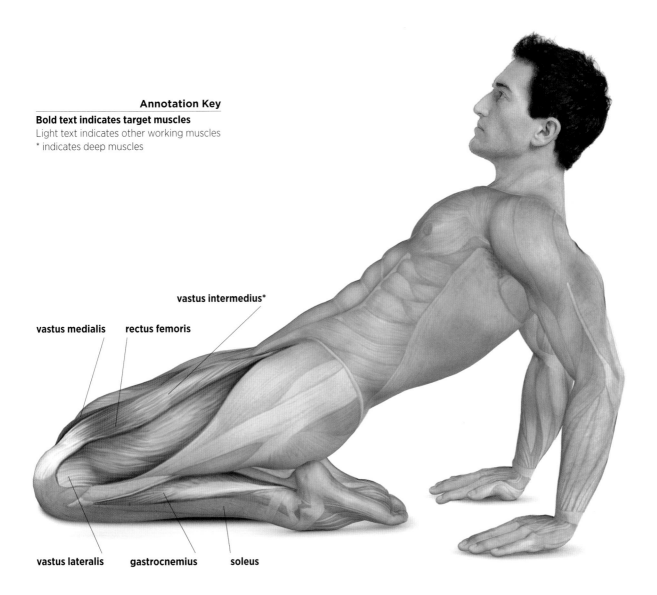

vastus intermedius*

vastus medialis   rectus femoris

vastus lateralis   gastrocnemius   soleus

Reclining Hero Pose

Reclining Hero Pose may be challenging, but it provides a strong stretch for your thighs, while loosening your quadriceps and opening the arches of your feet.

HOW TO DO IT

• Begin in Hero Pose (pages 224–25). Make sure that you are comfortable, sitting with your buttocks completely on the mat.

• Lean back gradually, and exhale, placing your hands on the mat behind you for support. Lower yourself onto your elbows.

• Recline all the way back until your back reaches the mat. Move your arms to your sides, relaxing them with your palms faceup. Squeeze your knees together so that they don't separate wider than your hips, and don't allow them to lift off the mat.

• Hold for the recommended breaths.

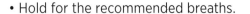

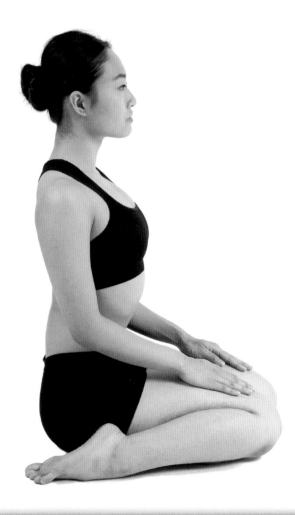

DO IT RIGHT

• If you are able to sit comfortably in Hero Pose but experience difficulty reclining onto the mat, place folded blankets underneath your back and neck for support.
• Avoid sliding your knees beyond the width of your hips.
• Do not push yourself down—relax into the pose.

FACT FILE

SANSKRIT
• Supta Virasana

TARGETS
• Hips
• Legs

BENEFITS
• Loosens thighs, knees, hip flexors, and ankles
• Stimulates digestion
• Alleviates arthritis
• Alleviates respiratory problems

CAUTIONS
• Knee injury
• Ankle injury
• Back issues
• Menstruation

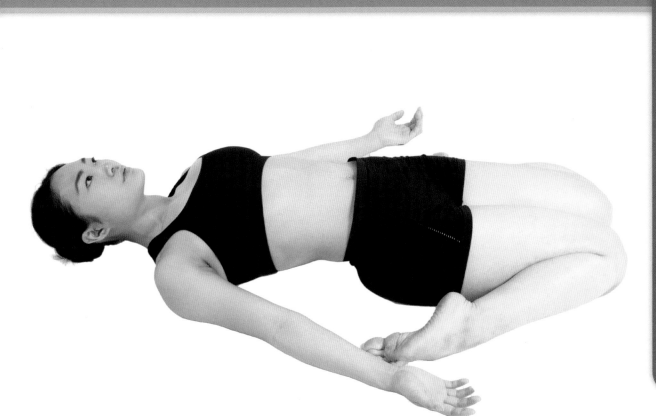

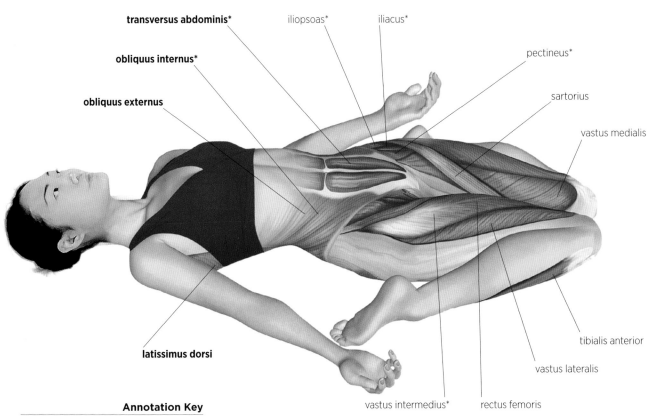

transversus abdominis*

obliquus internus*

obliquus externus

iliopsoas*

iliacus*

pectineus*

sartorius

vastus medialis

latissimus dorsi

tibialis anterior

vastus lateralis

vastus intermedius*

rectus femoris

Annotation Key

Bold text indicates target muscles
Light text indicates other working muscles
* indicates deep muscles

Reclining Bound Angle Pose

This is a classic restorative posture that can be modified to provide any level of hip and groin resistance. It is recommended for students of all levels.

HOW TO DO IT

- Lie on your back with your legs straight and your arms at your sides, with your palms faceup.

- Bend your knees, and step your heels toward your pelvis.

- Exhale and drop your knees out to your sides, pressing the soles of your feet together.

- Carefully ease your soles closer toward your pelvic area until you feel a good amount of resistance.

- Leave your arms relaxed at your sides with your hands on your inner thighs, or draw your arms overhead with your hands in prayer position.

DO IT RIGHT

- To deepen the stretch, keep the upper outside of your feet—your pinkie toes—on the mat and lift your heels upward.
- Avoid lifting your lower back off the mat.
- Do not bounce your legs open to achieve a deeper stretch.

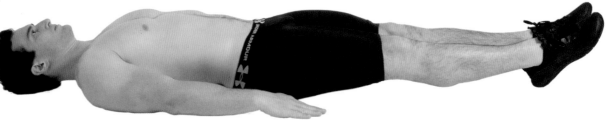

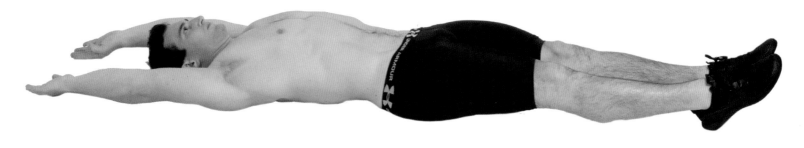

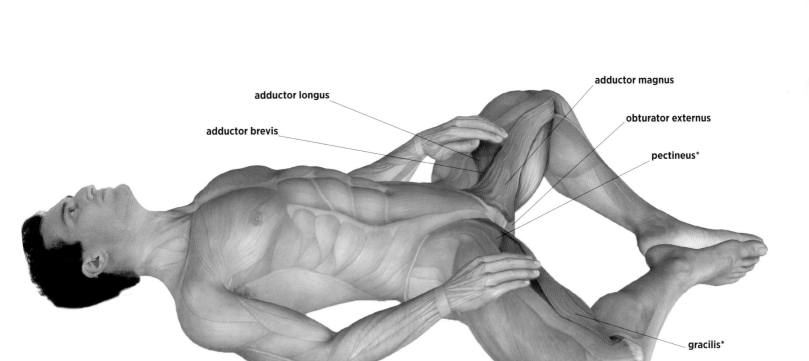

SANSKRIT
• Supta Baddha Konasana

TARGETS
• Groin
• Thighs
• Knees

BENEFITS
• Opens hips
• Restores energy

CAUTIONS
• Knee injury
• Groin issues

adductor longus

adductor brevis

adductor magnus

obturator externus

pectineus*

gracilis*

Annotation Key

Bold text indicates target muscles
Light text indicates other working muscles
* indicates deep muscles

Reclining Big Toe Prep

This preparatory pose safely lengthens your hamstrings and, when it is performed with a healthy lumbar curve, releases the lower back.

HOW TO DO IT

- Lie on your back with your legs extended, your feet flexed, and your arms resting at your sides.

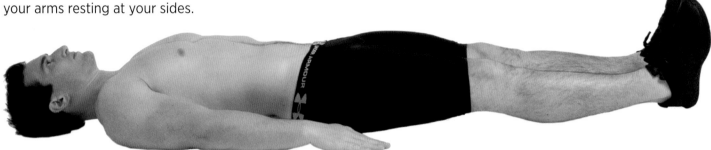

- With an exhalation, bend your right knee and hug your thigh to your chest. Keep your left leg extended along the mat.

- Exhale and straighten your right leg toward the ceiling. Keep the muscles in both legs engaged and strong.

- Draw your leg as close to your chest as you can while keeping it straight and maintaining a natural lumbar curve in your lower back. Hold this pose for the recommended breaths. Slowly release your right leg to the mat, and then repeat on the opposite side.

DO IT RIGHT

- Straighten your lifted leg completely, even if this causes the leg to move away from your head.
- Keep both hips on the floor throughout the exercise.
- Avoid allowing the hip on the side of your lifted leg to raise upward.
- Keep both feet flexed to really feel the stretch.

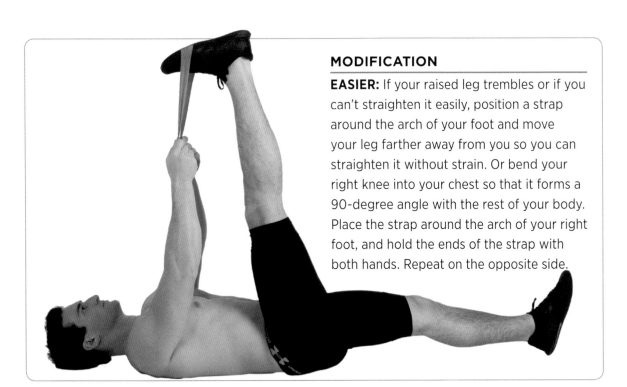

MODIFICATION

EASIER: If your raised leg trembles or if you can't straighten it easily, position a strap around the arch of your foot and move your leg farther away from you so you can straighten it without strain. Or bend your right knee into your chest so that it forms a 90-degree angle with the rest of your body. Place the strap around the arch of your right foot, and hold the ends of the strap with both hands. Repeat on the opposite side.

TARGETS
• Glutes
• Hamstrings
• Calves

BENEFITS
• Stretches hamstrings
• Strengthens abdomen
• Increases hip flexibility

CAUTION
• Groin issues

Annotation Key

Bold text indicates target muscles
Light text indicates other working muscles
* indicates deep muscles

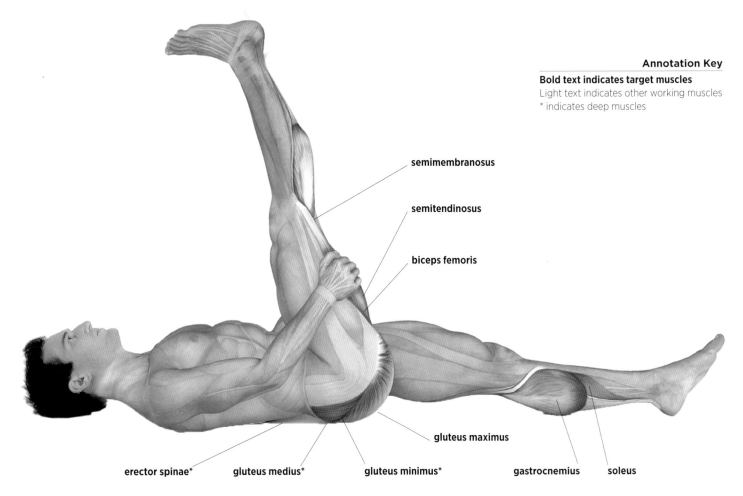

semimembranosus

semitendinosus

biceps femoris

gluteus maximus

erector spinae*   gluteus medius*   gluteus minimus*   gastrocnemius   soleus

Reclining Big Toe

The restorative Reclining Big Toe Pose will improve your flexibility, plus it provides a great foundation for the more demanding Big Toe Poses.

HOW TO DO IT

• Lie on your back with your legs outstretched. Raise and straighten your right leg up toward the ceiling so that your right heel is lined up with your right hip. If possible, continue to extend the leg over the top of your body.

• With your right hand, grasp your big toe in a yogi toe lock with your first two fingers wrapped around the inside of your big toe, and your thumb wrapped around the outside of your toe. If desired, bring your leg out to your right to get a deeper stretch in your hip or inner thigh, or cross your leg to your left to stretch your outer hip and IT band.

• Find a slight internal rotation in your right leg. Press your left thigh into the mat as you flex your foot to keep your leg active. Hold for the recommended breaths, gently drawing your right leg toward you to deepen the stretch. Repeat on the opposite side.

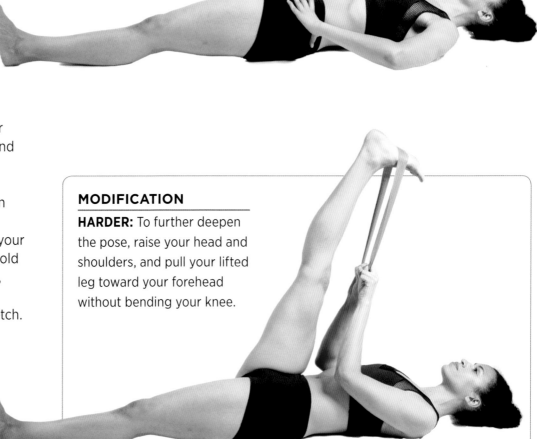

MODIFICATION

HARDER: To further deepen the pose, raise your head and shoulders, and pull your lifted leg toward your forehead without bending your knee.

FACT FILE

SANSKRIT
• Supta Padangusthasana

TARGETS
• Back
• Lower torso
• Legs

BENEFITS
• Stretches spine, groin, hamstrings, and calves
• Strengthens knees

CAUTIONS
• Hamstring issues
• Groin injury

DO IT RIGHT

• Straighten your lifted leg completely, even if this causes your leg to move away from your head.
• Keep both hips on the mat throughout the exercise.
• Avoid allowing the hip on the side of your lifted leg to raise upward.

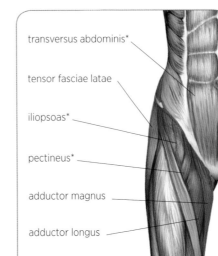

transversus abdominis*

tensor fasciae latae

iliopsoas*

pectineus*

adductor magnus

adductor longus

Annotation Key

Bold text indicates target muscles
Light text indicates other working muscles
* indicates deep muscles

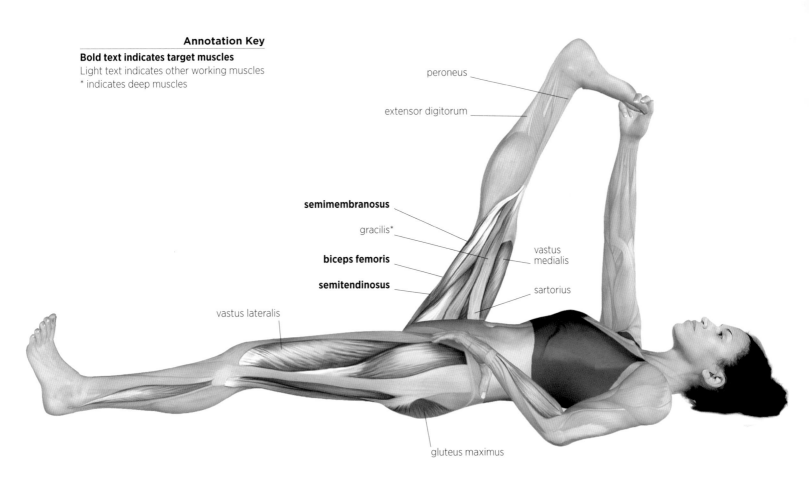

peroneus

extensor digitorum

semimembranosus

gracilis*

biceps femoris

semitendinosus

vastus medialis

sartorius

vastus lateralis

gluteus maximus

CHAPTER EIGHT

YOGA SEQUENCES

Yoga poses are effective for stretching and strengthening the body, stimulating circulation, increasing stamina, and improving balance. For many, they also calm the mind and enrich the spirit. By performing poses as a flowing series, you can multiply these benefits several times over. The recommended number of breaths for holding poses can be decreased to create a more cardio-based sequence or increased for a more strengthening experience.

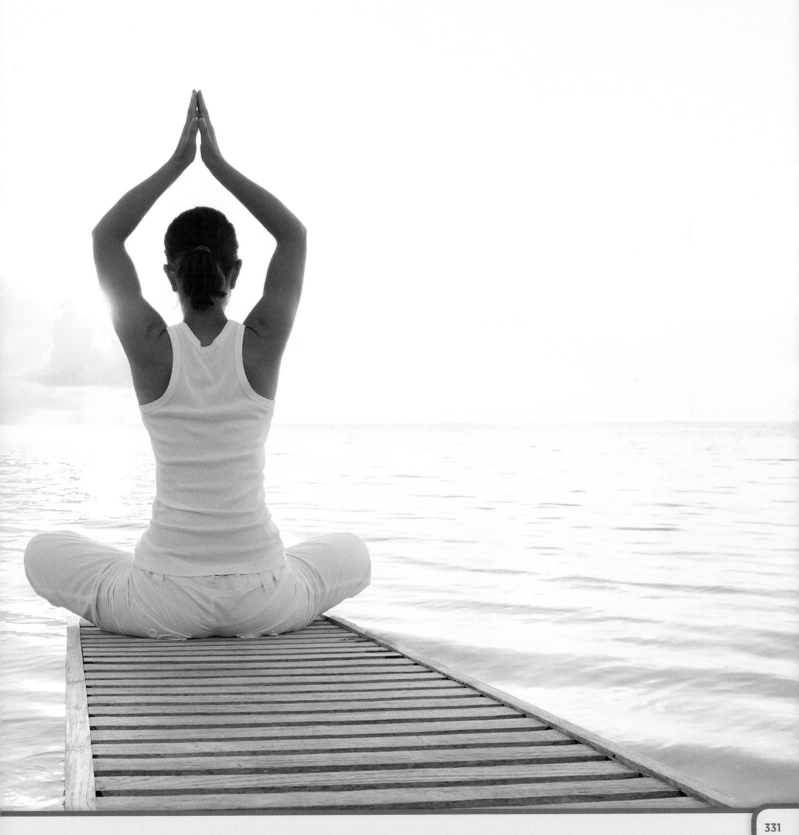

Beginner Sequence

This series of poses comprises a collection of gentle stretches, twists, backbends, and inversions that will prepare you for more complex positions.

1 MOUNTAIN POSE

Pages 32–33
Hold for 3 to 6 breaths.

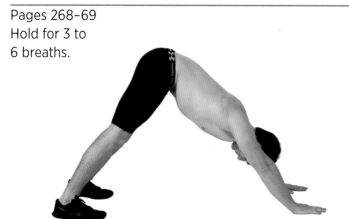

2 HIGH LUNGE

Pages 64–65
Hold for 3 to 6 breaths.

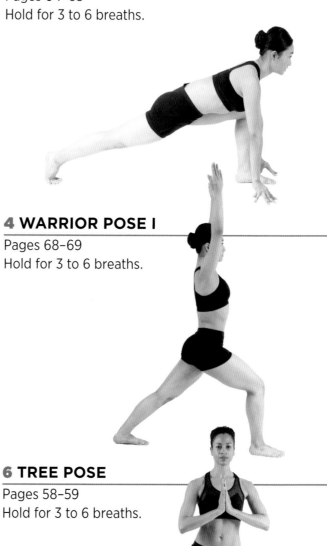

3 DOWNWARD-FACING DOG

Pages 268–69
Hold for 3 to
6 breaths.

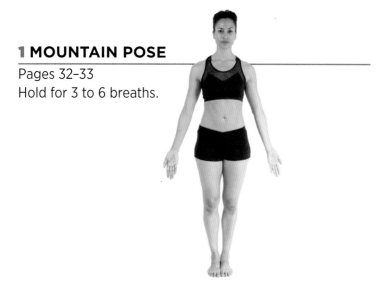

4 WARRIOR POSE I

Pages 68–69
Hold for 3 to 6 breaths.

5 INTENSE SIDE STRETCH POSE I

Pages 116–17
Hold for 3 to
6 breaths.

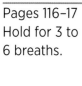
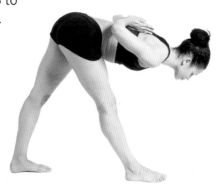

6 TREE POSE

Pages 58–59
Hold for 3 to 6 breaths.

7 CHAIR POSE

Pages 54-55
Hold for 3 to 6 breaths.

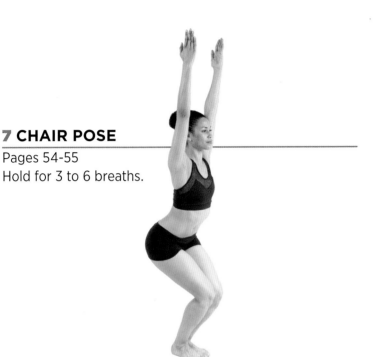

8 DOWNWARD-FACING DOG

Pages 268–69
Hold for 3 to 6 breaths.

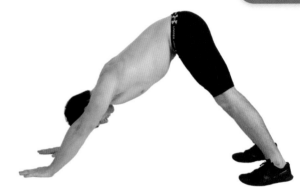

9 LOCUST POSE

Pages 174–75
Hold for 2 to 4 breaths.

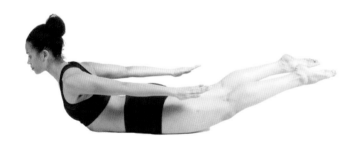

10 BOAT POSE

Pages 242–43
Hold for 2 to 4 breaths.

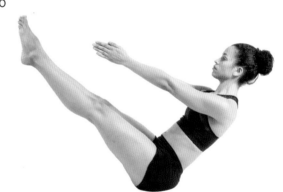

11 MARICHI'S POSE

Pages 226–27
Hold for 3 to 6 breaths.

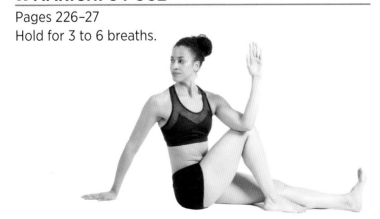

12 BOUND ANGLE POSE

Pages 222–23
Hold for 3 to 6 breaths.

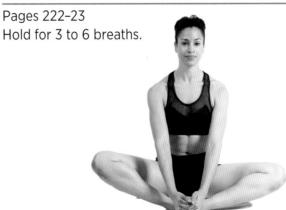

Beginner Sequence (continued)

13 BOUND ANGLE POSE WITH FORWARD BEND

Pages 138–39
Hold for 3 to 6 breaths.

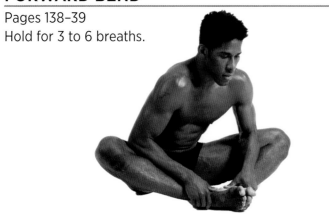

14 ONE-LEGGED KING PIGEON POSE PREP

Pages 198–99
Hold for 3 to 6 breaths.

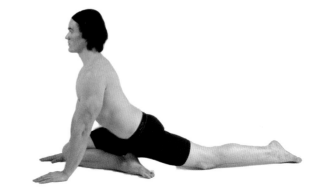

15 BRIDGE POSE

Pages 168–69
Hold for 3 to 6 breaths.

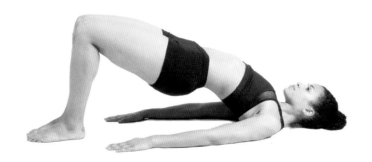

16 DOUBLE KNEE RECLINING TWIST

Pages 318–19
Hold for 3 to 6 breaths.

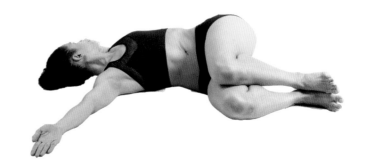

17 KNEES-TO-CHEST POSE

Pages 310–11
Hold for 3 to 6 breaths.

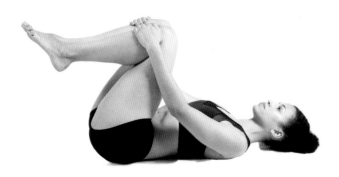

18 CORPSE POSE

Pages 308–09
Hold for several minutes.

Sun Salutation A

The Sun Salutation, Surya Namaskar in Sanskrit, is a series of gracefully linked asanas meant to warm, strengthen, and align the body. Inhale as you stretch, exhale as you fold or contract.

1 MOUNTAIN POSE

Pages 32-33
Hold for 3 to 6 breaths.

2 UPWARD SALUTE

Pages 36–37
Hold for 3 to 6 breaths.

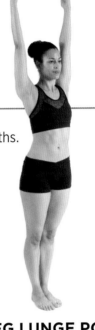

3 STANDING HALF FORWARD BEND TO FORWARD BEND

Pages 106–07
Hold for 3 to 6 breaths.

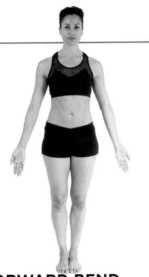

4 STRAIGHT-LEG LUNGE POSE

Pages 104–05
Hold for 3 to 6 breaths.

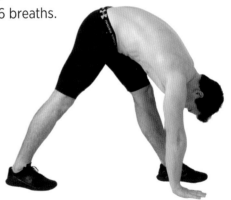

5 LOW LUNGE

Pages 62–63
Hold for 3 to 6 breaths.

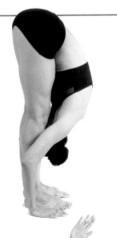
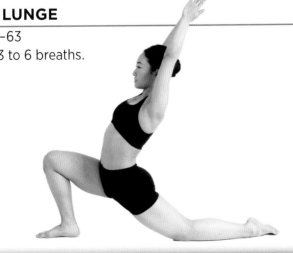

6 PLANK POSE

Pages 260–61
Hold for 3 to 6 breaths.

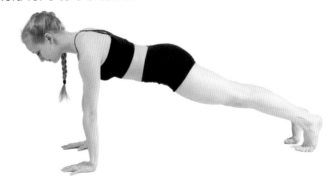

Sun Salutation A (continued)

7 FOUR-LIMBED STAFF POSE

Pages 262–63
Hold for 3 to 6 breaths.

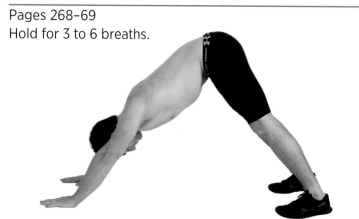

8 UPWARD-FACING DOG

Pages 170-71
Hold for 3 to 6 breaths.

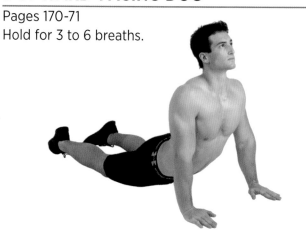

9 DOWNWARD-FACING DOG

Pages 268–69
Hold for 3 to 6 breaths.

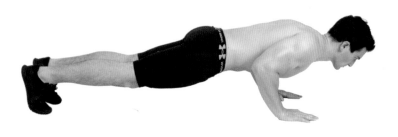

10 COW POSE

Pages 166–67
Hold for 3 to
6 breaths.

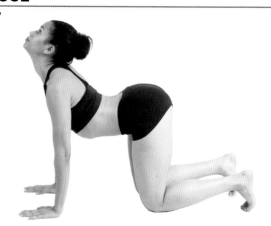

11 HALF CAMEL POSE

Page 184
Hold for 3 to
6 breaths.

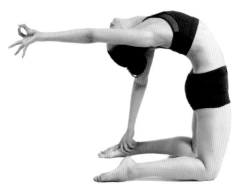

12 FOUR-LIMBED STAFF POSE

Pages 262–63
Hold for 3 to 6 breaths.

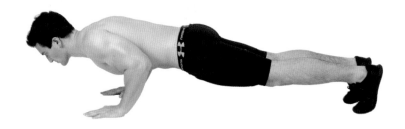

13 PLANK POSE

Pages 260–61
Hold for 3 to 6 breaths.

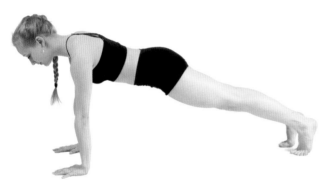

14 LOW LUNGE

Pages 62–63
Hold for 3 to 6 breaths.

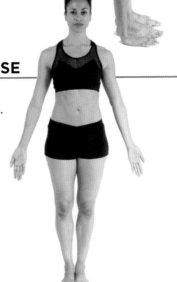

15 STRAIGHT-LEG LUNGE POSE

Pages 104–05
Hold for 3 to 6 breaths.

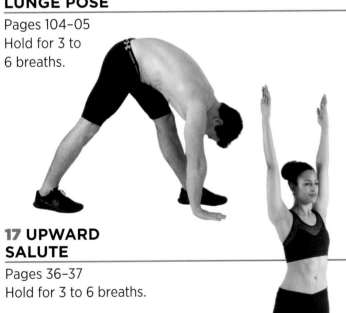

16 STANDING HALF FORWARD BEND TO FORWARD BEND

Pages 106–07
Hold for 3 to 6 breaths.

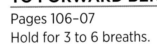
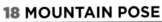

17 UPWARD SALUTE

Pages 36–37
Hold for 3 to 6 breaths.

18 MOUNTAIN POSE

Pages 32–33
Hold for 3 to 6 breaths.

Sun Salutation B

There are a number of Sun Salutation variations, and this one makes an excellent complement to—and can be flowed together with—Sun Salutation A.

1 MOUNTAIN POSE

Pages 32–33
Hold for 3 to 6 breaths.

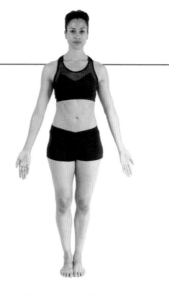

2 CHAIR POSE

Pages 54–55
Hold for 3 to 6 breaths.

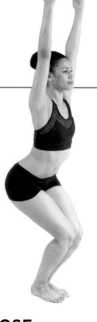

3 STANDING HALF FORWARD BEND TO FORWARD BEND

Pages 106–07
Hold for 3 to 6 breaths.

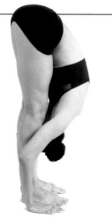

4 FOUR-LIMBED STAFF POSE

Pages 262–63
Hold for 2 to 4 breaths.

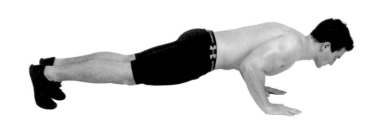

5 UPWARD-FACING DOG

Pages 170–71
Hold for 3 to 6 breaths.

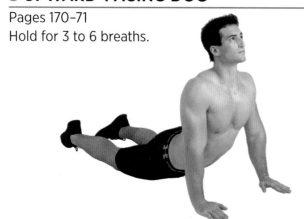

6 DOWNWARD-FACING DOG

Pages 268–69
Hold for 3 to 6 breaths.

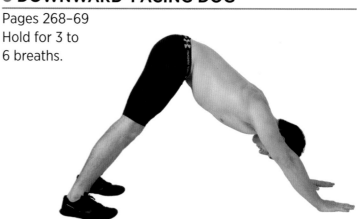

FACT FILE

LEVEL
• Beginner

TARGETS
• Lower Body
• Back
• Legs

BENEFITS
• Stimulates circulation
• Stretches spine
• Tightens abdominals

7 WARRIOR POSE I

Pages 68–69
Hold for 3 to 6 breaths.

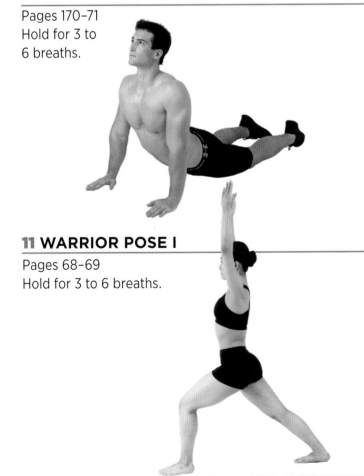

8 FOUR-LIMBED STAFF POSE

Pages 262–63
Hold for 2 to 4 breaths.

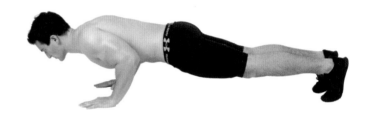

9 UPWARD-FACING DOG

Pages 170–71
Hold for 3 to 6 breaths.

10 DOWNWARD-FACING DOG

Pages 268–69
Hold for 3 to 6 breaths.

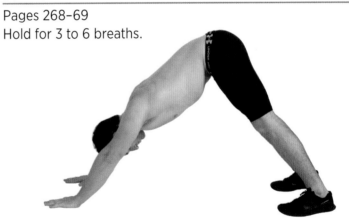

11 WARRIOR POSE I

Pages 68–69
Hold for 3 to 6 breaths.

12 FOUR-LIMBED STAFF POSE

Pages 262–63
Hold for 2 to 4 breaths.

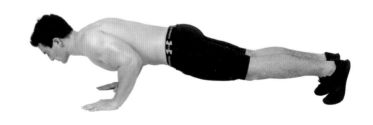

Sun Salutation B (continued)

13 UPWARD-FACING DOG

Pages 170–71
Hold for 3 to 6 breaths.

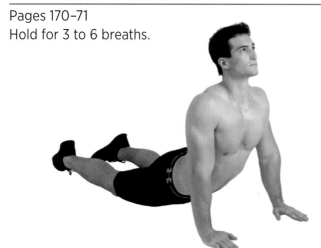

14 DOWNWARD-FACING DOG

Pages 268–69
Hold for 3 to 6 breaths.

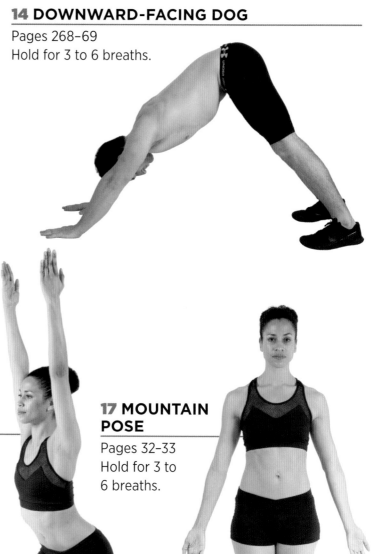

15 STANDING HALF FORWARD BEND TO FORWARD BEND

Pages 106–07
Hold for 3 to 6 breaths.

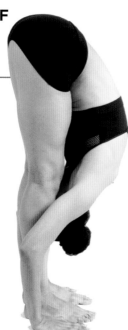

16 CHAIR POSE

Pages 54–55
Hold for 3 to 6 breaths.

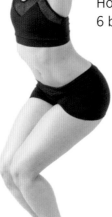

17 MOUNTAIN POSE

Pages 32–33
Hold for 3 to 6 breaths.

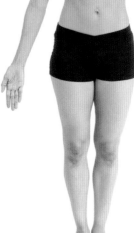

Simple Pose Flow

This gentle sequence uses backbends and inversions and begins to incorporate the twisting poses, which engage the muscles of the sides and the abdomen.

FACT FILE

LEVEL
• Beginner

TARGETS
• Back
• Core
• Thighs

BENEFITS
• Lengthens the spine
• Stretches the hamstrings
• Opens the chest

1 CAT POSE

Pages 102–03
Hold for 3 to 6 breaths.

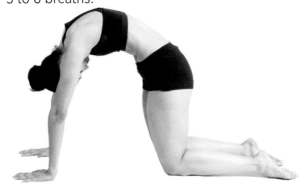

2 DOWNWARD-FACING DOG

Pages 268–69
Hold for 3 to 6 breaths.

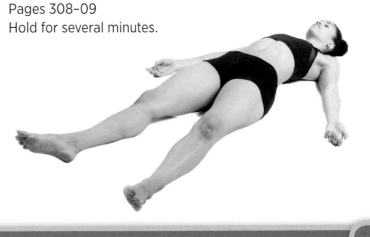

3 COBRA POSE

Pages 172–73
Hold for 2 to 4 breaths.

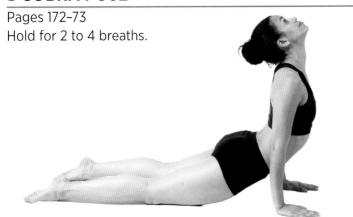

4 HALF LORD OF THE FISHES POSE

Pages 240–41
Hold for 3 to 6 breaths.

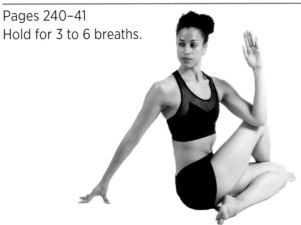

5 HEAD-TO-KNEE FORWARD BEND PREP

Pages 130–31
Hold for 3 to 6 breaths.

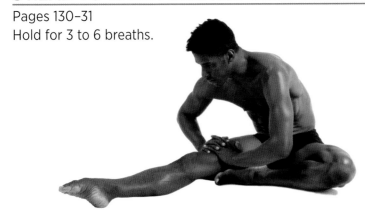

6 CORPSE POSE

Pages 308–09
Hold for several minutes.

Relaxing Flow

This is an excellent sequence to calm your mind and release tension; allow yourself to remain in Child's Pose at the end for at least 1 or 2 minutes.

1 STAFF POSE

Pages 218–19
Hold for 3 to
6 breaths.

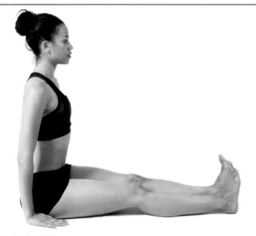

2 BOUND ANGLE POSE

Pages 222–23
Hold for 3 to 6 breaths.

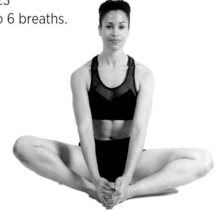

3 COW FACE POSE

Pages 234–35
Hold for 3 to
6 breaths.

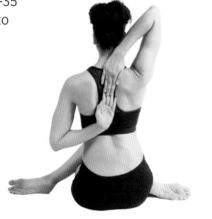

4 REVOLVED COW FACE POSE

Page 236
Hold for 3 to
6 breaths.

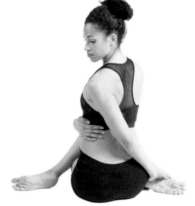

5 SEATED FORWARD BEND

Pages 140–41
Hold for 3 to 6 breaths.

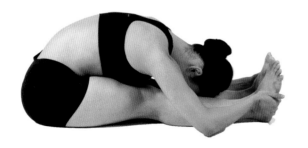

6 HEAD-TO-KNEE FORWARD BEND

Pages 142–43
Hold for 3 to 6 breaths.

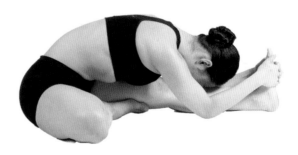

7 CAT POSE

Pages 102–03
Hold for 3 to
6 breaths.

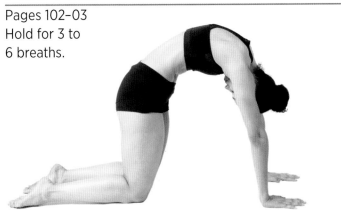

8 COW POSE

Pages 166–67
Hold for 3 to
6 breaths.

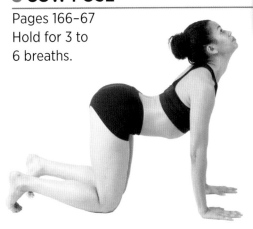

9 BOUND ANGLE POSE WITH FORWARD BEND

Pages 138–39
Hold for 3 to 6 breaths.

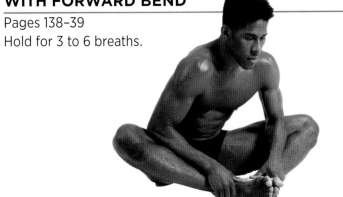

10 WIDE-ANGLE SEATED FORWARD BEND

Pages 156–57
Hold for 3 to 6 breaths.

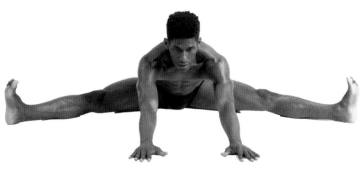

11 CHILD'S POSE WITH ARMS EXTENDED

Pages 134–35
Hold for 3 to 6 breaths.

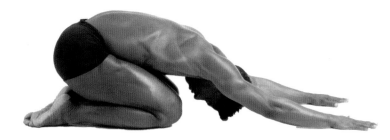

12 CHILD'S POSE

Pages 132–33
Hold for 1 or more minutes.

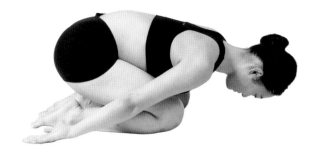

Well-Rounded Flow

This sequence—incorporating both floor work and standing poses—
can be performed with fewer breath holds for increased cardio
and circulatory benefits.

1 MOUNTAIN POSE

Pages 32–33
Hold for 3 to 6 breaths.

2 TREE POSE

Pages 58–59
Hold for 3 to 6 breaths.

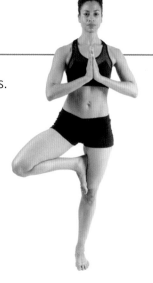

3 UPWARD SALUTE

Pages 36–37
Hold for 3 to 6 breaths.

4 STANDING HALF FORWARD
BEND TO FORWARD BEND

Pages 106–07
Hold for 3 to 6 breaths.

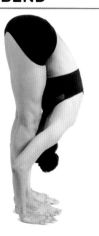

5 STRAIGHT-LEG LUNGE POSE

Pages 104–05
Hold for 3 to 6 breaths.

6 PLANK POSE

Pages 260–61
Hold for 3 to 6 breaths.

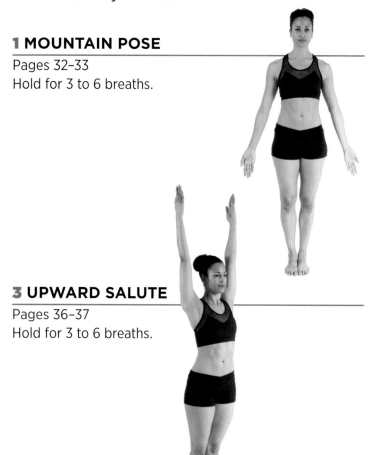

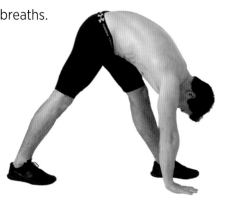

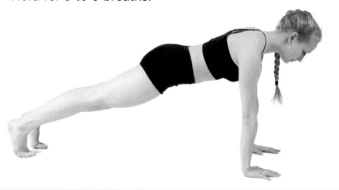

FACT FILE

LEVEL
• Beginner/ Intermediate

TARGETS
• Lower torso
• Spine
• Legs

BENEFITS
• Strengthens arms
• Stretches hamstrings
• Engages abdominals

7 FOUR-LIMBED STAFF POSE

Pages 262–63
Hold for 2 to 4 breaths.

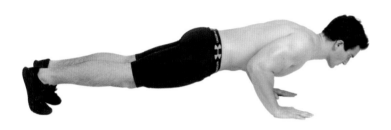

8 UPWARD-FACING DOG

Pages 170–71
Hold for 3 to 6 breaths.

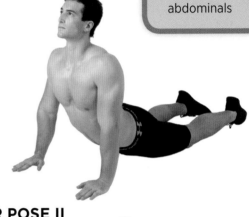

9 DOWNWARD-FACING DOG

Pages 268–69
Hold for 3 to 6 breaths.

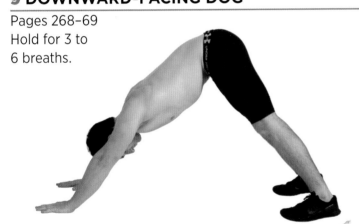

10 WARRIOR POSE II

Pages 72–73
Hold for 3 to 6 breaths.

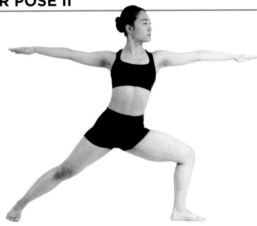

11 EXTENDED SIDE ANGLE POSE

Pages 82–83
Hold for 3 to 6 breaths.

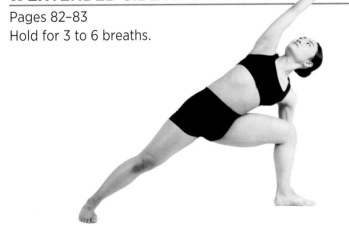

12 DOWNWARD-FACING DOG

Pages 268–69
Hold for 3 to 6 breaths.

Well-Rounded Flow (continued)

13 INTENSE SIDE STRETCH POSE I

Pages 116–17
Hold for 3 to
6 breaths.

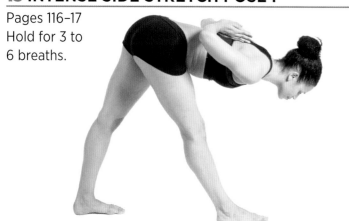

14 BRIDGE POSE

Pages 168–69
Hold for 3 to 6 breaths.

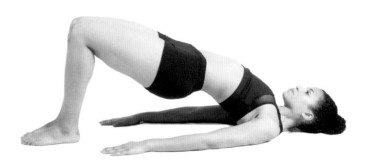

15 WHEEL POSE

Pages 194–95
Hold for 3 to
6 breaths.

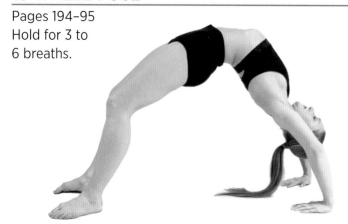

16 KNEES-TO-CHEST POSE

Pages 310–11
Hold for 3 to 6 breaths.

17 PLOW POSE

Pages 278–79
Hold for 3 to 6 breaths.

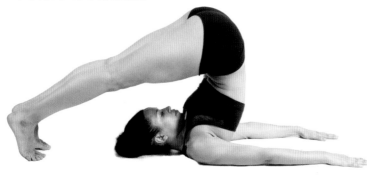

18 SUPPORTED SHOULDERSTAND

Pages 286–87
Hold for 2 to 4 breaths.

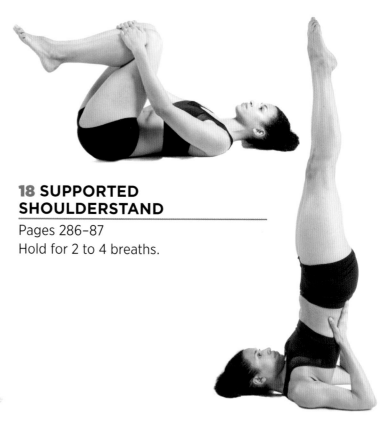

19 REVERSE TABLETOP POSE

Pages 280–81
Hold for 3 to 6 breaths.

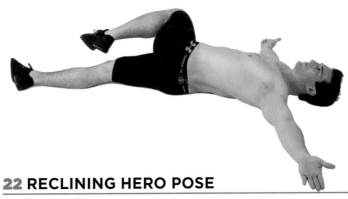

20 RECLINING SPINAL TWIST

Pages 316–17
Hold for 3 to 6 breaths.

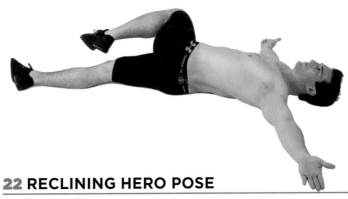

21 RECLINING BIG TOE PREP

Pages 326–27
Hold for 3 to 6 breaths.

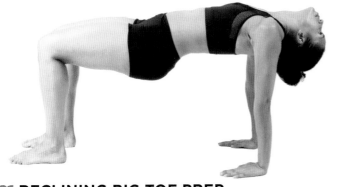

22 RECLINING HERO POSE

Pages 322–23
Hold for 3 to 6 breaths.

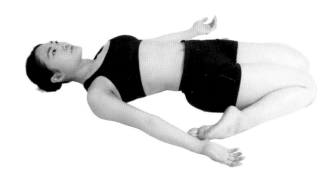

23 RECLINING BOUND ANGLE POSE

Pages 324–25
Hold for 3 to 6 breaths.

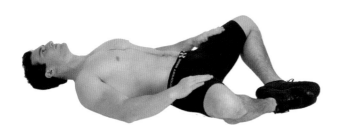

24 CORPSE POSE

Pages 308–09
Hold for several minutes.

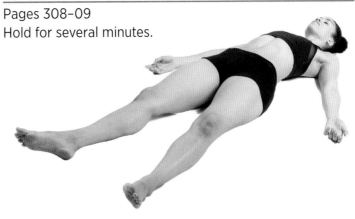

Moon Salutation

With its grounding qualities, this evening version of the Sun Salutation can be used to cool down the body and calm an anxious mind.

1 VOLCANO POSE

Page 38
Hold for 3 to 6 breaths.

2 PALM TREE SIDE BEND

Page 43
Hold for 3 to 6 breaths.

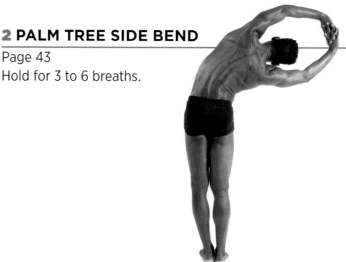

3 HORSE POSE

Pages 50–51
Hold for 3 to
6 breaths.

4 HORSE POSE WITH PALMS UP

Pages 52–53
Hold for 3 to
6 breaths.

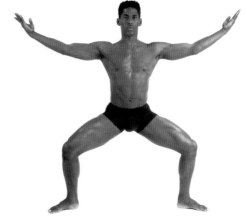

5 REVOLVED TRIANGLE POSE

Pages 78–79
Hold for 3 to 6 breaths.

6 STRAIGHT-LEG LUNGE POSE

Pages 104–05
Hold for 3 to
6 breaths.

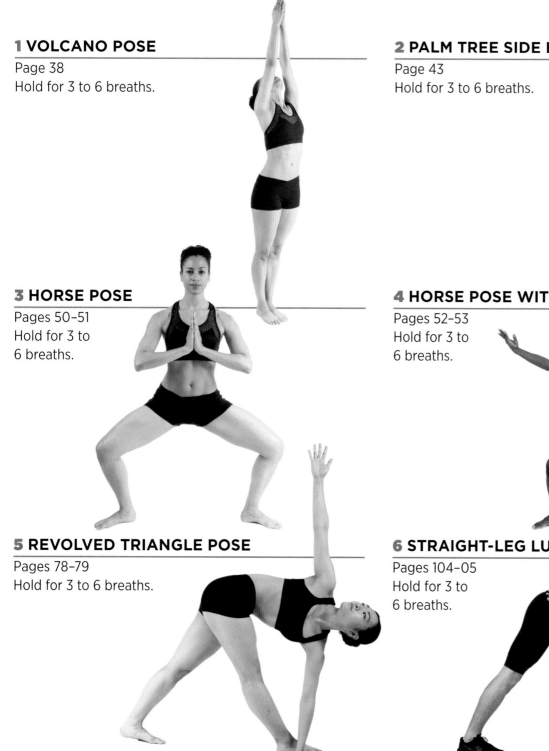

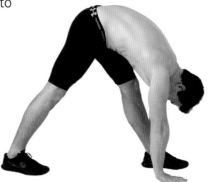

FACT FILE

LEVEL
• Beginner

TARGETS
• Upper Body
• Legs
• Spine

BENEFITS
• Opens shoulders and chest
• Stretches hips and groin
• Elongates lower back

7 LOW LUNGE

Pages 62–63
Hold for 3 to
6 breaths.

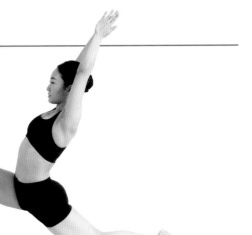

8 GARLAND POSE

Pages 48–49
Hold for 3 to
6 breaths.

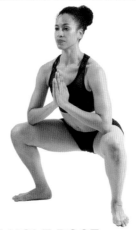

9 WIDE-ANGLE SEATED FORWARD BEND

Pages 156–57
Hold for 3 to 6 breaths.

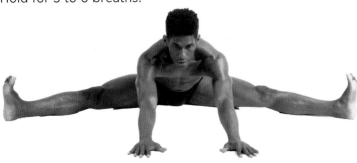

10 BOUND ANGLE POSE WITH FORWARD BEND

Pages 138–39
Hold for 3 to
6 breaths.

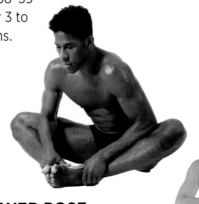

11 DOLPHIN POSE

Page 270
Hold for 3 to
6 breaths.

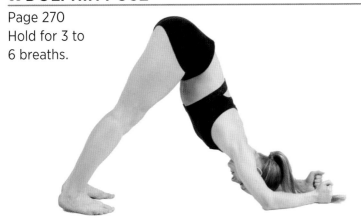

12 PRAYER POSE

Pages 34–35
Hold for 3 to 6 breaths.

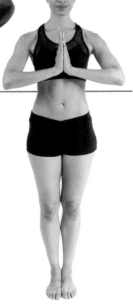

Gentle Flow

This mild sequence combines inversions, forward bends, and backbends to relax the spine and relieve lower-back pain.

1 CAT POSE

Pages 102–03
Hold for 3 to 6 breaths.

2 DOWNWARD-FACING DOG

Pages 268–69
Hold for 3 to 6 breaths.

3 CRESCENT LUNGE

Pages 70–71
Hold for 3 to 6 breaths.

4 WIDE-STANCE UPWARD SALUTE

Pages 40–41
Hold for 3 to 6 breaths.

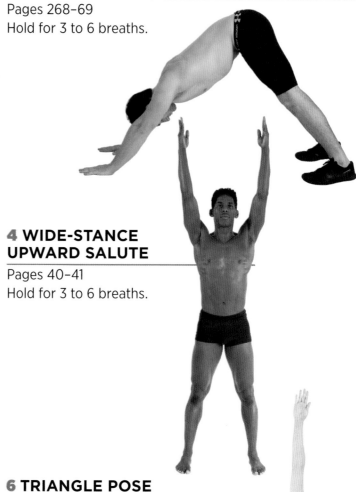

5 HORSE POSE WITH PALMS UP

Pages 52–53
Hold for 3 to 6 breaths.

6 TRIANGLE POSE

Pages 66–67
Hold for 3 to 6 breaths.

FACT FILE

LEVEL
• Beginner

TARGETS
• Spine
• Upper body
• Hamstrings

BENEFITS
• Stretches
  back and neck
• Flexes thighs
• Opens chest

7 EXTENDED TRIANGLE POSE

Pages 76–77
Hold for 3 to
6 breaths.

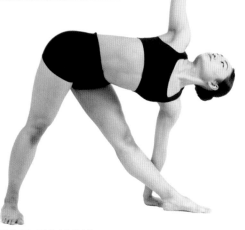

8 EAGLE POSE

Pages 60–61
Hold for 3 to 6 breaths.

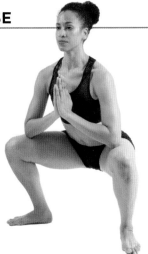

9 STANDING TOE TOUCH

Pages 110–11
Hold for 3 to
6 breaths.

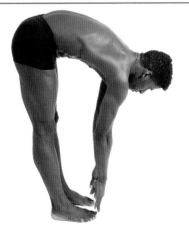

10 GARLAND POSE

Pages 48–49
Hold for 3 to 6 breaths.

11 SWIMMING LOCUST POSE

Pages 176–77
Hold for 3 to 6 breaths.

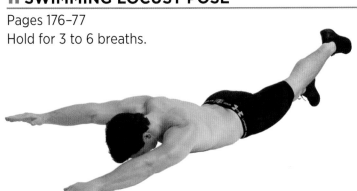

12 HALF FROG PREP

Pages 178–79
Hold for 3 to 6 breaths.

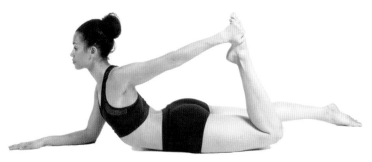

Gentle Flow (continued)

13 CHILD'S POSE WITH ARMS EXTENDED

Pages 134–35
Hold for 3 to 6 breaths.

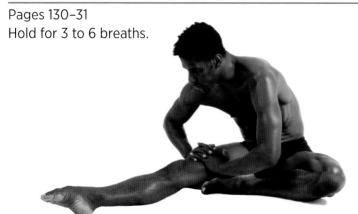

14 SEATED FORWARD BEND PREP

Pages 128–29
Hold for 3 to 6 breaths.

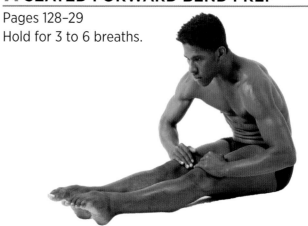

15 HEAD-TO-KNEE FORWARD BEND PREP

Pages 130–31
Hold for 3 to 6 breaths.

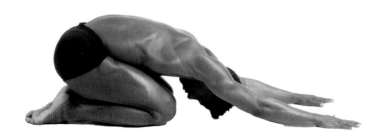

16 CHEST-TO-THIGH STRADDLE SPLIT

Pages 158–59
Hold for 2 to 4 breaths.

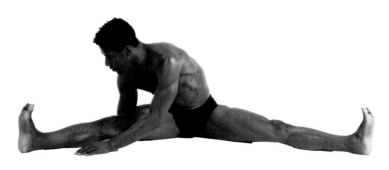

17 SEATED LEG CRADLE

Pages 150–51
Hold for 3 to 6 breaths.

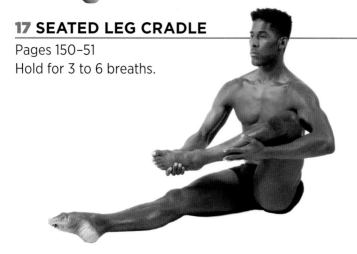

18 CORPSE POSE

Pages 308–09
Hold for several minutes.

Energized Flow

This sequence is sure to get your blood pumping as you switch from planks to upright poses, and even take on a few balance positions.

FACT FILE

LEVEL
• Beginner/ Intermediate

TARGETS
• Spine
• Legs
• Core

BENEFITS
• Stretches back
• Works abdominal and side muscles
• Improves stability

1 EXTENDED PUPPY POSE

Pages 136–37
Hold for 3 to 6 breaths.

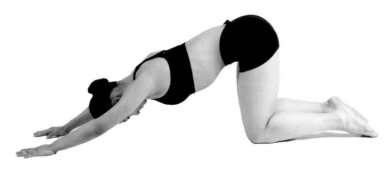

2 ONE-LEGGED PLANK

Pages 274–75
Hold for 3 to 6 breaths.

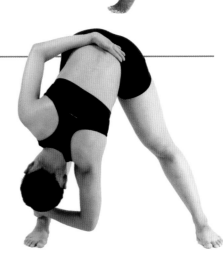

3 BIRD DOG POSE

Pages 276–77
Hold for 3 to 6 breaths.

4 CRESCENT LUNGE

Pages 70–71
Hold for 3 to 6 breaths.

5 TIPTOE INTENSE POSE II

Page 119
Hold for 3 to 6 breaths.

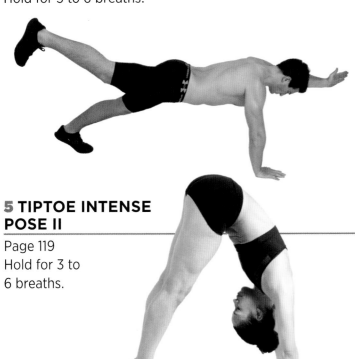

6 INTENSE SIDE STRETCH POSE II

Page 120
Hold for 3 to 6 breaths.

Energized Flow (continued)

7 SIDEWAYS INTENSE STRETCH POSE

Page 121
Hold for 3 to
6 breaths.

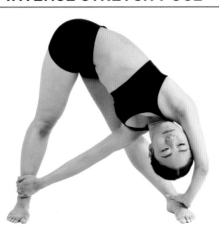

8 SIDE ANGLE POSE

Pages 74–75
Hold for 3 to 6 breaths.

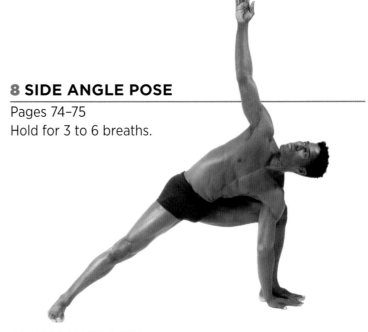

9 SIDE CRANE POSE

Pages 298–99
Hold for 2 to
4 breaths.

10 CRANE POSE

Pages 296–97
Hold for 2 to
4 breaths.

11 SIDE PLANK WITH TREE LEGS

Page 291
Hold for 3 to
6 breaths.

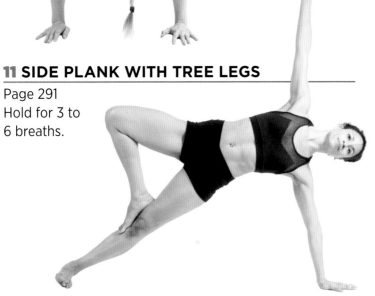

12 LIFTING UP

Page 258
Hold for 2 to 4 breaths.

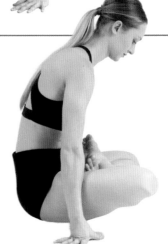

13 DOLPHIN PLANK POSE

Page 271
Hold for 3 to 6 breaths.

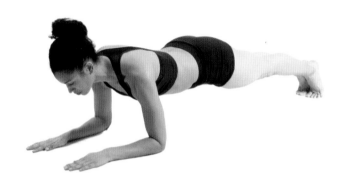

14 DOLPHIN PLANK WITH ARM REACH

Pages 272–73
Hold for 3 to 6 breaths.

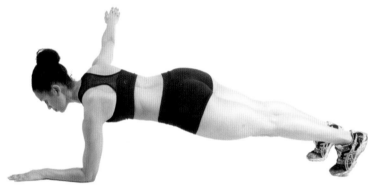

15 COBRA POSE

Pages 172–73
Hold for 2 to 4 breaths.

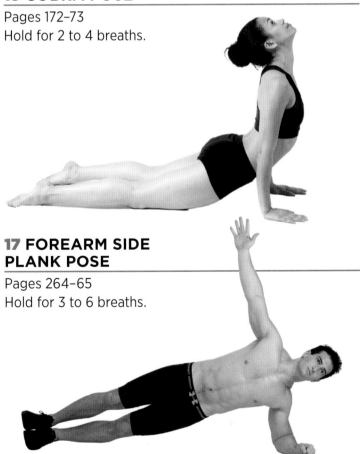

16 BRIDGE POSE EYE OF THE NEEDLE

Pages 186–87
Hold for 3 to 6 breaths.

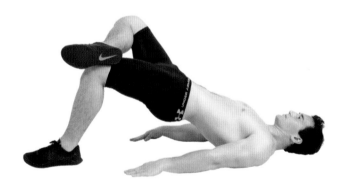

17 FOREARM SIDE PLANK POSE

Pages 264–65
Hold for 3 to 6 breaths.

18 CORPSE POSE

Pages 308–09
Hold for several minutes.

Hip-Opening Flow

This active sequence will help stretch your hips, and ease any tightness in your lower back, hamstrings, and glutes as well.

1 EASY POSE

Pages 220–21
Hold for 3 to
6 breaths.

2 CHILD'S POSE

Pages 132–33
Hold for 3 to 6 breaths.

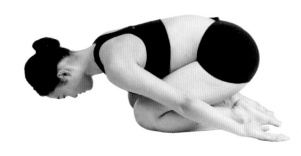

3 CAT POSE

Pages 102–03
Hold for 3 to 6 breaths.

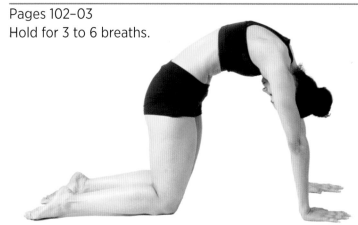

4 COW POSE

Pages 166–67
Hold for 3 to 6 breaths.

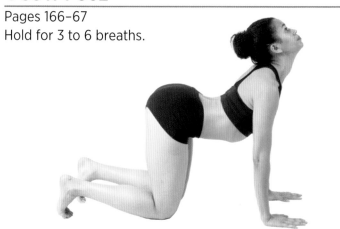

5 HALF FROG POSE

Pages 180–81
Hold for 2 to 4 breaths.

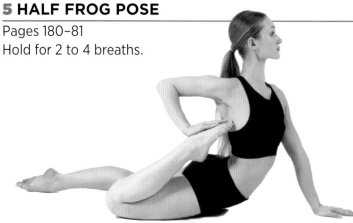

6 HALF CAMEL POSE

Page 184
Hold for 3 to
6 breaths.

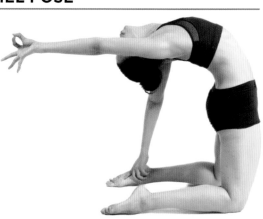

FACT FILE

LEVEL
• Intermediate

TARGETS
• Abdominals
• Obliques
• Hamstrings
• Lower back

TYPE
• Dynamic

BENEFITS
• Stretches back, leg, and core muscles
• Prepares you for more advanced routines

7 EXTENDED HAND-TO-TOE IN CAMEL POSE

Page 185
Hold for 2 to 4 breaths.

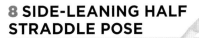

8 SIDE-LEANING HALF STRADDLE POSE

Pages 154–55
Hold for 3 to 6 breaths.

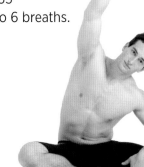

9 SIDE PLANK WITH TREE LEGS

Page 291
Hold for 3 to 6 breaths.

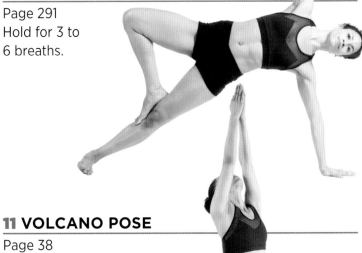

10 WARRIOR POSE III

Pages 92–93
Hold for 3 to 6 breaths.

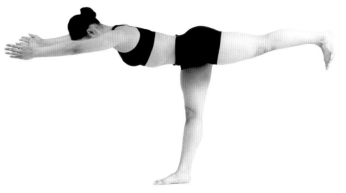

11 VOLCANO POSE

Page 38
Hold for 3 to 6 breaths.

12 DOWNWARD-FACING DOG

Pages 268–69
Hold for 3 to 6 breaths.

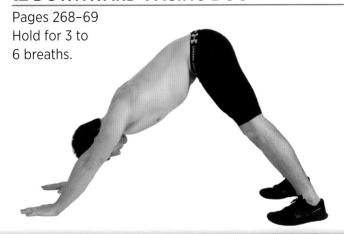

Hip-Opening Flow (continued)

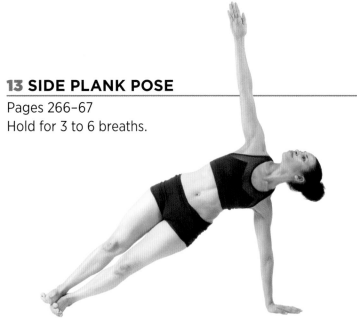

13 SIDE PLANK POSE
Pages 266–67
Hold for 3 to 6 breaths.

14 FLYING PIGEON POSE
Pages 302–03
Hold for 2 to
4 breaths.

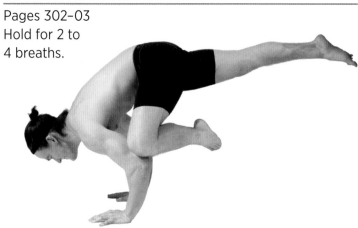

15 RECLINING HERO PREP
Pages 320–21
Hold for 3 to 6 breaths.

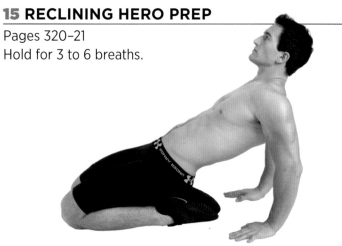

16 RECLINING HERO POSE
Pages 322–23
Hold for 3 to 6 breaths.

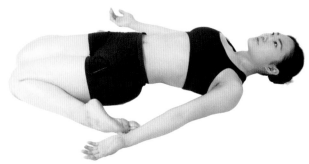

17 HAPPY BABY POSE
Pages 314–15
Hold for 3 to 6 breaths.

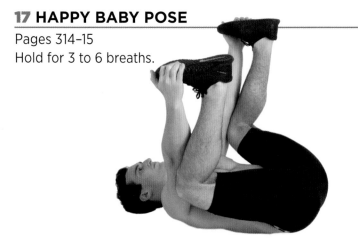

18 RECLINING PIGEON POSE
Pages 312–13
Hold for 3 to
6 breaths.

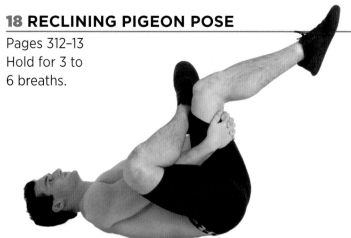

Hamstrings Flow

Get rid of those tight hammies with this effective series of poses that helps you stretch and extend the upper and lower legs.

FACT FILE

LEVEL
• Beginner/
  Intermediate

TARGETS
• Thighs
• Spine
• Glutes

BENEFITS
• Eases tense
  hamstrings
• Stretches
  entire back
• Tones glutes

1 BRIDGE POSE EYE OF THE NEEDLE

Pages 186–87
Hold for 3 to 6 breaths.

2 ONE-LEGGED BRIDGE I

Pages 188–89
Hold for 3 to
6 breaths.

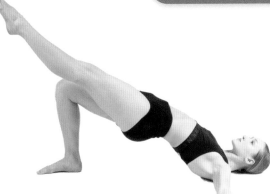

3 RECLINING BIG TOE

Pages 328–29
Hold for 3 to 6 breaths.

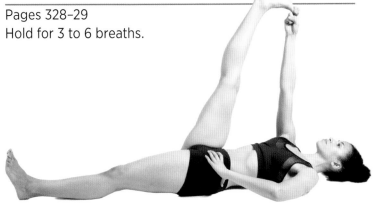

4 KNEES-TO-CHEST POSE

Pages 310–11
Hold for 3 to 6 breaths.

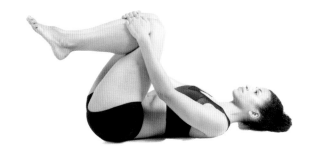

5 DOWNWARD-FACING DOG

Pages 268–69
Hold for 3 to
6 breaths.

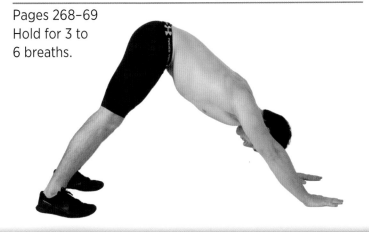

6 STANDING HALF FORWARD BEND TO FORWARD BEND

Pages 106–07
Hold for 3 to 6 breaths.

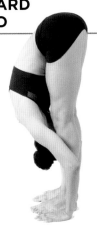

Hamstrings Flow (continued)

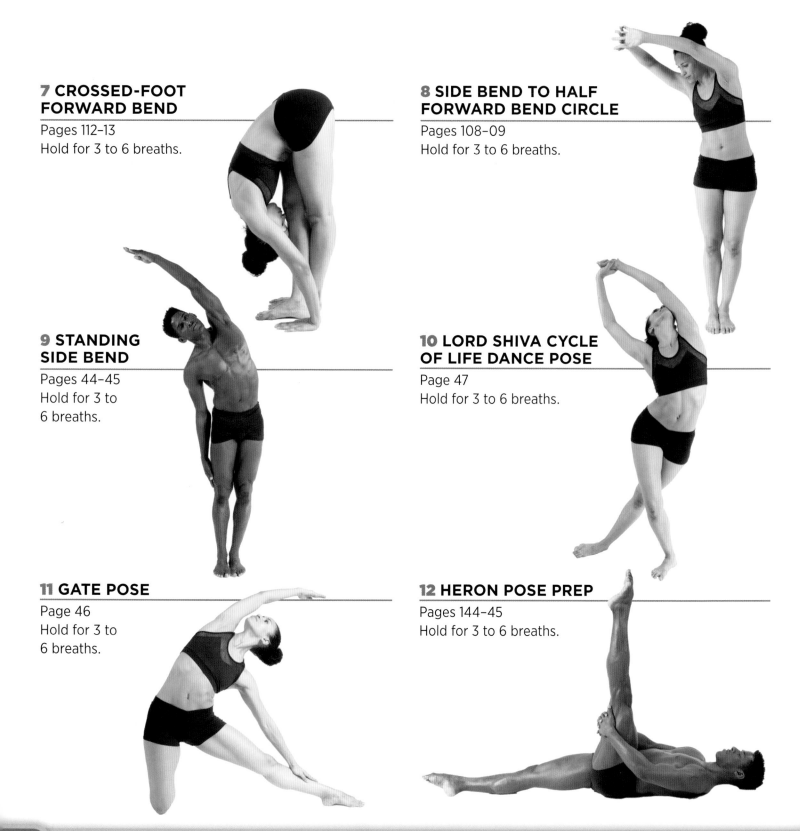

7 CROSSED-FOOT FORWARD BEND

Pages 112–13
Hold for 3 to 6 breaths.

8 SIDE BEND TO HALF FORWARD BEND CIRCLE

Pages 108–09
Hold for 3 to 6 breaths.

9 STANDING SIDE BEND

Pages 44–45
Hold for 3 to 6 breaths.

10 LORD SHIVA CYCLE OF LIFE DANCE POSE

Page 47
Hold for 3 to 6 breaths.

11 GATE POSE

Page 46
Hold for 3 to 6 breaths.

12 HERON POSE PREP

Pages 144–45
Hold for 3 to 6 breaths.

13 HERON POSE

Pages 146–47
Hold for 2 to 4 breaths.

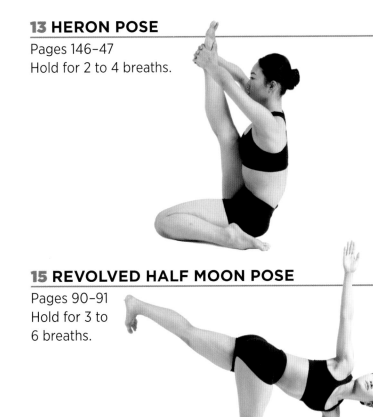

14 GATE POSE

Page 46
Hold for 3 to 6 breaths.

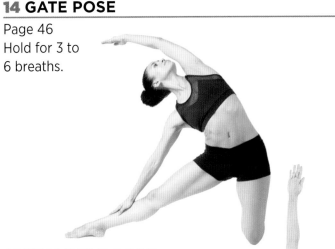

15 REVOLVED HALF MOON POSE

Pages 90–91
Hold for 3 to 6 breaths.

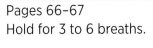

16 TRIANGLE POSE

Pages 66–67
Hold for 3 to 6 breaths.

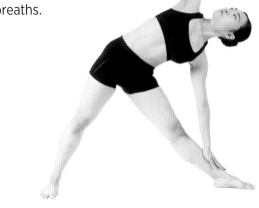

17 WARRIOR POSE III

Pages 92–93
Hold for 3 to 6 breaths.

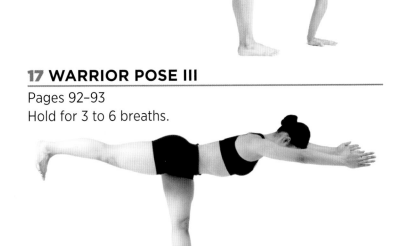

18 REVOLVED EXTENDED SIDE ANGLE POSE

Pages 84–85
Hold for 3 to 6 breaths.

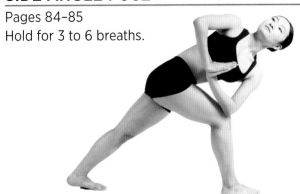

Hamstrings Flow (continued)

19 TIPTOE INTENSE POSE I

Page 118
Hold for 3 to 6 breaths.

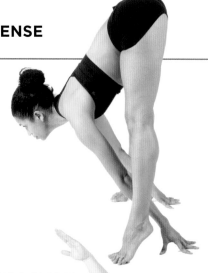

20 WIDE-ANGLE SEATED FORWARD BEND

Pages 156–57
Hold for 3 to 6 breaths.

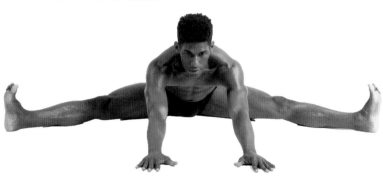

21 SIDE-LEANING HALF STRADDLE POSE

Pages 154–55
Hold for 3 to 6 breaths.

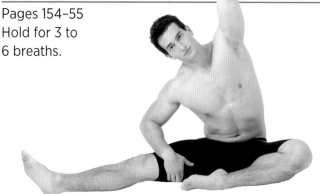

22 HALF STRADDLE POSE

Pages 152–53
Hold for 3 to 6 breaths.

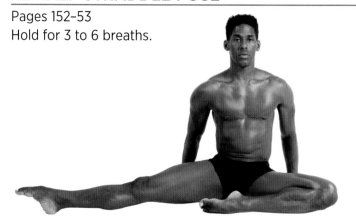

23 BOUND ANGLE POSE WITH FORWARD BEND

Pages 138–39
Hold for 3 to 6 breaths.

24 REVOLVED HEAD-TO-KNEE POSE

Pages 246–47
Hold for 3 to 6 breaths.

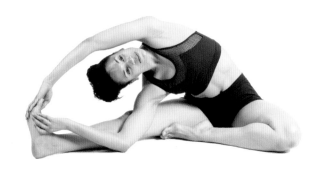

Twisting Flow

Limber up and gain increased flexibility with this series that focuses on stretching the muscles of the sides and abdomen.

1 HERO POSE

Pages 224–25
Hold for 3 to 6 breaths.

2 MERMAID POSE

Pages 238–39
Hold for 3 to 6 breaths.

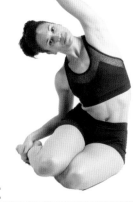

3 REVOLVED SUPPORTED BOAT POSE

Page 244
Hold for 2 to 4 breaths.

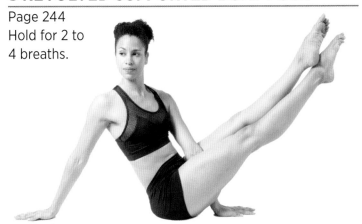

4 BIG TOE POSE

Page 250
Hold for 2 to 4 breaths.

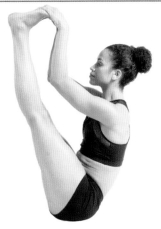

5 REVOLVED BOAT POSE WITH PRAYER HANDS

Page 245
Hold for 2 to 4 breaths.

6 CHILD'S POSE

Pages 132–33
Hold for 3 to 6 breaths.

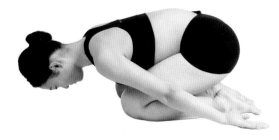

Twisting Flow (continued)

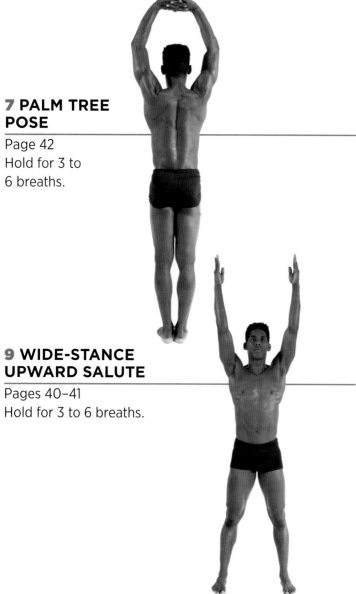

7 PALM TREE POSE

Page 42
Hold for 3 to
6 breaths.

8 PALM TREE SIDE BEND

Page 43
Hold for 3 to
6 breaths.

9 WIDE-STANCE UPWARD SALUTE

Pages 40–41
Hold for 3 to 6 breaths.

10 HORSE POSE

Pages 50–51
Hold for 3 to 6 breaths.

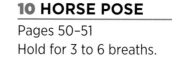

11 REVERSE TABLETOP POSE

Pages 280–81
Hold for 3 to 6 breaths.

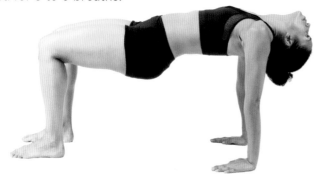

12 UPWARD PLANK POSE

Pages 282–83
Hold for 3 to 6 breaths.

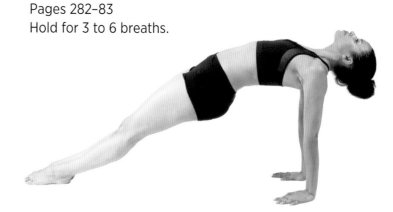

13 REVOLVED EXTENDED SIDE ANGLE POSE

Pages 84–85
Hold for 3 to 6 breaths.

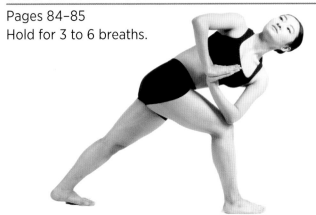

14 ONE-LEGGED SIDE PLANK PREP

Pages 288–89
Hold for 2 to 4 breaths.

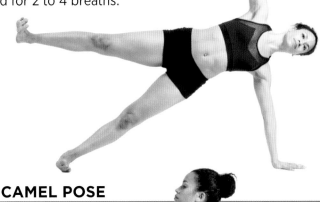

15 REVOLVED HEAD-TO-KNEE POSE

Pages 246–47
Hold for 2 to 4 breaths.

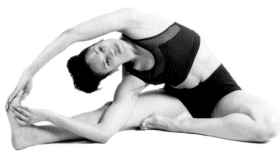

16 CAMEL POSE

Pages 182–83
Hold for 3 to
6 breaths.

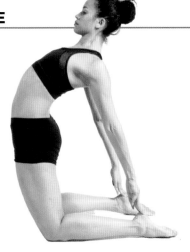

17 BHARADVAJA'S TWIST II

Page 230
Hold for 3 to 6 breaths.

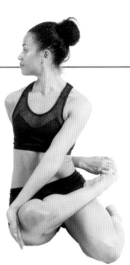

18 CHEST-TO-FLOOR STRADDLE SPLIT POSE

Pages 162–63
Hold for 3 to 6 breaths.

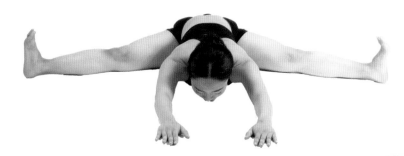

Shoulder-Opening Flow

This sequence will open up the shoulders and rib cage, and will increase flexibility in the back, thighs, and hamstrings.

1 DOWNWARD-FACING DOG

Pages 268–69
Hold for 3 to
6 breaths.

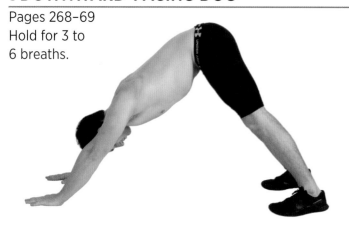

2 DOLPHIN POSE

Page 270
Hold for 3 to
6 breaths.

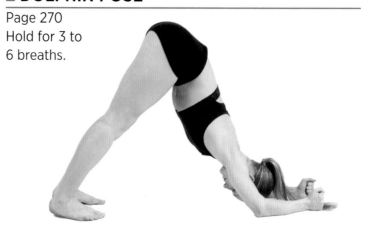

3 COW FACE POSE

Pages 234–35
Hold for 3 to 6 breaths.

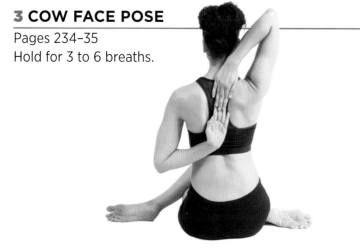

4 ONE-LEGGED KING PIGEON POSE I

Pages 200–01
Hold for 2 to
4 breaths.

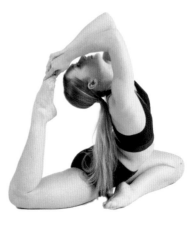

5 BIG TOE BOW POSE

Page 207
Hold for 2 to
4 breaths.

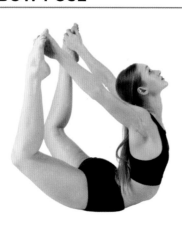

6 CHILD'S POSE WITH ARMS EXTENDED

Pages 134–35
Hold for 3 to 6 breaths.

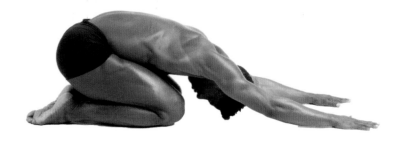

FACT FILE

LEVEL
• Intermediate

TARGETS
• Upper body
• Spine
• Legs

BENEFITS
• Opens chest
  and shoulders
• Elongates
  back
• Stretches
  hamstrings

7 EXTENDED PUPPY POSE

Pages 136–37
Hold for 3 to 6 breaths.

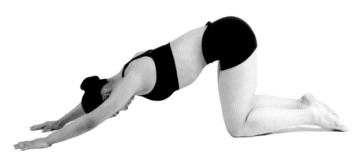

8 INTENSE SIDE STRETCH POSE I

Pages 116–17
Hold for 3 to
6 breaths.

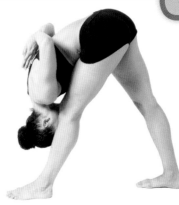

9 CAMEL POSE

Pages 182–83
Hold for 3 to
6 breaths.

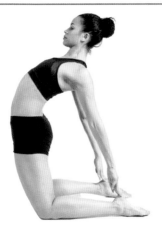

10 HALF CAMEL POSE

Page 184
Hold for 3 to
6 breaths.

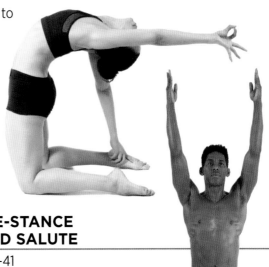

11 TOES-TO-ELBOW BOW POSE

Pages 208–09
Hold for 2 to
4 breaths.

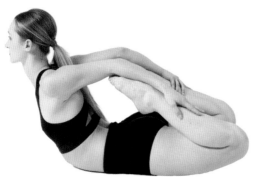

12 WIDE-STANCE UPWARD SALUTE

Pages 40–41
Hold for 3 to 6 breaths.

Intermediate Sequence

Now it's time to take the building-block poses you have mastered and put them together to create a slightly more demanding sequence.

1 MOUNTAIN POSE

Pages 32–33
Hold for 3 to 6 breaths.

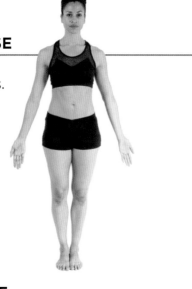

2 TWISTING CHAIR POSE

Pages 56–57
Hold for 3 to 6 breaths.

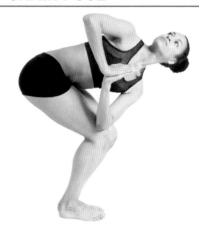

3 GARLAND POSE

Pages 48–49
Hold for 3 to 6 breaths.

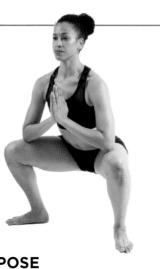

4 CROW POSE

Pages 294–95
Hold for 3 to 6 breaths.

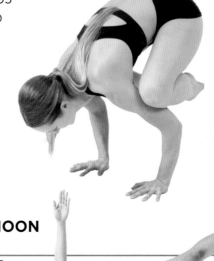

5 FLYING PIGEON POSE

Pages 302–03
Hold for 3 to 6 breaths.

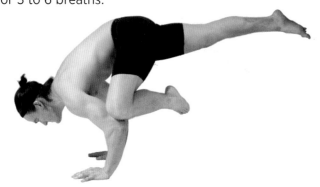

6 HALF MOON POSE

Pages 86–87
Hold for 3 to 6 breaths.

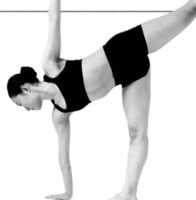

FACT FILE

LEVEL
• Intermediate

TARGETS
• Core
• Arms
• Legs

BENEFITS
• Tones abdominals
• Strengthens arms
• Stretches hamstrings and calves

7 TRIANGLE POSE

Pages 66–67
Hold for 3 to 6 breaths.

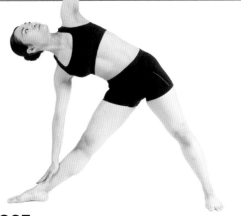

8 REVOLVED TRIANGLE POSE

Pages 78–79
Hold for 3 to 6 breaths.

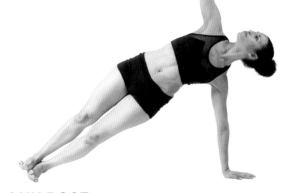

9 PLANK POSE

Pages 260–61
Hold for 3 to 6 breaths.

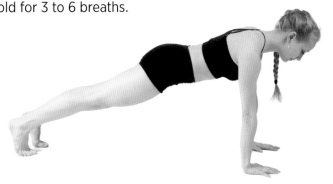

10 SIDE PLANK POSE

Pages 266–67
Hold for 3 to 6 breaths.

11 DOWNWARD-FACING DOG

Pages 268–69
Hold for 3 to 6 breaths.

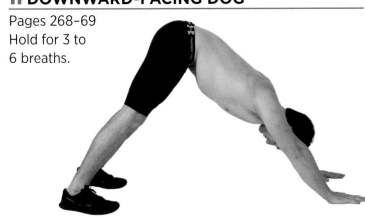

12 PLANK POSE

Pages 260–61
Hold for 3 to 6 breaths.

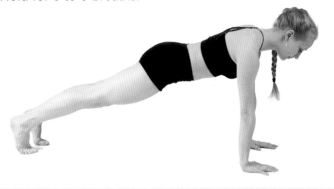

Intermediate Sequence (continued)

13 WHEEL POSE

Pages 194–95
Hold for 3 to
6 breaths.

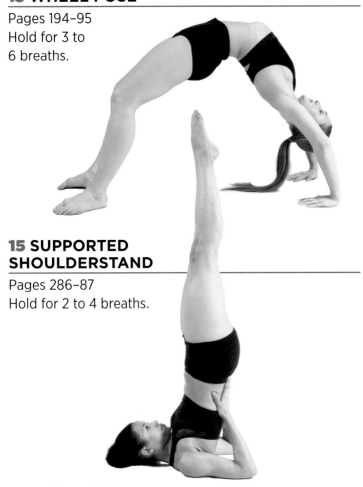

14 KNEES-TO-CHEST POSE

Pages 310–11
Hold for 3 to 6 breaths.

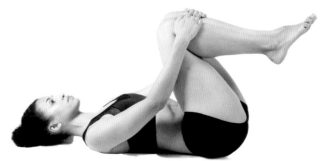

15 SUPPORTED SHOULDERSTAND

Pages 286–87
Hold for 2 to 4 breaths.

16 UPWARD PLANK WITH LIFTED LEG

Pages 284–85
Hold for 3 to
6 breaths.

17 FISH POSE

Pages 196–97
Hold for 3 to 6 breaths.

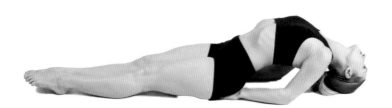

18 ONE-LEGGED KING PIGEON POSE PREP

Pages 198–99
Hold for 3 to
6 breaths.

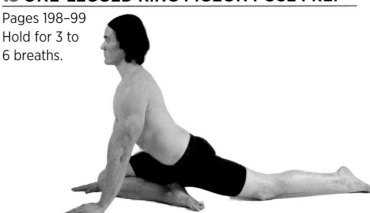

19 PLOW POSE

Pages 278–79
Hold for 3 to 6 breaths.

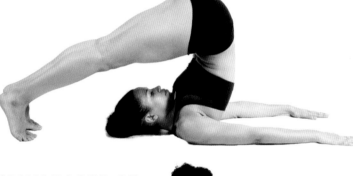

20 FIRE LOG POSE

Pages 232–33
Hold for 3 to 6 breaths.

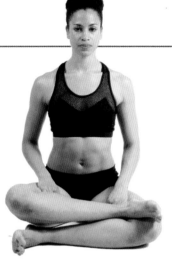

21 HALF LORD OF THE FISHES POSE

Pages 240–41
Hold for 3 to 6 breaths.

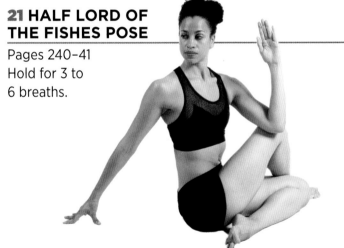

22 REVOLVED HEAD-TO-KNEE POSE

Pages 246–47
Hold for 2 to 4 breaths.

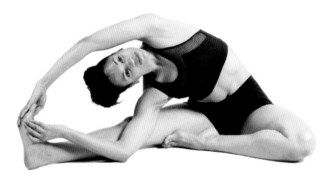

23 KING COBRA POSE

Page 206
Hold for 2 to 4 breaths.

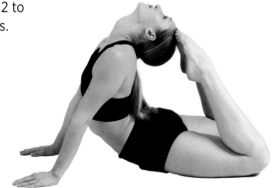

24 CORPSE POSE

Pages 308–09
Hold for several minutes.

Advanced Balance Flow

Balance poses can improve your core strength and general stability, and offer a chance for some extended stretching.

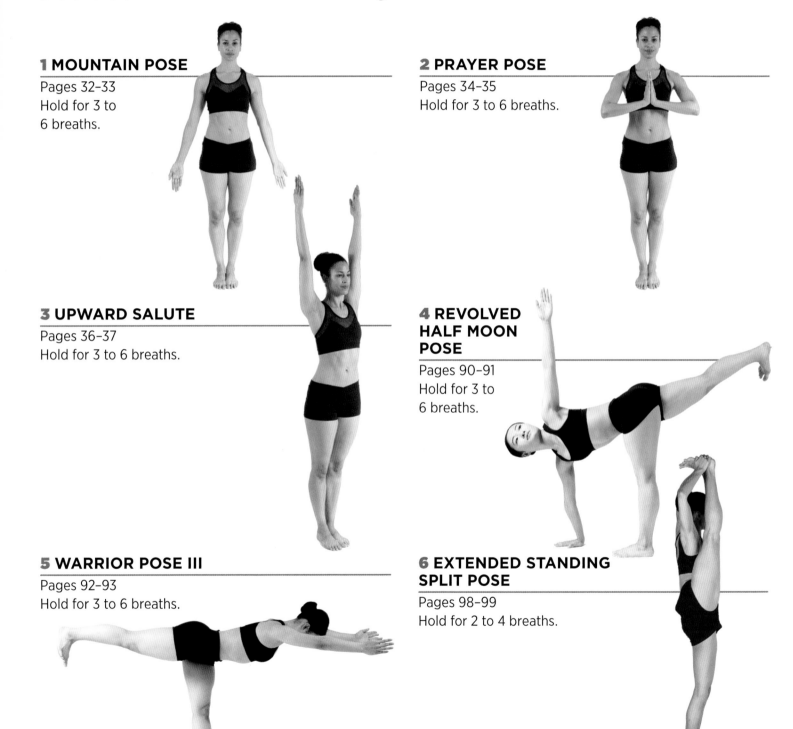

1 MOUNTAIN POSE

Pages 32–33
Hold for 3 to
6 breaths.

2 PRAYER POSE

Pages 34–35
Hold for 3 to 6 breaths.

3 UPWARD SALUTE

Pages 36–37
Hold for 3 to 6 breaths.

4 REVOLVED HALF MOON POSE

Pages 90–91
Hold for 3 to
6 breaths.

5 WARRIOR POSE III

Pages 92–93
Hold for 3 to 6 breaths.

6 EXTENDED STANDING SPLIT POSE

Pages 98–99
Hold for 2 to 4 breaths.

FACT FILE

LEVEL
• Intermediate/Advanced

TARGETS
• Abdominals
• Upper Legs
• Back

BENEFITS
• Increases sense of balance
• Stretches arms and legs
• Tightens abdominal and side muscles

7 BOWING WITH RESPECT POSE

Page 94
Hold for 2 to 4 breaths.

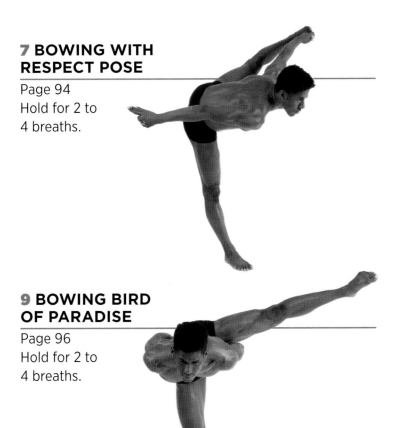

8 BOWING BIRD OF PARADISE PREP

Page 95
Hold for 2 to 4 breaths.

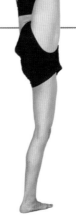

9 BOWING BIRD OF PARADISE

Page 96
Hold for 2 to 4 breaths.

10 EXTENDED STANDING SPLIT POSE

Pages 98–99
Hold for 2 to 4 breaths.

11 MOUNTAIN POSE

Pages 32–33
Hold for 3 to 6 breaths.

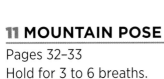

12 UPWARD SALUTE

Pages 36–37
Hold for 3 to 6 breaths.

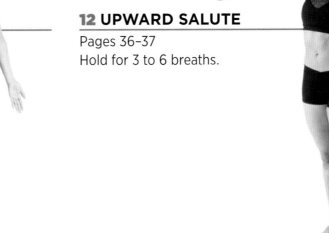

Advanced Balance Flow (continued)

13 WARRIOR POSE III

Pages 92–93
Hold for 3 to 6 breaths.

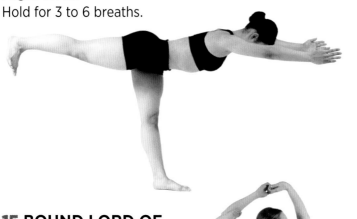

14 LORD OF THE DANCE POSE

Pages 210–11
Hold for 3 to 6 breaths.

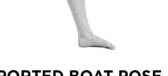

15 BOUND LORD OF THE DANCE POSE

Page 212
Hold for 2 to 4 breaths.

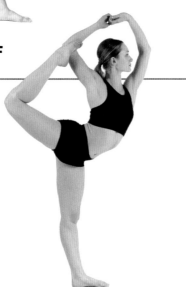

16 HAND-TO-FOOT LORD OF THE DANCE POSE

Page 213
Hold for 2 to 4 breaths.

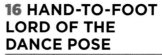

17 STAFF POSE

Pages 218–19
Hold for 3 to 6 breaths.

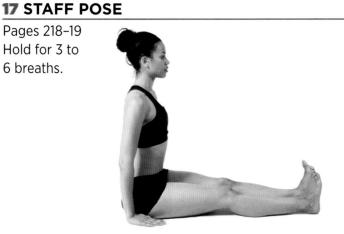

18 REVOLVED SUPPORTED BOAT POSE

Page 244
Hold for 2 to 4 breaths.

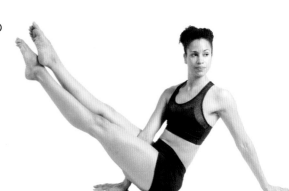

19 REVOLVED BOAT POSE WITH PRAYER HANDS

Page 245
Hold for 2 to
4 breaths.

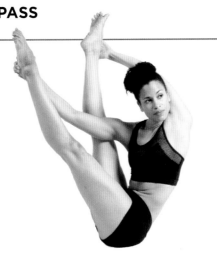

20 BOAT POSE

Pages 242–43
Hold for 3 to
6 breaths.

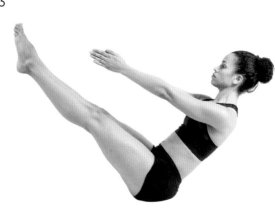

21 DOUBLE COMPASS POSE

Page 251
Hold for 3 to
6 breaths.

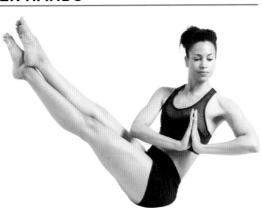

22 RECLINING PIGEON POSE

Pages 312–13
Hold for 3 to 6 breaths.

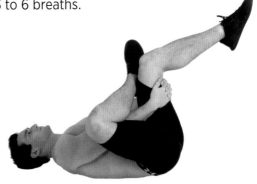

23 RECLINING HERO PREP

Pages 320–21
Hold for 3 to
6 breaths.

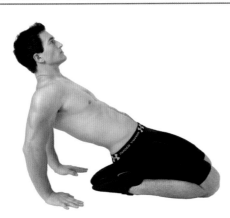

24 RECLINING HERO POSE

Pages 322–23
Hold for 3 to 6 breaths.

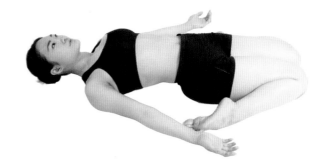

Advanced Backbend Flow

Backbends provide an ideal way to loosen tight spine and shoulder muscles while at the same time opening up the hips and rib cage.

1 EASY POSE

Pages 220–21
Hold for 3 to
6 breaths.

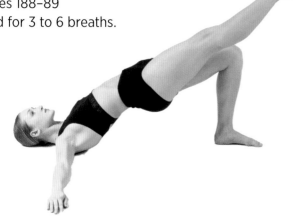

2 BRIDGE POSE

Pages 168–69
Hold for 3 to 6 breaths.

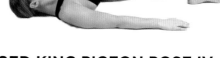

3 ONE-LEGGED BRIDGE I

Pages 188–89
Hold for 3 to 6 breaths.

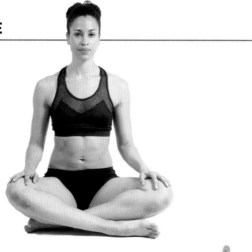

4 ONE-LEGGED BRIDGE II

Pages 190–91
Hold for 3 to 6 breaths.

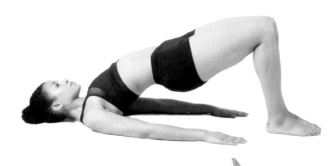

5 ONE-LEGGED KING PIGEON POSE III

Page 204
Hold for 2 to 4 breaths.

6 ONE-LEGGED KING PIGEON POSE IV

Page 205
Hold for 2 to 4 breaths.

FACT FILE

LEVEL
• Intermediate/
  Advanced

TARGETS
• Shoulders
• Spine
• Hips

BENEFITS
• Eases lower
  back stiffness
• Loosens hip
  muscles and
  glutes
• Opens the
  chest

7 KING COBRA POSE

Page 206
Hold for 2 to 4 breaths.

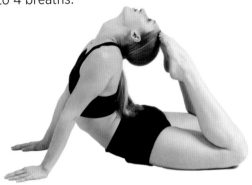

8 BIG TOE BOW POSE

Page 207
Hold for 2 to
4 breaths.

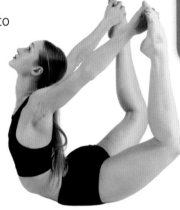

9 TOES-TO-ELBOW BOW POSE

Pages 208–09
Hold for 2 to 4 breaths.

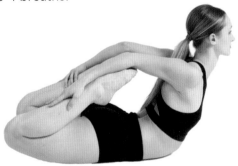

10 ONE-LEGGED KING PIGEON POSE I

Pages 200–01
Hold for 2 to
4 breaths.

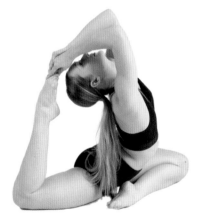

11 ONE-LEGGED KING PIGEON POSE II

Pages 202–03
Hold for 2 to
4 breaths.

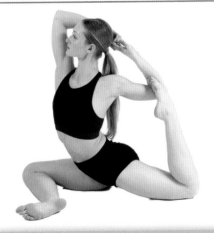

12 FISH POSE

Pages 196–97
Hold for 3 to 6 breaths.

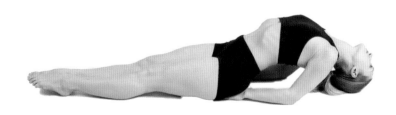

APPENDICES

Within this section, you will find a glossary to help explain terms that may be unfamiliar to you; an index of icons that show the different yoga poses featured in the book; an index of all the topics covered by the book; and the credits for the photos.

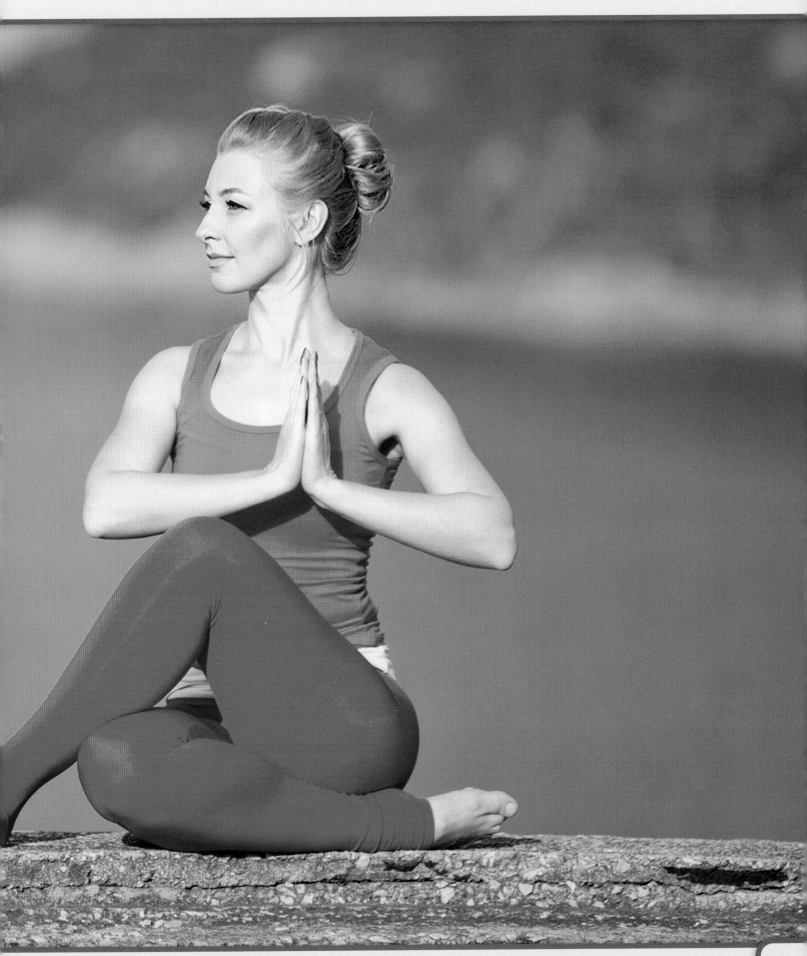

Glossary

GENERAL TERMS

abduction: Movement away from your body.

adduction: Movement toward your body.

aerobic exercise: A type of exercise involving aerobic metabolism in which your body uses oxygen to create energy; refers to sustained activity.

anaerobic exercise: A type of exercise involving anaerobic metabolism in which your muscles do not use oxygen to create energy; refers to short bursts of activity.

anterior: Located in the front of your body.

asana: A physical posture of yoga; literally, a "seat."

Ashtanga: The eight-limbed yogic path.

ayurveda: The ancient Indian science of health.

bhakti: Devotion, as in bhakti yoga.

cardiovascular exercise: Any exercise that increases your heart rate, making oxygen and nutrient-rich blood available to working muscles.

bandha: Internal muscular "locks" that, when engaged, support the toning and lifting of strategic areas of your body.

cooldown: An exercise performed at the end of the workout session that works to cool and relax your body.

core: Refers to the deep muscle layers that lie close to your spine and provide structural support for your entire body. The core is divided into two groups: the major and the minor muscles. The major core muscles reside in the abdominal area and in the middle and lower back. This area encompasses the pelvic floor muscles (levator ani, pubococcygeus, iliococcygeus, puborectalis, and coccygeus), the abdominals (rectus abdominis, transversus abdominis, obliquus externus, and obliquus internus), the spinal extensors (multifidus spinae, erector spinae, splenius, longissimus thoracis, and semispinalis), and the diaphragm. The minor core muscles include the latissimus dorsi, gluteus maximus, and trapezius. The minor core muscles assist the major muscles when your body engages in activities or movements that require added stability.

core stabilizer: An exercise that calls for resisting motion along your lumbar spine through activation of your abdominal muscles and deep stabilizers; improves core strength and endurance.

core strengthener: An exercise that allows for motion in your lumbar spine, while working your abdominal muscles and deep stabilizers; improves core strength.

drishti: Focal point of gazing during meditation or yoga practice—and quite useful during balancing poses.

extension: The straightening of a joint.

extensor muscle: A muscle that extends a limb, or other body part, away from your body.

flexion: The bending of a joint.

flexor muscle: A muscle that decreases the angle between two bones, as when bending your elbow or raising your thigh toward your abdomen.

guru: A teacher or master; literally, "one who illuminates the darkness."

hamstrings: The three muscles at the back of your thigh (semitendinosus, semimembranosus, and biceps femoris) that flex your knee and extend your hip.

hatha yoga: From ha ("sun") and tha ("moon"), hatha yoga seeks to unify opposites—body and mind—and describes any of the physical practices of yoga.

hyperextension: An exercise that works your lower back as well as your middle and upper back, specifically the erector spinae, which usually involves raising your torso and/or lower body from the floor while keeping your pelvis firmly anchored.

internal rotation: The act of moving a part of your body toward the center of your body.

interval: A period of activity or rest.

isolation exercise: A movement that focuses on only one muscle or muscle group.

iliotibial band (IT band): A thick band of fibrous tissue that runs down the outside of your thigh, beginning at your hip and extending to the outer side of your tibia, just below your knee joint. The band functions in concert with several of your thigh muscles to provide stability to the outside of your knee joint.

lateral: Refers to the outer side of your body; the opposite of medial.

lunge: A group of lower-body exercises in which one leg is positioned forward with your knee bent and foot flat on the floor, while your other leg is positioned behind you.

mantra: A tool or instrument of thought involving sounds, syllables, words, or groups of words that are repeated with the goal of creating a positive transformation; a sacred thought or a prayer.

medial: Refers to the middle of your body; the opposite of lateral.

meditation: The focusing and calming of your mind, often through breath work to reach deeper levels of consciousness.

mudra (a seal): Hand gestures that influence the energies of your body or mood. Most often, your hands and fingers are held in a mudra to aid concentration, focus, and connection to yourself.

nadis: The energy channels through which prana, or life force, flows. Pranayama uses your breath to direct and expand the flow of prana in the nadis.

namaste: Sanskrit word commonly spoken at the end of yoga class. One thoughtful interpretation: "I honor that place in you where the whole universe resides. And when I am in that place in me and you are in that place in you, there is only one of us."

neutral: Describes the position of your legs, pelvis, hips, or other part of your body that is neither arched nor curved forward.

neutral position: A position in which the natural curve of your spine is maintained, typically adopted when lying on your back with one or both feet on the mat.

om: A mantra usually chanted at the beginning and end of yoga class. It is said to be the origin of all sounds and the seed of creation, and it is often referred to as the "universal sound of consciousness."

posterior: Refers to the back of your body.

posterior chain: Your gluteals, hamstrings, and back.

prana: Life energy, or life force.

pranayama: Breath awareness used to facilitate inner stillness and awareness.

props: Tools such as mats, blocks, blankets, and straps used to extend your range of motion or facilitate achieving a pose.

pulling muscles: The primary muscle groups associated with pulling movements: abdominals, biceps, forearms, latissimus dorsi, hamstrings, obliques, and trapezius.

pushing muscles: The primary muscle groups associated with pushing movements: calves, deltoids, gluteals, pectorals, quadriceps, and triceps.

quadriceps: A large muscle group that includes the four prevailing muscles at the front of your thigh: rectus femoris, vastus intermedius, vastus lateralis, and vastus medialis; the main extensor muscles of your knee that surround the front and sides of your femur muscle.

range of motion: The distance and direction a joint can move between the flexed and the extended positions.

resistance: The weight your muscles are working against to complete a movement, whether your own body weight or added weight, such as dumbbells.

rotator muscle: One of a group of muscles that assists the rotation of a joint, such as your hip or shoulder.

samadhi: The state of complete enlightenment.

Savasana: The ultimate relaxation pose, typically at the end of yoga class; literally, "corpse pose."

scapula: The protrusion of bone in your middle to upper back known as your shoulder blade.

Shakti: Female energy.

shanti: A term meaning "peace," it is often chanted three times in yoga class.

Shiva: Male energy; a Hindu deity.

stretch: Refers to the straightening or extending of your body, or a part of your body, to full length.

Surya Namaskar, or Sun Salutations: A sequence of dynamic asanas, often used to warm up your body at the beginning of yoga class.

swami: A Hindu ascetic or religious leader; literally, a "master."

Tantra: A meditative yoga that unites your mind and body.

Ujjayi or Hissing Breath, Victorious Breath: A type of pranayama in which your lungs are fully expanded and your chest is puffed out; especially associated with the vinyasa style.

Upanishads: Texts of a religious and philosophical nature, expounding the Vedas, written in Sanskrit in India probably between 800 BC and 500 BC.

Veda: One of the ancient Hindu scriptures written in Sanskrit, consisting of hymns, philosophy, and guidance on rituals for Vedic priests.

ventral aspect: The front of your body.

vinyasa: Movements linked with breath; postures are strung together to create a short or a long flow.

warm-up: Any form of light exercise of short duration that prepares your body for more intense exercises.

Yang yoga: A style of yoga that is rhythmic, repetitive, and energetic, and helps build strength and fitness.

Yin yoga: A series of passive floor poses that are held for several minutes and that target the fascia, or connective tissue, in your body. A combination of Yin and Yang keeps students balanced and healthy.

yoga: From the Sanskrit yug ("yoke"), meaning "union." Yoga is an ancient discipline in which physical postures, breath practice, meditation, and philosophical study are used as tools for achieving liberation.

yogi/yogini: A male/female practitioner of yoga.

LATIN TERMS

The following glossary explains the Latin scientific terminology used to describe the muscles of the human body. Certain words are derived from Greek, which is indicated in each instance.

CHEST

coracobrachialis: Greek *korakoeidés*, "ravenlike," and *brachium*, "arm"

pectoralis (major and minor): *pectus*, "breast"

ABDOMEN

obliquus (externus and internus): *obliquus*, "slanting"

rectus abdominis: *rego,* "straight, upright," and *abdomen,* "belly"

serratus anterior: *serra*, "saw," and *ante*, "before"

transversus abdominis: *transversus*, "athwart," and *abdomen*, "belly"

NECK

scalenus: Greek *skalénós*, "unequal"

semispinalis: *semi*, "half," and *spinae*, "spine"

splenius: Greek *spléníon*, "plaster, patch"

sternocleidomastoideus: Greek *stérnon*, "chest," Greek *kleís*, "key," and Greek *mastoeidés*, "breastlike"

BACK

erector spinae: *erectus*, "straight," and *spina*, "thorn"

latissimus dorsi: *latus*, "wide," and *dorsum*, "back"

multifidus spinae: *multifid*, "to cut into divisions," and *spinae*, "spine"

quadratus lumborum: *quadratus*, "square, rectangular," and *lumbus*, "loin"

rhomboideus: Greek *rhembesthai*, "to spin"

trapezius: Greek *trapezion*, "small table"

SHOULDERS

deltoideus (anterior, medialis, and posterior): Greek *deltoeidés*, "delta-shaped"

infraspinatus: *infra*, "under," and *spina*, "thorn"

levator scapulae: *levare*, "to raise," and *scapulae*, "shoulder [blades]"

subscapularis: *sub*, "below," and *scapulae*, "shoulder [blades]"

supraspinatus: *supra,* "above," and *spina*, "thorn"

teres (major and minor): *teres*, "rounded"

UPPER ARM

biceps brachii: *biceps*, "two-headed," and *brachium*, "arm"

brachialis: *brachium*, "arm"

triceps brachii: *triceps*, "three-headed," and *brachium*, "arm"

LOWER ARM

anconeus: Greek *anconad*, "elbow"

brachioradialis: *brachium*, "arm," and *radius*, "spoke"

extensor carpi radialis: *extendere*, "to extend," Greek *karpós*, "wrist," and *radius*, "spoke"

extensor digitorum: *extendere*, "to extend," and *digitus*, "finger, toe"

flexor carpi pollicis longus: *flectere*, "to bend," Greek *karpós*, "wrist," *pollicis*, "thumb," and *longus*, "long"

flexor carpi radialis: *flectere*, "to bend," Greek *karpós*, "wrist," and *radius*, "spoke"

flexor carpi ulnaris: *flectere*, "to bend," Greek *karpós*, "wrist," and *ulnaris*, "forearm"

flexor digitorum: *flectere*, "to bend," and *digitus*, "finger, toe"

palmaris longus: *palmaris*, "palm," and *longus*, "long"

pronator teres: *pronate*, "to rotate," and *teres*, "rounded"

HIPS

gemellus (inferior and superior): *geminus*, "twin"

gluteus maximus: Greek *gloutós*, "rump," and *maximus*, "largest"

gluteus medius: Greek *gloutós*, "rump," and *medialis*, "middle"

gluteus minimus: Greek *gloutós*, "rump," and *minimus*, "smallest"

iliopsoas: *ilium,* "groin," and Greek *psoa*, "groin muscle"

obturator externus: *obturare*, "to block," and *externus,* "outward"

obturator internus: *obturare*, "to block," and *internus*, "within"

pectineus: *pectin*, "comb"

piriformis: *pirum*, "pear," and *forma,* "shape"

quadratus femoris: *quadratus*, "square, rectangular," and *femur*, "thigh"

UPPER LEG

adductor longus: *adducere*, "to contract," and *longus*, "long"

adductor magnus: *adducere*, "to contract," and *magnus*, "major"

biceps femoris: *biceps*, "two-headed," and *femur*, "thigh"

gracilis: *gracilis*, "slim, slender"

rectus femoris: *rego*, "straight, upright," and *femur*, "thigh"

sartorius: *sarcio*, "to patch" or "to repair"

semimembranosus: *semi*, "half," and *membrum*, "limb"

semitendinosus: *semi*, "half," and *tendo*, "tendon"

tensor fasciae latae: *tenere*, "to stretch," *fasciae*, "band," and *latae*, "laid down"

vastus intermedius: *vastus*, "immense, huge," and *intermedius*, "between"

vastus lateralis: *vastus*, "immense, huge," and lateralis, "side"

vastus medialis: *vastus*, "immense, huge," and *medialis*, "middle"

LOWER LEG

adductor digiti minimi: *adducere*, "to contract," *digitus*, "finger, toe," and *minimum* "smallest"

adductor hallucis: *adducere*, "to contract," and *hallex*, "big toe"

extensor digitorum longus: *extendere*, "to extend," *digitus*, "finger, toe," and *longus*, "long"

extensor hallucis longus: *extendere*, "to extend," *hallex*, "big toe," and *longus*, "long"

flexor digitorum longus: *flectere*, "to bend," *digitus*, "finger, toe," and *longus*, "long"

flexor hallucis longus: *flectere*, "to bend," *hallex*, "big toe," and *longus*, "long"

gastrocnemius: Greek *gastroknémía*, "calf [of the leg]"

peroneus: *peronei*, "of the fibula"

plantaris: *planta*, "the sole"

soleus: *solea*, "sandal"

tibialis (anterior and posterior): *tibia*, "reed pipe"

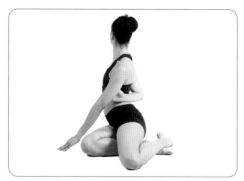

Bharadvaja's Twist I
Pages 228–29

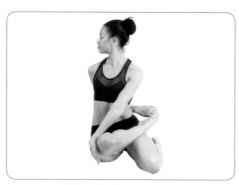

Bharadvaja's Twist II
Page 230

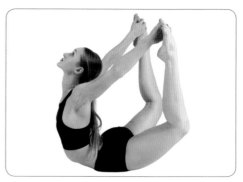

Big Toe Bow Pose
Page 207

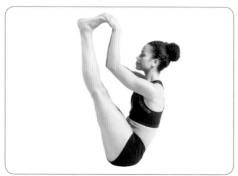

Big Toe Pose
Page 250

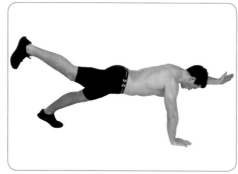

Bird Dog Pose
Pages 276–77

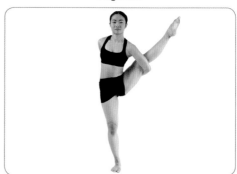

Bird Of Paradise Pose
Page 97

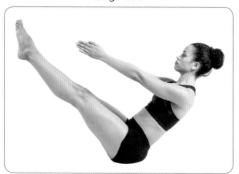

Boat Pose
Pages 242–43

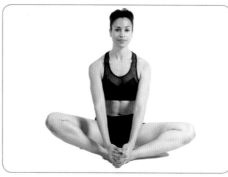

Bound Angle Pose
Pages 222–23

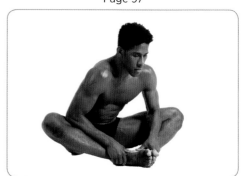

Bound Angle Pose with Forward Bend
Pages 138–39

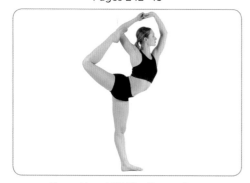

Bound Lord Of The Dance Pose
Page 212

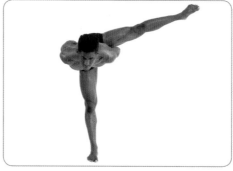

Bowing Bird of Paradise
Page 96

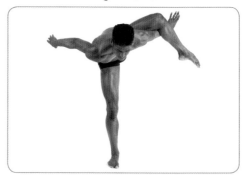

Bowing Bird of Paradise Prep
Page 95

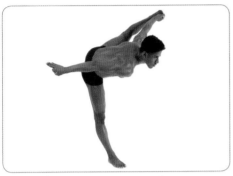

Bowing with Respect Pose
Page 94

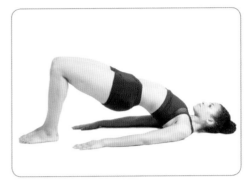

Bow Pose
Pages 192–93

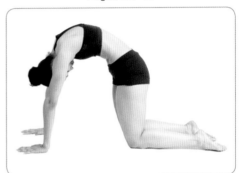

Bridge Pose
Pages 168–69

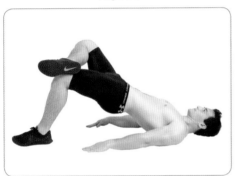

Bridge Pose Eye of the Needle
Pages 186–87

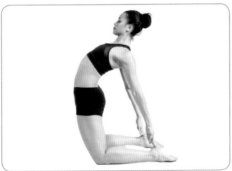

Camel Pose
Pages 182–83

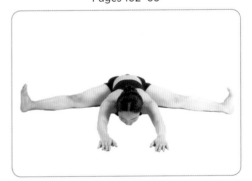

Cat Pose
Pages 102–03

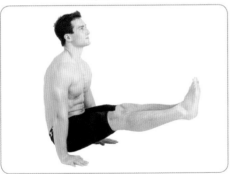

Celibate's Pose
Pages 292–93

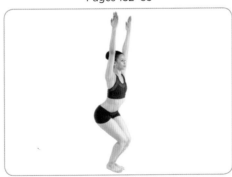

Chair Pose
Pages 54–55

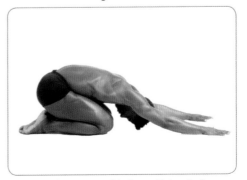

Chest-to-Floor Straddle Split Pose
Pages 162–63

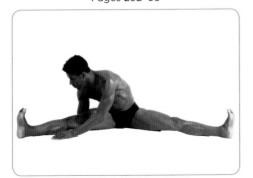

Chest-to-Thigh Straddle Split
Pages 158–59

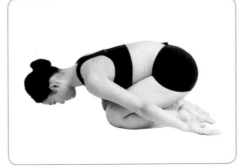

Child's Pose
Pages 132–33

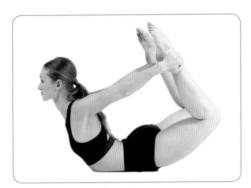

Child's Pose with Arms Extended
Pages 134–35

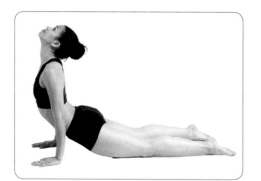

Cobra Pose
Pages 172–73

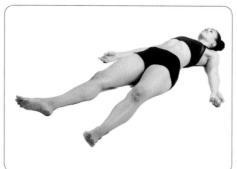

Corpse Pose
Pages 308–09

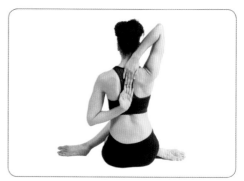

Cow Face Pose
Pages 234–35

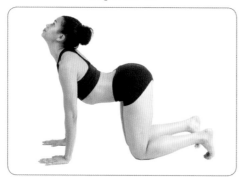

Cow Pose
Pages 166–67

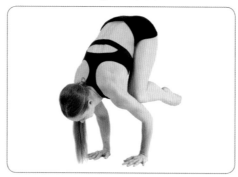

Crane Pose
Pages 296–97

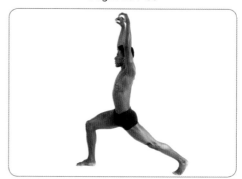

Crescent Lunge
Pages 70–71

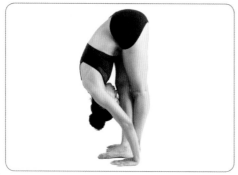

Crossed-Foot Forward Bend
Pages 112–13

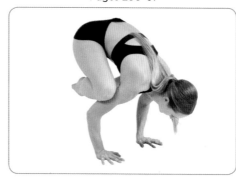

Crow Pose
Pages 294–95

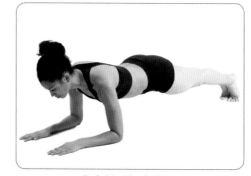

Dolphin Plank Pose
Page 271

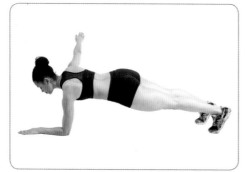

Dolphin Plank with Arm Reach
Pages 272–73

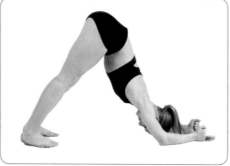

Dolphin Pose
Page 270

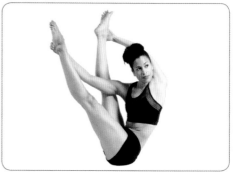

Double Compass Pose
Page 51

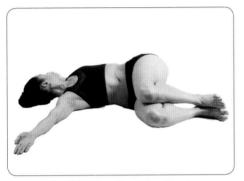
Double Knee Reclining Twist
Pages 318–19

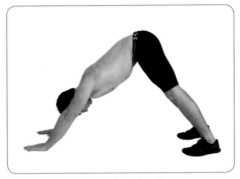
Downward-Facing Dog
Pages 268–69

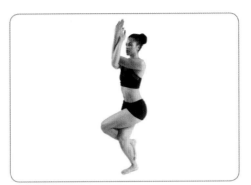
Eagle Pose
Pages 60–61

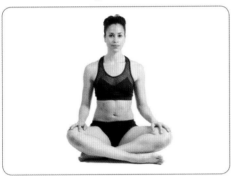
Easy Pose
Pages 220–21

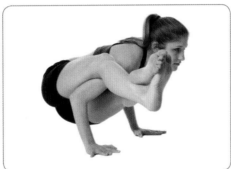
Eight-Angle Pose
Pages 300–01

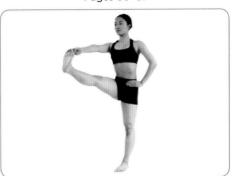
Extended Hand-to-Big-Toe Pose
Pages 88–89

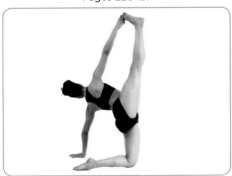
Extended Hand-to-Toe in Camel Pose
Page 85

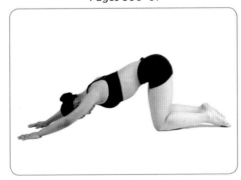
Extended Puppy Pose
Pages 136–37

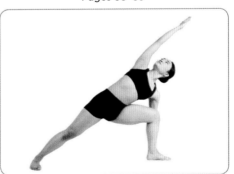
Extended Side Angle Pose
Pages 82–83

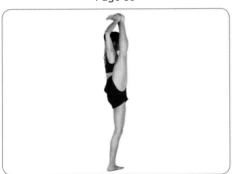
Extended Standing Split Pose
Pages 98–99

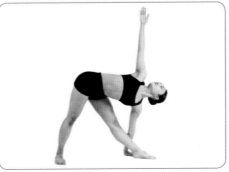
Extended Triangle Pose
Pages 76–77

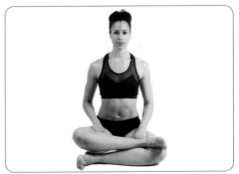
Fire Log Pose
Pages 232–33

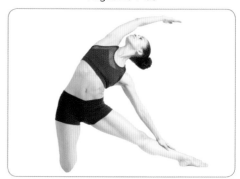

Fish Pose
Pages 196–97

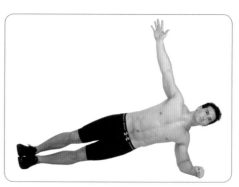

Flying Pigeon Pose
Pages 302–03

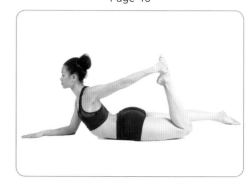

Forearm Side Plank Pose
Pages 264–65

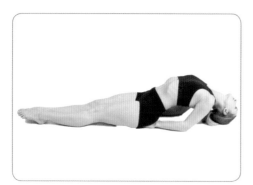

Four-Limbed Staff Pose
Pages 262–63

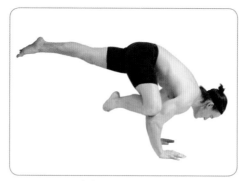

Garland Pose
Pages 48–49

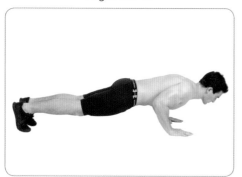

Gate Pose
Page 46

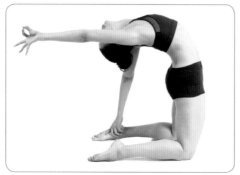

Half Camel Pose
Page 184

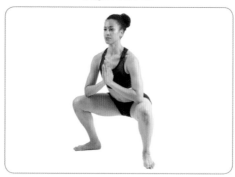

Half Frog Pose
Pages 180–81

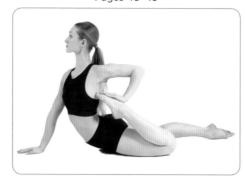

Half Frog Prep
Pages 178–79

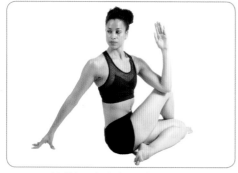

Half Lord of the Fishes Pose
Pages 240–41

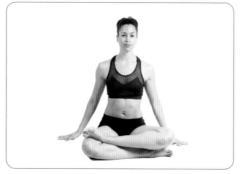

Half Lotus Pose
Page 231

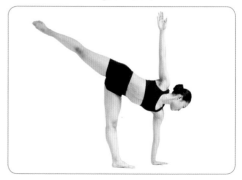

Half Moon Pose
Pages 86–87

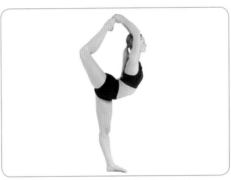

Half Straddle Pose
Pages 152–53

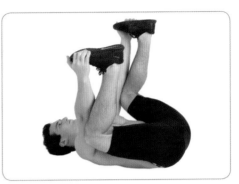

Hand-to-Foot Lord of the Dance Pose
Page 213

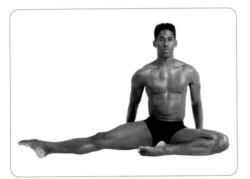

Happy Baby Pose
Pages 314–15

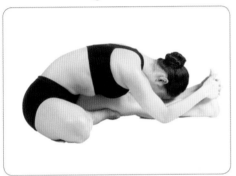

Head-to-Knee Forward Bend
Pages 142–43

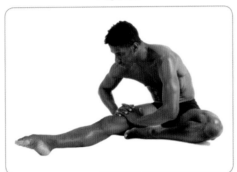

Head-to-Knee Forward Bend Prep
Pages 130–31

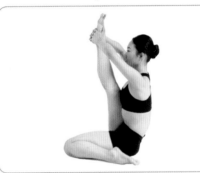

Heron Pose
Pages 146–47

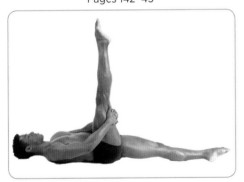

Heron Pose Prep
Pages 144–45

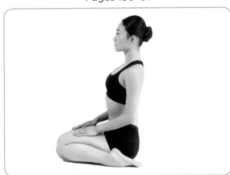

Hero Pose
Pages 224–25

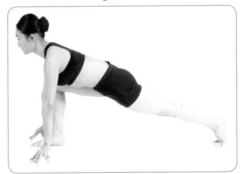

High Lunge
Pages 64–65

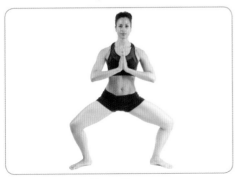

Horse Pose
Pages 50–51

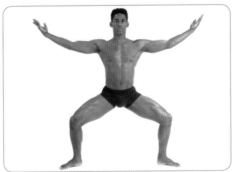

Horse Pose with Palms Up
Pages 52–53

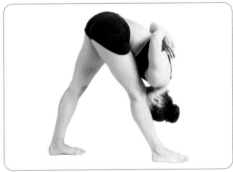

Intense Side Stretch Pose I
Pages 116–17

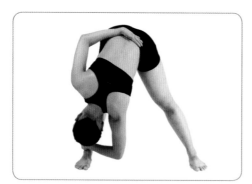

Intense Side Stretch Pose II
Page 120

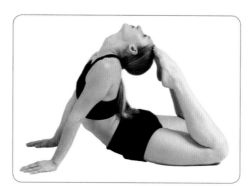

King Cobra Pose
Page 206

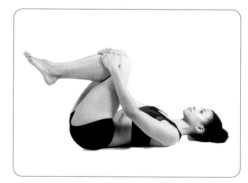

Knees-to-Chest Pose
Pages 310–11

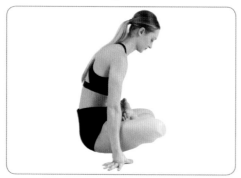

Lifting Up
Page 258

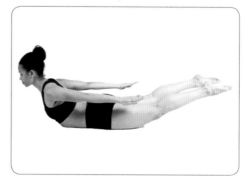

Locust Pose
Pages 174–75

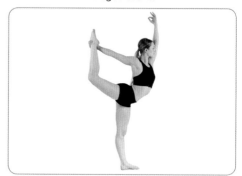

Lord of the Dance Pose
Pages 210–11

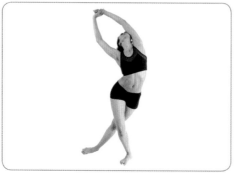

Lord Shiva Cycle of Life Dance Pose
Page 47

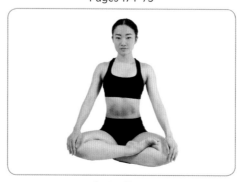

Lotus Pose
Pages 248–49

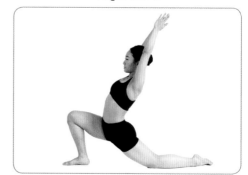

Low Lunge
Pages 62–63

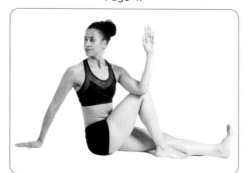

Marichi's Pose
Pages 226–27

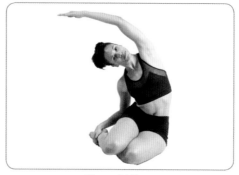

Mermaid Pose
Pages 238–39

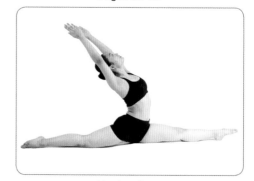

Monkey Pose
Pages 252–53

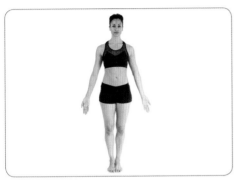

Mountain Pose
Pages 32–33

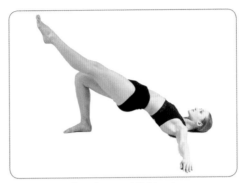

One-Legged Bridge I
Pages 188–89

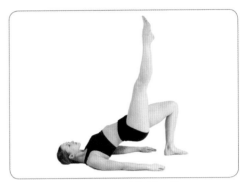

One-Legged Bridge II
Pages 190–91

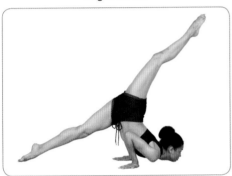

One-Legged Inverted Locust Pose
Page 214

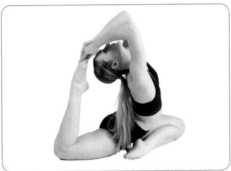

One-Legged King Pigeon Pose I
Pages 200–01

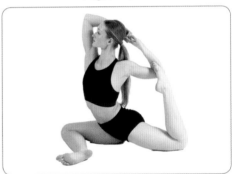

One-Legged King Pigeon Pose II
Pages 202–03

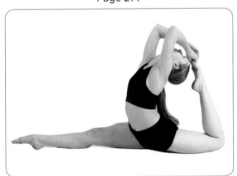

One-Legged King Pigeon Pose III
Page 204

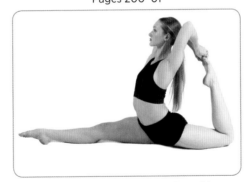

One-Legged King Pigeon Pose IV
Page 205

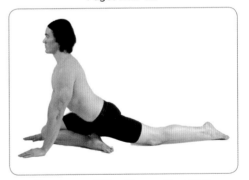

One-Legged King Pigeon Pose Prep
Pages 198–99

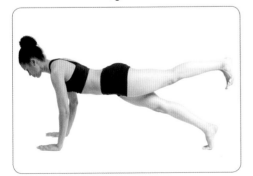

One-Legged Plank
Pages 274–75

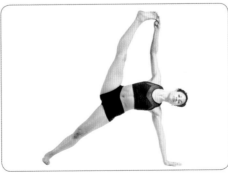

One-Legged Side Plank Pose
Page 90

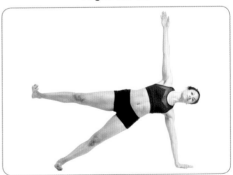

One-Legged Side Plank Prep
Pages 288–89

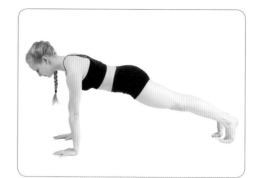

Palm Tree Pose
Page 42

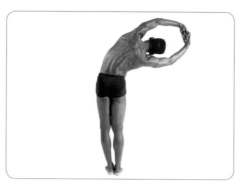

Palm Tree Side Bend
Page 43

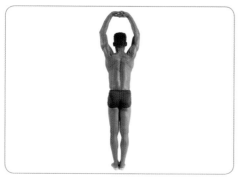

Plank Pose
Pages 260–61

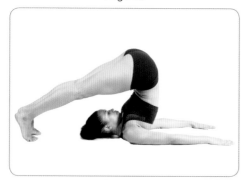

Plow Pose
Pages 278–79

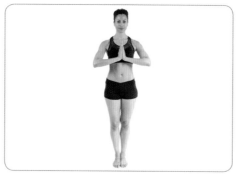

Prayer Pose
Pages 34–35

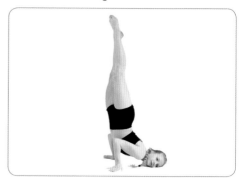

Raised Inverted Locust Pose
Page 215

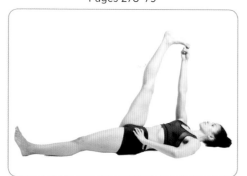

Reclining Big Toe
Pages 328–29

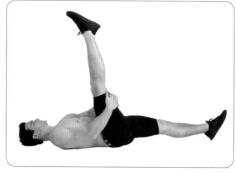

Reclining Big Toe Prep
Pages 326–27

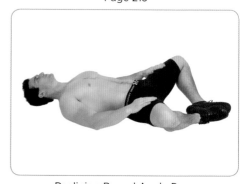

Reclining Bound Angle Pose
Pages 324–25

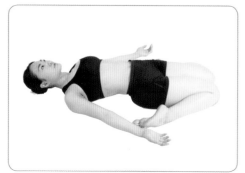

Reclining Hero Pose
Pages 322–23

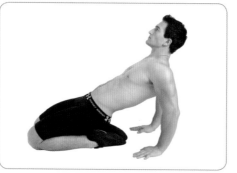

Reclining Hero Prep
Pages 320–21

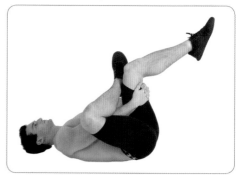

Reclining Pigeon Pose
Pages 312–13

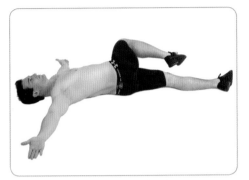

Reclining Spinal Twist
Pages 316–17

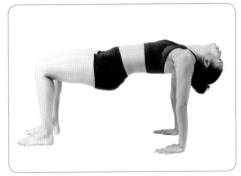

Reverse Tabletop Pose
Pages 280–81

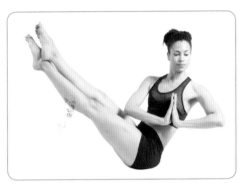

Revolved Boat Pose with Prayer Hands
Page 245

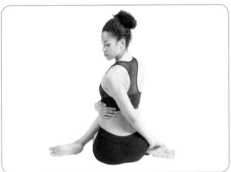

Revolved Cow Face Pose
Page 236

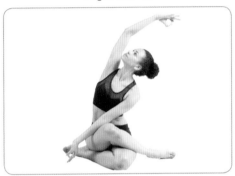

Revolved Cow Face Side Bend
Page 237

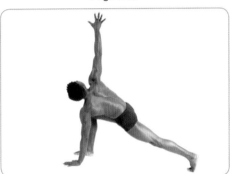

Revolved Crescent Lunge
Pages 80–81

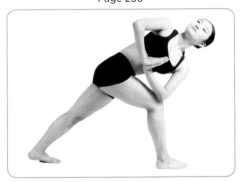

Revolved Extended Side Angle Pose
Pages 84–85

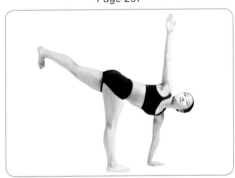

Revolved Half Moon Pose
Pages 90–91

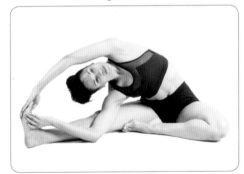

Revolved Head-to-Knee Pose
Pages 246–47

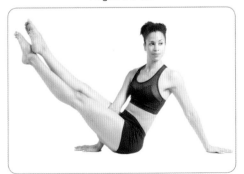

Revolved Supported Boat Pose
Page 244

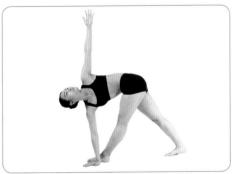

Revolved Triangle Pose
Pages 78–79

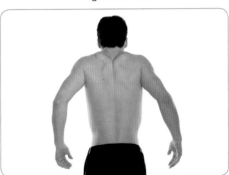

Scapular Range of Motion
Pages 256–57

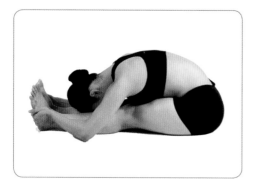

Seated Forward Bend
Pages 140–41

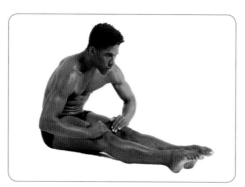

Seated Forward Bend Prep
Pages 128–29

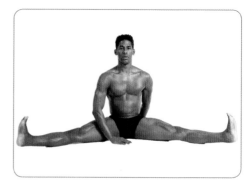

Seated Straddle Split
Pages 160–61

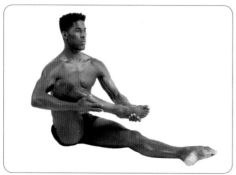

Seated Leg Cradle
Pages 150–51

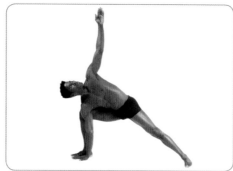

Side Angle Pose
Pages 74–75

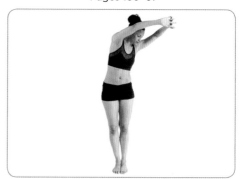

Side Bend to Half Forward Bend Circle
Pages 108–09

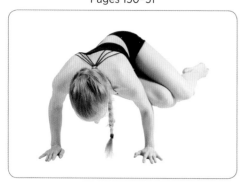

Side Crane Pose
Pages 298–99

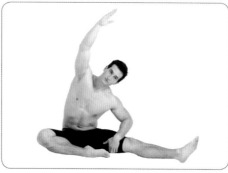

Side-Leaning Half Straddle Pose
Pages 154–55

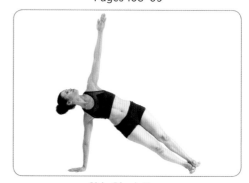

Side Plank Pose
Pages 266–67

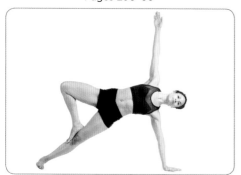

Side Plank with Tree Legs
Page 291

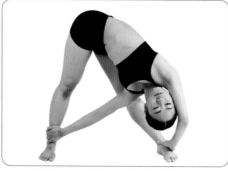

Sideways Intense Stretch Pose
Page 21

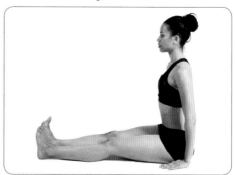

Staff Pose
Pages 218–19

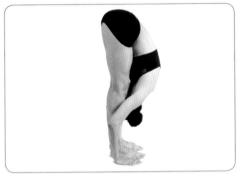

Standing Half Forward Bend to Forward Bend
Pages 106–07

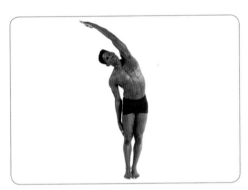

Standing Side Bend
Pages 44–45

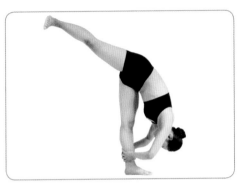

Standing Split Pose
Pages 124–25

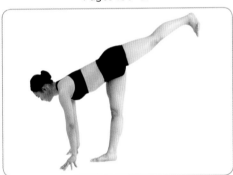

Standing Split Pose Prep
Pages 122–23

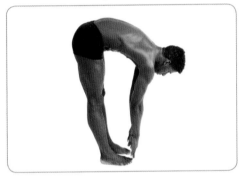

Standing Toe Touch
Pages 110–11

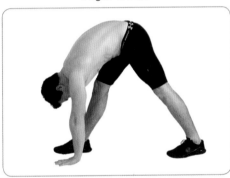

Straight-Leg Lunge Pose
Pages 104–05

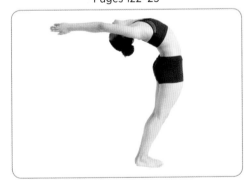

Sun Salutation A
Page 39

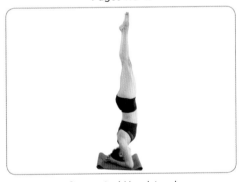

Supported Headstand
Pages 304–05

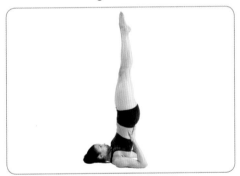

Supported Shoulderstand
Pages 286–87

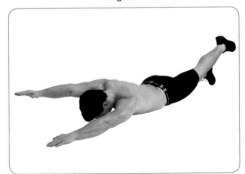

Swimming Locust Pose
Pages 176–77

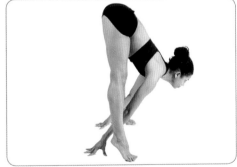

Tiptoe Intense Pose I
Page 18

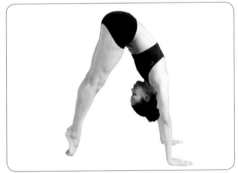

Tiptoe Intense Pose II
Page 119

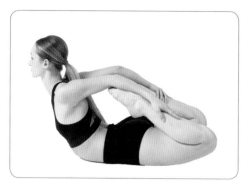

Toes-to-Elbow Bow Pose
Pages 208–09

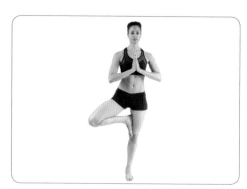

Tree Pose
Pages 58–59

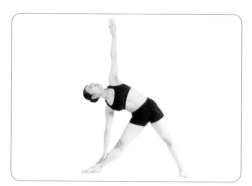

Triangle Pose
Pages 66–67

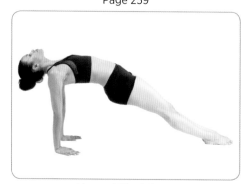

Turtle Neck
Page 259

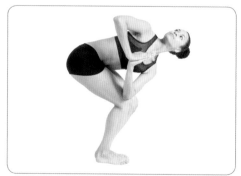

Twisting Chair Pose
Pages 56–57

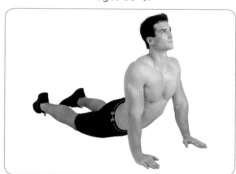

Upward-Facing Dog
Pages 170–71

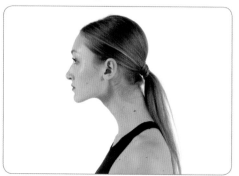

Upward Plank Pose
Pages 282–83

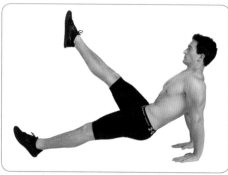

Upward Plank with Lifted Leg
Pages 284–85

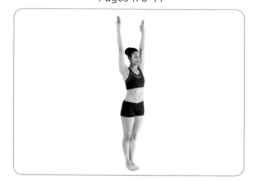

Upward Salute
Pages 36–37

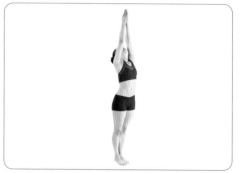

Volcano Pose
Page 38

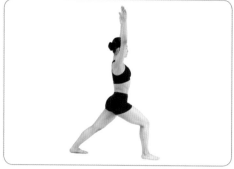

Warrior Pose I
Pages 68–69

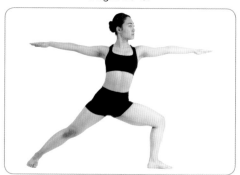

Warrior Pose II
Pages 72–73

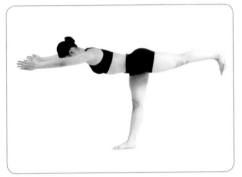

Warrior Pose III
Pages 92–93

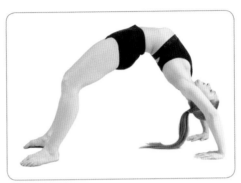

Wheel Pose
Pages 194–95

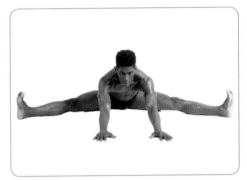

Wide-Angle Seated Forward Bend
Pages 156–57

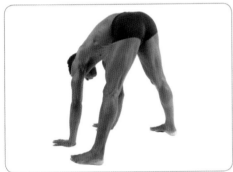

Wide-Legged Forward Bend
Pages 114–15

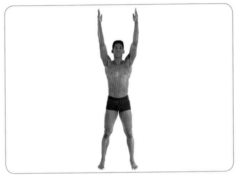

Wide-Stance Upward Salute
Pages 40–41

Index